Wisconsin Publications i
History of Science and Me____
Number 7

General Editors

William Coleman
David C. Lindberg
Ronald L. Numbers

Rima D. Apple

Mothers and Medicine
A Social History of Infant Feeding,
1890–1950

The University of Wisconsin Press

Published 1987

The University of Wisconsin Press
114 North Murray Street
Madison, Wisconsin 53715

The University of Wisconsin Press, Ltd.
1 Gower Street
London WC1E 6HA, England

First printing

Printed in the United States of America

For LC CIP information see the colophon

ISBN 0-299-11480-5 cloth; 0-299-11484-8 paper

For Michael, Paul, and Peter,
with love and appreciation

First we nursed our babies; then science told us not to. Now it tells us we were right in the first place. Or were we wrong then but would be right now?

—Mary McCarthy, The Group (1954), p. 228

Contents

Table and Figures

Table

Figures

Acknowledgments

This book has been many years in the making, years during which I was fortunate to meet many people and organizations who provided invaluable assistance along the way. I am grateful to have this opportunity to thank them publicly for all they have done.

My research would have been impossible without the special facilities of several libraries and the kind assistance of their thoughtful librarians. In particular I would like to thank Dorothy Hanks of the National Library of Medicine, B. Joseph O'Neil of the Boston Public Library, Wendy Shadwell of the New York Historical Society, and John N. Hoffman of the National Museum of American History, Smithsonian Institution, for insuring that my brief stays with them would be as productive as possible. Priscilla Neill and her staff at the Interlibrary Loan Department of Memorial Library, University of Wisconsin–Madison, were always ready to help me track down elusive publications. In the Middleton Health Sciences Library, University of Wisconsin–Madison, Dorothy Whitcomb, Librarian of the Historical Collection, and Blanche Singer, formerly the interlibrary loan librarian there, helped me decipher and locate sometimes obscure sources. Their expertise and efforts greatly enhanced my research.

Archivists too gave freely of their time and knowledge. Josephine M. Elliott and Helen Reed of the Special Collections Department, Indiana State University-Evansville, made available the Mead Johnson Collection. The staff of the State Historical Society of Wisconsin helped me use the many resources of their institution. R. C. Stribley, Nutrition Director, Wyeth Laboratories, and Jane Engates, Public Affairs Research, Smith Kline Corporation, graciously answered my many questions and sent me materials from the files of their companies.

Parts of this study were funded by Maurice L. Richardson Research

Grants of the University of Wisconsin Medical School and a Woodrow Wilson Research Grant in Women's Studies. I appreciate the financial assistance of these agencies.

I am grateful to the editors at the Johns Hopkins University Press and the *Journal of the History of Medicine and Allied Sciences* for permission to reprint in a different form material previously published in " 'To be used only under the direction of a physician': Commercial infant feeding and medical practice, 1870–1940," *Bulletin of the History of Medicine, 54* (1980), 402–417; and " 'Advertised by our loving friends': The infant-formula industry and the creation of new pharmaceutical markets, c.1870–1910," *Journal of the History of Medicine, 41* (1986), 3–23. I would also like to thank Appleton & Lange for permission to reprint the chart in figure 10.1.

Marge Berlow, Colonial Club, Sun Prairie, Wisconsin; Dorothy Clover and Norma Starkweather, Westside Coalition on Aging, Madison, Wisconsin; Kay Ahren, Segoe Terrace, Madison, Wisconsin; Virginia Stoeber and Marge Shaffer, the South Madison Coalition, Madison, Wisconsin; Liba Daub, the 60+ Club of the First Baptist Church, Madison, Wisconsin; and the staff of the Wisconsin State Medical Society helped me contact potential interviewees. Thanks to the many friends who have patiently listened to me for years discussing infant feeding; I appreciate their tolerance and their assistance in locating other interviewees and pertinent sources. A special note of gratitude to the mothers and doctors who talked to me about their infant feeding practices. Their experiences have added immeasurably to this study.

James Harvey Young has frequently and willingly discussed ideas about the infant-food industry and directed me to likely collections of ephemera. His comments are always helpful and always appreciated. I thank Rosemary Sullivant for her insightful comments on earlier drafts of the manuscript and Regina Markell Morantz-Sanchez and an anonymous reviewer for their useful criticism and comments of the book in an earlier stage.

For many years, the Department of the History of Medicine and the Women's Studies Program, both of the University of Wisconsin–Madison, have provided significant intellectual stimulation and encouragement in an atmosphere of collegiality and support within which I have been able to discuss and clarify my ideas. I especially want to thank Judith Walzer Leavitt and Ronald L. Numbers. From the time I began studying infant feeding as my dissertation topic, they have encouraged and supported me, giving generously of their time and expertise to read earlier drafts of this book. Their demand for rigor and clarity, and their enthusiasm for the historical undertaking and their example have all helped shape my views of history. In the truest sense of the term, they are mentors.

To Diane Mary Chase Worzala I owe a special debt of gratitude. She has read and perceptively critiqued numerous drafts of this manuscript over many years. Her thought-provoking suggestions stimulated new ideas and have undeniably improved this book. She is a special colleague and friend.

Finally I gratefully acknowledge the critical role my family played. My husband Michael has always shared my excitement for history. I cannot begin to describe the many ways in which he has sustained me and given me the strength and space to persevere with this study. Our sons, Paul and Peter, have been part of this project since they were infants. Though I fed them in the last third of the twentieth century, my infant-care experiences taught me much about situations faced by mothers of an earlier era. As the boys have grown, their understanding of the pressures of historical scholarship and their willingness to help alleviate the tensions that arise have given me the time and energy to complete the manuscript. I could not have researched and written this book without the support and confidence of Michael, Paul, and Peter.

Infant Feeding in the Nineteenth Century

I

"The Grand Prerogative of Woman"

"Every mother ought to nurse her own child, if she is fit to do it," counseled the author of a nineteenth-century home medical manual. Furthermore, he continued, "no woman is fit to have a child who is not fit to nurse it," a commonly voiced assertion of the period.[1] A century later, in a similar publication, L. Emmett Holt, Jr., comfortingly assured his readers, "under good medical guidance. . . . [a] bottle mother may still be a perfect mother."[2] The gulf between these two observations indicates a dramatic shift in American child-care practices: the profound transformation of infant feeding and of mothers' nurturing role. Women in the earlier period stood at the center of the domestic sphere; infants were commonly breast-fed. Yet within barely three generations—between the late nineteenth century and the mid-twentieth century—mothers lost their singular position; babies regularly were bottle-fed under medical supervision.

Now that development is under attack as in recent years critiques of the medical profession's dominant role in society have appeared with increasing frequency. Consumers have challenged a wide range of medical practices and pronouncements that affect our lives. Women's groups in particular have argued that the profession significantly contributed to women's relative loss of power over their lives and their bodies. In attempting to uncover the roots of our present circumstances, historical studies often portray women as passive in the face of medical expertise, (male) physicians as engaged in conscious manipulation of (female) patients, or both. Although such analyses illuminate some aspects of today's situation, they ignore many important dynamics. This is especially the case for an issue of historical and contemporary importance—infant feeding.

A mother today deciding between bottle feeding and breast feeding her infant does not make her choice in isolation. The media, and to some extent

4

the medical profession, exhort women to nurse their babies. Other, often more subtle influences, such as advertising, peer-group pressure, and societal expectations, promote the ease, efficacy, and acceptability of artificial infant feeding. The option of generally successful bottle feeding and many of the other factors that in our society affect a woman's decision about infant feeding did not exist even ninety years ago. Focusing on the history of infant feeding in this country, we can clarify the major elements involved in the complex and sometimes contradictory interaction between women and the medical profession, an interaction that reveals much about the changing roles of mothers and physicians in American society.

In the nineteenth century, the overwhelming majority of infants received their nourishment at the breast; many people considered bottle feeding a death warrant for the unfortunate baby whose mother could not, or would not, breast feed; and few physicians concerned themselves with infant feeding. Mothers who did not breast feed depended upon wet-nurses to nourish their children, or they prepared paps or cow's-milk mixtures from recipes listed in home medical manuals or supplied by friends and relatives. During the second half of the century, concern for the high rate of infant mortality stimulated interest in the question of infant feeding, since a high proportion of infant deaths were blamed on inadequate nutrition, due either to deficient breast milk or to poor artificial food. Using the findings of contemporary science, research-oriented physicians fashioned theories of healthful infant feeding. Faced with breast-fed infants who did not thrive and mothers who could not or would not nurse their children, practitioners too wanted a satisfactory substitute for mother's milk. Commercial infant-food products, typically devised by chemists, appeared on the market, providing alternatives to maternal nursing. Furthermore, women who feared that their milk was deficient wanted an artificial food that they could use safely.

Subsequently, the actions and interests of the medical profession, manufacturers, and mothers reached far beyond the development of efficacious artificial feeding for ill children and babies deprived of breast milk. Manufacturers of infant food, condensed milk, and, later, evaporated milk found bottle feeding highly profitable. Based on increasingly sophisticated analyses of human and cow's milk, the creation of "scientific" infant formulas provided a rationale for growing medical intervention in child care. Once their research had disclosed the variable nature of breast milk, some physicians promoted artificial feeding with a food compounded of known ingredients in preference to the uncertainty of maternal nursing. For medical practitioners, artifical feeding came to represent an important and lucrative aspect of medical practice. Moreover, as increasing numbers of mothers worried that they could not successfully nurse their infants, women sought out healthful substitutes for mother's milk. Mothers' changing perceptions coupled with developments in medical practice, the growth of infant-food manufacture, and scientific research resulted in American mothers' typically bottle feeding their infants under medical supervision.

By the middle of this century, most infants were bottle-fed by mothers who believed that medically directed artificial infant feeding was equal to, if not better than, breast feeding. This book analyzes how and why infant feeding patterns changed so dramatically from the 1890s to the 1940s. It investigates women's active attempts to use the information and facilities available to them to better their lives and those of their children. Simultaneously, this study illuminates the growing importance in our society of medical and scientific expertise and the impact of advertising and commercialization on mothers' practices. In the movement from condemnation to whole-hearted acceptance of bottle feeding, mothers reacted to and interacted with a variety of changes influencing American society in general and infant-care practices in particular. The roots of this transformation lay in the nineteenth century.

"The cult of domesticity," or "the cult of true womanhood," which crystallized in the first half of the nineteenth century, placed women at the center of the family and exalted the role of mother. In one of the most popular early nineteenth-century home medical books, William Buchan explained: "The more I reflect on the situation of a mother, the more I am struck with the extent of her powers, and the inestimable value of her services."[3] Nineteenth-century American culture entrusted woman with the nurturance and maintenance of the family and the domestic realm. Through maternity, women were to find their identity and meaning in their lives. As one home health manual proclaimed in 1866: "The reproduction of the species—their nurture in the womb, and their support and culture during infancy and childhood—is the grand prerogative of woman. It is a noble and a holy office, to which she is appointed by God; and the duty is both pure and sacred."[4]

Women writing in the same period agreed. Motherhood conscientiously undertaken ennobled women; it also gave them significance and power within a limited arena. Marion Harland, a popular writer, declared that "if it be a 'queendom to be a simple wife,' THE MOTHER is a Lady of Kingdoms, the bane or blessing of whose dominion will outlast the stars."[5] Harland's claim suggests the awesome responsibility that accompanied women's maternal "power," a burden specifically addressed by many writers in the nineteenth century:

> Here then lies your power; you can mould them [children] at your will. Your
> work commences ere the light dawns upon the little buds of immortality
> that are blossoming in your homes, ere you press "the first kiss upon their
> brow," the elements for a long, useful, and happy life, or the seeds that will
> cause an early death are there implanted.[6]

Maternal power, then, meant maternal responsibility. Practically the entire burden of childrearing rested on the shoulders of the mother, who had to supervise the well-being of her family and, in particular, "preserve the life of [her] children."[7]

Yet women were not without advisors who sought to instruct them in child-care techniques. In the nineteenth century pediatrics did not have the status of a defined medical specialty,[8] and few American physicians devoted any time to pediatric research; but doctors were not totally uninterested in or oblivious to child health. In popular medical manuals physicians covered a wide range of health topics, sometimes including a section on infant feeding. A few physicians began to construct theories of infant feeding and to devise "scientifically" correct infant formulas.

Medical writers and research-oriented physicians attracted to pediatric studies focused much of their attention on the problem of infant feeding and infant foods. They attributed the infant death rate in large part to improper food and the resulting intestinal disturbances such as inflammation of the bowels, "summer complaint" or cholera infantum, and diarrhea.[9] In discussions and analyses of infant mortality, physicians assumed the superiority of breast milk in infant nutrition, noting that difficulties arose most often with infants denied their "natural food." Yet, they pointed out, breast milk was the proper food only when it was "in proper condition." Despite the general admonition that every mother should breast feed her children, not every mother could nourish "her child as a wise Creator intended," because the mammary gland was a sensitive mechanism.[10] Certain physical impediments precluded breast feeding: a breast that was inactive, diseased, or lacking a nipple; scrofula, consumption, syphilis, or puerperal fever; and pregnancy. In some cases nursing ostensibly "overtaxed" the mother's system, causing a "general weariness and fatigue," "a want of refreshment from sleep," "headaches and vertigo," and other, even more debilitating side-effects. Any hint of mental instability hindered suckling, as did "fretful temper" or "emotional upset."[11] Describing the potentially deadly effect of emotions on breast milk, one domestic medical manual told of a woman who saw her husband attacked by a soldier. At first "she trembled with fear" but then threw herself into the fight and helped overcome the assailant. Shortly afterward, while still in an excited state, she began to nurse her child. "In a few minutes, it stopped nursing, became restless, panted, and expired on its mother's bosom."[12]

Believing that breast milk was the best infant food, but that in actuality "the ideal breast milk is rare," some physicians recommended that mothers protect and improve their milk supply through exercise, wholesome diet, and a serene disposition.[13] If a mother was incapable of nursing her child, then, given the superiority of breast milk, the next best food was the milk of another woman. Most physicians, however, rejected the option of wet-nursing. They thought it difficult, if not impossible, to procure a wet-nurse who was perfect physically, psychologically, and morally. Doctors therefore preferred to employ a bottle, since "the physical defects of the bottle we understand pretty well, and can, to a great extent, guard against them. Its moral qualifications, compared with those of the wet-nurse, are simply sublime."[14] A handful of research-oriented physicians devoted themselves to improving substitutes for human milk.[15]

The preparation usually recommended in the nineteenth century consisted of cow's milk diluted with water and sweetened with a small amount of sugar. Empirical observation and pragmatism prompted the employment of this mixture. Cow's milk was widely available in the United States. Human milk appeared thinner and tasted slightly sweeter than the bovine fluid. As chemical comparisons of human and cow's milks became more and more detailed, physicians introduced additional ingredients. At mid-century William H. Cumming, an Atlanta physician, recognized that diluting cow's milk with water produced a mixture too low in "butter" or, as he put it, with a "deficiency of nerve food." Thus he advocated augmenting the diluted bovine fluid with top-milk or cream.[16] Noting that human milk was alkaline and bovine milk acid, some physicians suggested that lime-water be added to any cow's-milk formula in order to correct the acidity and make the mixture more digestible.[17]

In 1884 Dr. A. V. Meigs of Philadelphia published the chemical analyses of human and cow's milk that have served as the basis for modern infant feeding. Using more refined laboratory techniques than had previously been available, Meigs determined that human milk contained approximately 87.1 percent water, 4.2 percent fat, 7.4 percent sugar, 0.1 percent inorganic matter (salts or ash), and only 1 percent casein (or protein). Cow's milk, on the other hand, contained approximately 88 percent water, 4 percent fat, 5 percent sugar, 0.4 percent ash, and 3 percent casein. Meigs also observed that the casein of cow's milk coagulated more easily and more firmly; the resultant coagulum was more difficult to digest than that of human milk. To produce a mixture that closely resembled human milk, Meigs suggested diluting cow's milk with lime-water to reduce the casein and to make the resultant fluid alkaline. To increase the fat to the correct proportion, he added cream; to augment the sugar, he used milk sugar.[18] During the last third of the nineteenth century, other physicians proposed similar recipes to transform cow's milk into human milk, but the formulas of Cumming and Meigs were among the most popular.

Cow's milk and human milk differed in more than chemical composition. Nursing mothers fed their infants directly from the breast, whereas cow's milk, especially that sold in cities, passed through many hands, and the product bought by the consumer often was not pure.[19] Moreover, by the 1870s physicians and public officials aware of contemporary bacteriological research also worried about bacterial contamination. In the last quarter of the nineteenth century, the process recommended to eliminate the problem of germ-laden milk was sterilization, a term often used in a loose generic sense to connote any form of heating or cooking the food. The application of heat would destroy disease germs, physicians believed, and would also make the milk more digestible. Others warned that the dangers of sterilization far outweighed its benefits, claiming that heat "devitalized" the milk and that only raw milk was nutritious. The condition most often blamed on heated milk was scurvy. Only fresh food, physicians believed, contained "that single mysterious, unknown antiscorbutic element." Medical practitioners who frequently saw cases of infantile scurvy insisted on using raw milk; other physicians preferred the safety of heated milk.[20]

By the 1890s medical science had produced few clear-cut answers to the problem of infant feeding. Cow's milk was the best and most widely available substitute for mother's milk, but one had to modify it. Cow's milk often carried disease germs, but milk heated to eliminate bacterial contamination opened the door to innutrition, particularly scurvy. In addition, medical practitioners recommended many different cow's-milk preparations.

Alternatives to maternal nursing were also created by chemists, under whose aegis the infant-food industry grew rapidly. The first commercial infant foods resulted in large measure from the nutritional research of Justus von Liebig, the acclaimed German chemist who in 1846 had described all living tissue, including food, as composed of different proportions of fats, carbohydrates, and proteins. Over the succeeding decades, chemists added mineral elements and salts, sometimes called "ash," to the list of food

No More Wet Nurses !

Liebe's, Baron von Liebig's, *Soluble* Food—the most perfect substitute for *Mother's* milk. Prepared by T. Paul Liebe, Chemist, Dresden.

This food dissolves easily in warm milk, and is *at once ready* for the use of babies.

At all druggists. $1 per bottle.

Depot,   HEIL & HARTUNG,
390 PEARL STREET,
Wholesale Druggists, New-York.

Figure 1.1. Liebig's Food advertisement. Source: *Hearth & Home, 1* (1869), 207

constituents. Concerned for the health of infants deprived of breast milk, Liebig in the 1860s constructed what he considered the perfect infant food. The product consisted of wheat flour, some cow's milk, and malt flour with a little bicarbonate of potash to reduce the acidity of the flours. As a result of his chemical and physiological studies, Liebig determined that these ingredients provided the infant with all the nutritive elements of human milk. He claimed not only that this formula was more nutritious than other mixtures, but also that it was more digestible. In the cooking process the malt converted the starch of the wheat flour into dextrin and glucose, two elements that the immature digestive system of the infant could more easily assimilate than the flour itself. By 1869 Liebig's Food was on sale in the United States (figure 1.1).[21]

Other chemists, particularly Europeans, entered the infant-food industry in increasing numbers. Henri Nestlé, a Swiss merchant with a passion for chemistry, and an interest in the problem of infant mortality, determined that the solution lay in "placing within the reach of all" the "good Swiss milk" of cows fed on nutritious Alpine grass. Because cow's milk differed from human milk in "plastic and respiratory aliments," he combined milk, sugar, and wheat flour and cooked the wheat with malt to convert the indigestible starch into more easily digested dextrin. Nestlé described his Milk Food as "good Swiss milk and bread, cooked after a new method of my invention, mixed in proportion, scientifically correct, so as to form a food which leaves nothing to be desired." By the early 1870s the Nestlé's Milk Food Company was distributing its product throughout Europe, Australia, and the Americas.[22]

Though Nestlé's Milk Food resembled Liebig's Food, Henri Nestlé often stressed the originality of his product and never mentioned specific medical or chemical sources from which he might have drawn the theoretical basis for it. In contrast, other companies marketing infant-food products in the United States at this time proudly announced their indebtedness to Justus von Liebig. But while Liebig's theory was widely respected, Liebig's Food was difficult to prepare. Several other chemists attempted to manufacture Liebig-type foods that mothers could prepare more easily. The best-known and most widely used of these products was Mellin's Food.

In the late 1860s the English chemist Gustav Mellin concluded that "correct and ingenious as were the principles which Liebig followed, the difficulty of preparation was so great as to make it impossible for every busy mother to prepare the food at home." He therefore undertook to create a more convenient infant food based on the same chemical theories. Unlike Nestlé's, which was a "complete" infant food and needed the addition of water only, Mellin's, a "milk modifier," called for dilution in milk and water. Americans imported Mellin's Food in the late 1870s, and by the early 1880s the Doliber-Goodale Company, an American firm, was manufacturing and distributing it in the United States. For many years the company continued to emphasize that its product "fulfills the requirements of Liebig's principles."[23]

Throughout the 1870s and 1880s other manufacturers entered the infant-food market in the United States. There was Dr. J. S. Hawley, who originally named his product "Liebig's Food for Infants," but later changed its name to Hawley's Food. William C. Wagner developed "Wagner's Infant Food" to nourish his infant daughter, and John Carnrick concocted "Carnrick's Soluble Food" for a son who had frequent attacks of "stomach and bowel ailments" with both milk from a wet-nurse and other prepared infant foods. Similarly, the impetus for Gail Borden's invention of condensed milk grew out of his concern for infant health. According to company tradition, during a trans-Atlantic crossing Borden noted with despair the illness of children who were fed milk from seasick cows, and realized that comparable problems existed in cities where pure milk was not available. After years of experimentation he devised a method of preserving milk with the addition of sugar. Sales of this sweetened condensed milk expanded during the Civil War as the government ordered it as a regular field ration. By the end of the war, the Borden Company was advertising Eagle Brand for feeding infants and for general home use. Later in the century, a Philadelphia druggist, Frank Baum, devised a milk modifier that he named Albumenized Food. The product so impressed the pharmaceutical firm Smith Kline & French that in the 1890s the company contracted with Baum to manufacture and sell the renamed Eskay's Albumenized Food.[24] Yet the most famous American product in the late nineteenth century was Horlick's Malted Milk.

James Horlick, an English pharmacist who had worked for Mellin's in England, came to the United States in 1875 at the urging of his brother, William Horlick, who wished to manufacture a Liebig-type infant food. Though they were successful, James Horlick quickly recognized the major drawback in their product: bad milk could spoil its usefulness. He developed a new product that had "for its object, first, to provide a non-farinaceous highly-nutritious food for infants and invalids by combining the nutritive parts of the cereals with milk; and secondly, to render such food free from all souring tendency irrespective of the climate or state of the atmosphere to which it may be subjected, and yet of such a nature as to be readily soluble in water." In the early 1880s the company patented this combination of dry milk and milk modifiers, Horlick's Malted Milk.[25]

Although the infant-food companies stressed the uniqueness of their products, asserting that they and they alone were "the perfect food," or "the only perfect substitute for mother's milk," or "the best of all foods for infants," the manufacturers all approached potential medical and non-medical audiences with substantially the same techniques. Most companies advertised widely in women's and other popular magazines. They almost invariably offered consumers free booklets on infant care and infant feeding as well as free samples of their products. In advertisements and brochures, companies published testimonials from satisfied mothers and physicians. Typical was "Mellin's Food for Infants and Invalids," a twenty-page pamphlet distributed by the Doliber-Goodale Company. The first three pages discussed the scientific rationale for the infant food, quoting from Liebig; the remaining seventeen reproduced letters written by mothers, physicians, and directors of institutions such as the Woman's Hospital and Foundling's Home of Detroit, Michigan, and reprinted newspaper articles that extolled the virtues of Mellin's.[26]

Infant feeding was a very minor part of medical practice and research in the 1870s and 1880s, yet infant-food companies cultivated medical patronage. Though Nestlé directed many of his promotional efforts to mothers, contending that "mothers will do my publicity for me," he also attempted to garner support from physicians and chemists. By 1868 he had sought and won the approval of a Dr. Barthey, a physician to the Prince Imperial, who then introduced Nestlé's Milk Food into the aristocratic circles of Paris.[27] Hawley presented his product to the Medical Society of the County of Kings, New York, and then published a pamphlet of his presentation.[28] In 1887 William Horlick formally announced Horlick's Malted Milk to the medical profession at medical meetings and in journal advertisements.[29] Most infant-food companies extensively advertised in medical journals, as well as non-

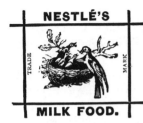

NESTLÉ'S FOOD

Is Especially Suitable for Infants in Hot Weather.

Requires no Milk in its Preparation, and is very Effective in the Prevention of Cholera Infantum.

"Ziemssen's Cyclopedia of the Practice of Medicine," Vol. VII., the standard authority, says: **"In cases of Cholera-Infantum Nestlé's Milk Food is alone to be recommended."** Because the gastro-intestinal disorders to which infants are so subject are provided for by presenting only the *nourishing* properties of cow's milk in a digestible form. "Cow's milk produces a coagulated mass of curd or cheese, which the immature gastric juice is **utterly unable to dispose of.**"

This is one of several reasons why infant foods requiring the **addition** of cow's milk fail as a diet in hot weather.

Pamphlet by Prof. Lebert and sample sent on application.

THOS. LEEMING & CO., Sole Agents, New York.

Figure 1.2. Nestlé's Food advertisement. Sources: *Babyhood*, 4 (44) (1888), viii, and *American Analyst*, 4 (1888), 178

medical magazines, and often invited physicians to send for free booklets and free samples. They sometimes directed the same advertisements to medical and nonmedical readers (figure 1.2).

The firm of Reed and Carnrick invited physicians and chemists to visit its "laboratory" in Goshen, New York, to witness "every detail connected with the production of Carnrick's Soluble Food." "All expenses from New York to Goshen," they promised, "will be paid by us."[31] This invitation pleased some physicians. Dr. Charles Warrington Earle, professor of diseases of children, Woman's Medical College, Chicago, "carefully examined the process of manufacture" and recommended the use of the product. Dr. Simon Baruch, physician to the New York Juvenile Asylum, reported that Carnrick had adopted suggestions made by leading physicians.[32] The Doliber-Goodale Company's invitation to the editors of *American Analyst* resulted in a two-page article with "illustrations descriptive of the extensive laboratory" and praise for Mellin's Food.[33] Several illustrations and much of the prose are taken directly from material Doliber-Goodale itself published for distribution to physicians and mothers. Through these multifaceted promotional campaigns, infant-food companies hoped to attract medical support for their products at a time when some physicians appeared to be developing an interest in the problem of artificial infant feeding.

Debates within the medical profession provided the rationale for several different products. For physicians and consumers worried about the local milk supply, several companies advised that their products contained sterilized, safe milk. "No milk is required in preparing Nestlé's Food, only water used," the company emphasized, so that the use of Nestlé's Food avoided the possibility of contaminated milk.[34] At least one physician found this the most telling advantage of Nestlé's, since

> bottle feeding is made difficult . . . by the changes that milk undergoes either at the hands of the milk man, or under atmospheric influences, or from want of care between the time when it leaves the cow and when the last of the evening's or morning's supply is given to the baby.[35]

Similarly, advertisements characterized Carnrick's Soluble Food as "the Only Food that thoroughly nourishes the child without the addition of cow's milk," and Horlick's patent application discussed the same point. (Neither companies nor physicians stressed the danger of contaminated water, but both often directed consumers to mix the product with water that had been boiled.) However, not all physicians preferred sterilized foods; some recommended uncooked milk for infant feeding. In these cases the Doliber-Goodale Company emphasized that one should mix Mellin's Food with fresh, raw milk.[36]

Companies bolstered their claims with statements from respected physicians and researchers and were not above quoting out of context. For example, Professor Alfred R. Leeds of the Stevens Institute of Technology published an analysis of eighteen infant foods in which he assiduously avoided recommending any one product. Yet the Doliber-Goodale Company announced in its advertising copy that "he had a Favorable Report upon Mellin's Food" and implied that Leeds had chosen this product over all the others. The company did offer to send a copy of the report to any physician who requested it, but still the Mellin's advertisement leaves the reader with the false impression that a specific highly respected individual had recommended its product.[37]

How much influence this type of testimonial advertising had is difficult to ascertain. It is certain, however, that some physicians felt strongly enough about products to recommend them in their writings. Dr. Abraham Jacobi, America's leading nineteenth-century pediatrician, favored the original

Liebig's Food but found that "the attention required in preparing the food is the source of failure in most cases."[38] In an 1882 analysis of various infant foods, the editor of the Department of Diseases of Children of the *American Journal of Obstetrics,* Dr. George B. Fowler, concluded that some of the products could be satisfactory substitutes for mother's milk. In particular he appreciated Nestlé's Milk Food, which "possesses a high degree of nutritive value, and is an ingenious and elegant article." With Horlick's, in contrast, he found that "the irritating effects and indigestible character of the bran in this food is an objection."[39] Several physicians praised Mellin's Food, including Dr. I. N. Love, one-time vice-president of the American Medical Association and professor of diseases of children, clinical medicine, and hygiene at Marion-Sims College of Medicine, who thought there was "no better agent."[40] Obviously physicians had reached no consensus.

The 1888 report of the Sub-Committee on Infant Feeding of the AMA shows most clearly the lack of unanimity among physicians. The committee directed to "leading authorities" in the field the question "Will any of the ordinary 'infant foods' now in the market thoroughly nourish the child without the addition of cow's milk?" Some physicians responded in the negative: "No artificial food will efficiently nourish an infant unless cow's milk is added; for all preserved foods want the living antiscorbutic principle, which is to be found in fresh foods" and "None of those which I have studied, either theoretically or practically, seem to me to fulfill the indication." Others accepted the commercial infant milk-foods: "Yes, provided you include milk foods, as ——'s and ——'s," and "I think a good milk food answers the requirements very successfully."[41]

Mothers too were puzzled about the most healthful alternative to mother's milk. Which was better for the baby: a cow's-milk mixture or a commercial infant food? Should a wet-nurse be hired? Women used their own experience and those of others to find satisfactory answers to these questions. Mothers wrote letters of advice to their daughters, nieces, and friends who moved away. Women recorded in their diaries the suggestions they were given as well as their own infant-feeding practices.[42] Through the print media also, women reached out to help new mothers. For instance, "A lady, who was unable to suckle her babes, reared a large family of healthy children according to the plan so carefully laid down by Dr. Cummings [*sic*]," reported *Herald of Health,* in 1871. Unfortunately the work, originally published in 1859, was out of print, and the woman's copy was "nearly worn out in service." For her own use and for "the benefit of those needing such information," the mother outlined the doctor's book and submitted her summary to the journal, which gladly published it for its readers.[43]

In describing their practices and offering advice to other readers in women's journals, mothers often stimulated extended discussions of infant feeding. The popular journal *Babyhood* published just such a transcontinental exchange in 1886–1887.[44] Fanny B. Workman of Worcester, Massachusetts, wrote a scathing letter condemning the practice of wet-nursing. Since she could not nurse her infant, her doctor had recommended artificial feeding, which she attempted for three weeks with disastrous results. Next she tried a wet-nurse, whose own infant the Workmans boarded out in the country. But when the nurse's child became ill, the nurse "became greatly agitated, and consequently her milk had a decidedly bad effect" on the Workmans' infant. The second nurse hired "proved quite as untrustworthy as the other." Finally, several months later, Baby Workman was thriving on Mellin's Food:

> A great burden fell from my shoulders. For four months and a half those two nurses had required my hourly superintending, and then I never felt sure the food the child received was not impure. In one respect, at least, the milk of the gentle cow has the advantage over that of the wet-nurse—it is not affected by indulgence in peanuts, cucumbers, and ice-cream.

In a later issue of *Babyhood,* Louise J. of San Francisco wrote that given a choice she would prefer a wet-nurse to artificial feeding, a decision applauded by the journal's editor, who, however, advised that since "wet-nurses are not selected from the highly-intelligent classes," they must be carefully watched. A.B.C., of Boston, concurred:

> I wish to enter a plea for wet-nurses. Although many and manifold have been my trials and tribulations, I thoroughly believe in them. In twenty months I have had seven. . . . and I have never seen the slightest ill-effect from changing wet-nurses.

Despite this praise, and probably because of its "trials and tribulations," wet-nursing remained a minor aspect of infant feeding in the United States in the nineteenth century.

Rather than face the problems and difficulties of dealing with wet-nurses, nonnursing mothers apparently preferred to bottle feed their infants. Women's requests to journals for information about successful bottle formulas and commercial foods show growing interest in artificial infant feeding. Descriptions of mothers' experiences demonstrate fears about the inadequacy of maternal nursing and their own knowledge of bottle feeding. Explained one mother, Helen Maxwell, in the *Ladies' Home Journal:*

If fed from your breast, be sure that the quantity and quality supply his demands. If you are weak and worn out, your milk cannot contain the nourishment a babe needs, and good cow's milk, or some food that contains the same elements as human milk, should be at least partially substituted. You will soon feel the advantage yourself, and see it in the child.

While praising breast feeding, another mother described how to manage the uncertainties inherent in artificial infant feeding. First, she advised, obtain fresh milk both in the morning and in the afternoon; in warm weather scald the milk, but Eagle Brand Condensed Milk was convenient also. Second, she acknowledged that physicians recommended various foods, but asserted, "I have used "Mellin's" with excellent results. Experience only can determine a choice. A few trials will show whether the kind in use agrees with that particular child."[45]

The comments of these mothers, as well as the longevity of many infant-food products such as Nestlé's, Mellin's, and Horlick's, demonstrate that manufacturers had successfully identified and were astutely cultivating a previously unrecognized market. Some mothers in need of a substitute for maternal nursing turned to wet-nursing with all its perplexities. Others, however, preferred to employ the bottle, at times acknowledging the advice of physicians but usually selecting without medical assistance from the growing list of cow's-milk formulations and commercial foods.

In sum, then, although American babies commonly received breast milk in the late nineteenth century, artifical feeding was not unknown. Over the next several decades, preference for bottle feeding strengthened. Discoveries in bacteriology, physiology, and nutrition effected a new understanding of infants' diets. Coupled with analyses of high infant death rates that often demonstrated the inadequacy of mother's milk, these scientific advances suggested how to protect children's lives through new "scientific" modes of infant feeding. These, in turn, were used to establish and maintain successful business enterprises—both manufacturing concerns and medical practices. Employment of these new methods also enhanced the prestige of their users by denoting such medical practitioners as "scientific" and such mothers as "modern."

It is not surprising that physicians, manufacturers, and mothers all looked to science to answer the perplexing problem of healthful artificial infant feeding. Science held a special place in American society in the late nineteenth and early twentieth centuries. Indeed, according to the historian Charles Rosenberg, "Almost every American social problem in the nineteenth century attracted scientific discussion: the role of women, ethnic differences, appropriate sexual behavior, the logic of class, the effects of urban life, for example."[46] Bacteriological studies led to the development of new, more effective treatments and preventatives. Increasingly sophisticated nutritional studies disclosed the importance of various newly discovered food elements in the diets of humans and other animals. Medical researchers used scientific findings to produce new diagnostic tools with which the physician could better explain and predict the course of disease. The application of these discoveries significantly contributed to the success and prestige of medicine, particularly in the arenas of public health and surgery. The latest discoveries were celebrated in the popular press as well as medical journals, fostering a general awareness of science. Commentators especially discussed bacteriological research or germ theory, in which science not only explained disease causation but also held the hope of future curative and preventive techniques. Science represented progress.

The growth in scientific knowledge affected the professional identity of medical practitioners. Physicians viewed science as the foundation and symbol of medical authority, and increasingly so too did the public. New diagnostic tools unveiled to the physician, but not to the patient, the hidden mysteries of the human body. In providing physicians with information not directly available to the patient, these instruments accentuated the esoteric nature of medical-scientific knowledge, thereby altering the doctor-patient relationship and strengthening the authority of the physician. Moreover, physicians needed more extensive training in order to use the new technology proficiently; consequently medical education changed as medical schools became increasingly science-oriented.

At the turn of the century, scientific knowledge held a privileged status. The terms "science" and "scientific" were rarely defined specifically. Yet groups frequently appropriated the terms in order to add prestige and lend a note of authority to their work, creating labels as diverse as "scientific management," "scientific social work," and "scientific housekeeping." In many areas "science" became practically synonymous with progress and reform. This evocation of "science" dovetailed neatly with the Progressive view that saw salvation in the rise of the professional, the expert. Physicians emphasized a close identity between science and medicine; similarly, they stressed that they, as medical practitioners, were the experts who held knowledge unavailable to the laity. Over the years this claim to special knowledge created an ever-growing gulf between physicians and mothers. As the "experts," physicians strove to replace traditional knowledge with the latest scientific discoveries. Through the next decades more and more mothers and others convinced of the progressiveness of science turned away from older sources of information, such as female relatives, neighbors, and friends, and instead increasingly sought out the advice of scientific experts—namely, the physicians.

The rise of artificial infant feeding resulted both from a new theoretical understanding of diet and nutrition and from changes in medical practice and women's lives. To explicate more clearly the forces influencing the emergence of medically directed artificial infant feeding in the late nineteenth and twentieth centuries, the remainder of this book is divided into four major sections. Section I documents developments in medical theory that provided the basis for the rise of scientific bottle feeding, and it outlines how infant-food manufacturers used science to promote their products. Section II focuses on how practitioners employed this medical theory to establish and maintain infant feeding as an important aspect of general practice. It also investigates practitioners' attempts to maintain and extend their position as experts in infant feeding by controlling the activities of infant-food companies. Section III discusses the development of the ideology of scientific motherhood and its promulgation, including the dissemination of the latest scientific theories on nutrition and the advertising of infant foods. Section IV analyzes how contemporary medical practices and the ideology of scientific motherhood crucially influenced mothers' perceived ability and desire to breast feed or bottle feed and examines the pragmatic reasons underlying the willingness of mothers to accept, and even actively seek out, the control of medical advisors on infant feeding.

The book's structure is not meant to imply that theory and practice can be easily separated or that they should be considered divorced from one another. Nor did medical practice and women's experiences develop independently of one another. In a sense the four sections represent, to use Nancy Cott's terms, the "informers of consciousness," or prescriptions (Sections I and III), and the "reflections of consciousness," or descriptions (Sections II and IV).[47] We can draw no sharp distinctions between the two. Theory undoubtedly shaped practice; yet practice in turn altered theory. Theoretically based pronouncements proscribed certain practices, but the successful employment of these same practices modified medical theory and research. Moreover, a single historical source often embodies prescription and description. Thus mothers writing articles in women's magazines both "informed" other readers and "reflected" their own experiences. Similar conflations appear in medical texts.

However, only by disentangling the overlapping concerns of mothers, physicians, and manufacturers—the realms of theory-building and practical experience—can we comprehend the complex interactions of science, medicine, economics, and culture that transformed infant-feeding practices in the United States. In their desire to provide the best care for their children, American mothers relied increasingly on experts. A combination of sophisticated advertising techniques, the aura of scientific motherhood, and the vaunted expertise of the medical profession—an interplay of ideology and material factors—created an atmosphere that motivated many women to seek out commercial products and medical advice. The commercialization and medicalization of infant care established an environment that made artificial feeding not only acceptable to many mothers but also "natural" and "necessary."

PART ONE

Infant-Feeding Theories and Infant-Food Products

II

"Establishing Rules for Substitute Feeding" 1890–1915

The "frightful and criminal" infant mortality rate of the 1890s galvanized medical researchers. It was frightful because so many babies died (in many cities more than one-third of all infants died before their fifth birthday), and criminal because, as Dr. E. A. Wood wrote in the *Journal of the American Medical Association,* "nine-tenths [of these deaths] are from preventable causes."[1] Poor diet was the most significant cause of infant deaths, argued many physicians:

> The preventive medicine of early life is pre-eminently the intelligent management of the nutriment which enables young human beings to breathe and grow and live. In fact, it is a proper or an improper nutriment which makes or mars the perfection of the coming race.
>
> Infant feeding, then, is the subject of all others which should interest and incite to research all who are working in the preventive medicine of early life.[2]

Not surprisingly, infant-feeding studies became the *raison d'être* of pediatric research.[3]

Since medical researchers specifically linked improper nutrition with commercial infant foods, to some extent the development and the very success of the infant-food industry helped focus the profession's attention on artificial infant feeding. Physicians analyzed, and sometimes evaluated, patent infant foods in relation to the newest chemical and physiological knowledge.[4] Though such research may have unintentionally attracted a wider audience to these products, many physicians looked askance at proprietary foods.

Promotion and distribution of infant foods directly to the public meant that mothers could, and did, feed their infants without medical supervision.

Since manufacturers advertised their infant foods to both the medical profession and the laity, medical researchers indicted the industry on two counts. The lack of medical oversight in infant feeding, physicians contended, contributed to the infant death rate at a time when concerned researchers regarded the prevention of infant mortality through medically directed feeding as the keynote of the nascent specialty of pediatrics. Similarly, widespread nonmedical use of infant foods placed the physician in an awkward position. While physicians were attempting to bring infant feeding into the province of the medical profession, the actions of the manufacturers suggested that nonmedical personnel knew as much as, if not more than, physicians.

Both humanitarian sentiments and considerations of status spurred these physicians to delve more deeply into the science of infant feeding. A prime mover in these developments was Thomas Morgan Rotch. His work and writings both mirrored the concerns expressed by many of his contemporaries and defined the role medicine was to play in infant feeding. From his position on the faculty of Harvard Medical School and through numerous publications and presentations, he influenced more than a generation of physicians. During the period from 1890 to 1915, the many researchers who discussed infant feeding, whether they agreed or disagreed with Rotch's theories, had, at the very least, to respond to his "scientific approach" to the problem.[5] Infant-food manufacturers too were affected by his pronouncements.

Rotch was particularly upset with the role of these manufacturers in artificial infant feeding:

> It would seem hardly necessary to suggest that the proper authority for establishing rules for substitute feeding should emanate from the medical profession, and not from non-medical capitalists. Yet when we study the history of substitute feeding as it is represented all over the world, the part which the family physician plays, in comparison with numberless patent and proprietary foods administered by the nurses, is a humiliating one, and one which should no longer be tolerated.[6]

The medical profession must "rescue" infant feeding from "the pretensions of proprietary foods."[7]

From the beginning Rotch stressed the importance of human milk for infant health, especially in the first few months of life. Human milk must be the standard for any infant nutrient. Research demonstrating that milk contained casein, fat, sugar, and salts had also shown that human milk contained varying proportions of these nutritive elements. Moreover, many conditions could affect the quality and quantity of a woman's milk supply. From these data, Rotch and others concluded that even maternal nursing gave no assurance that the infant would receive the most healthful nutriment. A mother's milk could be totally unfit for her infant if, for example, the woman did not nurse at regular intervals, or if her temperament was "undisciplined," or if she was not "willing to regulate her diet, her exercise, and her sleep according to the rule which [would] best fit her for her task." Medical intervention in infant feeding meant, first of all, the responsibility to explain to a mother how to fulfill her nursing duty by regulating her life.[8]

Researchers such as Rotch believed not that human milk per se was the preeminent infant food, but rather that a varied combination of the different elements of the milk made it the best food during the first year.[9] Because mother's milk varied from individual to individual—and even the milk of a given mother varied at different times and under different conditions—and because infants were individuals, no one combination of fat, protein, and sugar could satisfy all. Rotch clearly saw that the solution to the problem of artificial infant feeding lay in a method by which physicians could supply to each and every infant the food uniquely suited to that individual's digestion and development. And because the needs of infants change over time, the procedure should be flexible enough to allow the physician to alter the proportions of the various constituents as required.

Rotch began his search for a flexible infant food with a mixture of cow's milk, lime-water, milk sugar, and cream similar to that recommended by Meigs. Agreeing that this formulation resulted in "an alkaline mixture with the percentage of its ingredients closely corresponding to that of human milk," Rotch cautioned that creams in which the proportion of fat was unknown could produce formulas with incorrect fat content. He therefore recommended using cream removed from whole milk by a "centrifugal machine." Such cream contained an "almost unvarying percentage" of fat and could be confidently employed in mixing infant formulas.[10]

The variability of human milk inspired two other recommendations. First, the physician should have on hand analyses of each mother's milk, "in case, as so frequently happens, something should occur to end the nursing at an early period." With these control records the physician would know at once the correct percentages of the various components that suited the infant's digestion.[11] Second, believing that "slight changes in the percentages of the three elements of milk of which we have most accurate knowledge, namely: the fat, sugar and albumenoids [proteins], have an important bearing upon the management of the digestion and nutrition of infants," Rotch devised a "more exact system" for constructing infant formulas. Physicians could use Rotch's percentage method to calculate formulas with the exact proportions desired.

In addition, Rotch insisted that an infant's artificial food "should be written as precisely for by prescription as the combinations of drugs which we are continually sending to the pharmacist." To be certain that the formula in the bottle was the formula prescribed by the physician, the food should be compounded as carefully as a drug prescription, using only pure materials of known composition. To this end Rotch established a milk laboratory in Boston in 1891, a facility of which he made good use.[12]

In publications that combined theory-building and case studies, Rotch often discussed cases in which slight modifications in the prescribed formulas were necessary and successful. Called in to see a three-month-old baby with colic who cried constantly, Rotch determined that the mother's milk had a superabundance of proteids and that the woman was "worried by some trivial family matter and did not take much exercise." He advised that she "lessen the amount of mental disturbance" and exercise more. The infant's symptoms abated but they returned a few days later because the mother did not exercise or reduce the tension in her life. Over the next several weeks, as the infant's conditions changed, Rotch prescribed a series of formulas, varying the proportions of the ingredients by as little as one-half of one percent. He was pleased with the child's progress on the prescribed milk formulas. The baby lost weight, however, and the parents insisted that a wet-nurse be tried. Rotch examined the milks of various wet-nurses and could find none he considered satisfactory. Against medical advice, the family hired a wet-nurse. This woman had successfully fed other children, but in this case her milk upset the infant's digestion, and colic again developed. Once more Rotch was called upon to prescribe another series of formulas, and the infant's condition improved.[13]

In Rotch's opinion, this case substantiated his theory that "while there are many varieties of good milk, there are also many infants who cannot thrive on them all, but only upon such as suit their individual digestive powers." The best way to accommodate the individual infant's idiosyncrasies was a milk laboratory that gave physicians the means of prescribing "even slight changes in the percentages" and of making these changes as often as necessary, even "day by day as well as month by month." The laboratory also saved the physician time and ensured that the infant's bottle contained exactly what the doctor had prescribed.[14]

Rotch's percentage method proved to be the foundation for infant-feeding research in the period. Many investigators and teachers enthusiastically embraced the method, commending Rotch for "providing us with a rational method of feeding babies." To Rotch's supporters, its "greatest value" was in teaching physicians to think in terms of percentages and individual infants.[15] In particular, these physicians praised the creation of the milk laboratory as "not only a great scientific achievement in itself," in the words of Dr. Thompson S. Westcott of the University of Pennsylvania Hospital, but also "the means of changing the whole trend of professional thought upon the subject and of establishing this science of infant feeding upon an exact and rational basis."[16]

Unfortunately not everyone had access to a milk laboratory. As an alternative, Rotch developed a form of "home modification." For the cream he instructed mothers to let a quart jar of milk stand undisturbed for six hours and then siphon off the bottom 24 ounces, leaving 8 ounces of 10 percent cream (gravity cream). He constructed tables listing the amounts of siphoned milk, 10 percent cream, milk sugar (available at drug stores), lime-water, and boiled water needed to produce formulas of desired percentages. For example, if the physician determined that the infant needed a formula of 1.00 percent fat, 5.00 percent sugar, and 0.75 percent proteids, then the mother would be instructed to dissolve two 3.375-drachm measures of milk sugar in 20 ounces of water and to mix this sugar-water with 2 ounces of cream, 2 ounces of milk, and 1 ounce of lime-water.[17]

In the years following the introduction of the percentage method, other physicians produced elaborate charts detailing the proportions of gravity cream, milk, lime-water, water, and milk sugar necessary to produce formulas with given percentages of fat, sugar, and proteids. L. Emmett Holt, a staunch proponent of Rotch's method, published a series of increasingly complex formulations. In 1897 he suggested ten formulas to feed infants from birth to age eighteen months. To compound these formulas, the physician would order mixtures of various quantities of 12 percent cream with a 6 or 7 percent sugar solution, or 8 percent cream with a 5, 7, or 10 percent sugar solution. By 1902 Holt was recommending thirteen different formulas composed of 10 percent milk, 7 percent milk, or plain milk mixed with milk sugar, lime-water, and water. Seven years later he listed nineteen possible formulas for birth to one year of age and in 1911 presented his most detailed table (figure 2.1). Early twentieth-century pediatric textbooks and medical journals reprinted innumerable charts from other researchers as well.[18]

Other proponents of the percentage method feared that tables such as these disregarded important characteristics of Rotch's system. With these charts practitioners would merely memorize a few mixtures and would not think in terms of percentages; according to William Baner, a New York physician, this practice ignored the "great principle" of Rotch's method. If

A New Method of Calculating Milk Percentages. L. Emmett Holt, New York.

Formula obtained from milk containing different percentages of fat.

		A 7% Milk	B 6%	C 5%	D 4%	E 3%	F 2%	G 1%	Per cent.		Per cent.
I	1 ounce in 20 has Fat.	0.35	0.30	0.25	0.20	0.15	0.10	0.05	with Protein	0.175	Sugar 0.225
II	2 ounces in 20 has Fat.	0.70	0.60	0.50	0.40	0.30	0.20	0.10	with Protein	0.35	Sugar 0.45
III	3 ounces in 20 has Fat.	1.05	0.90	0.75	0.60	0.45	0.30	0.15	with Protein	0.50	Sugar 0.65
IV	4 ounces in 20 has Fat.	1.40	1.20	1.00	0.80	0.60	0.40	0.20	with Protein	0.70	Sugar 0.90
V	5 ounces in 20 has Fat.	1.75	1.50	1.25	1.00	0.75	0.50	0.25	with Protein	0.85	Sugar 1.30
VI	6 ounces in 20 has Fat.	2.10	1.80	1.50	1.20	0.90	0.60	0.30	with Protein	1.05	Sugar 1.35
VII	7 ounces in 20 has Fat.	2.45	2.10	1.75	1.40	1.05	0.70	0.35	with Protein	1.20	Sugar 1.55
VIII	8 ounces in 20 has Fat.	2.80	2.40	2.00	1.60	1.20	0.80	0.40	with Protein	1.40	Sugar 1.80
IX	9 ounces in 20 has Fat.	3.05	2.70	2.25	1.80	1.35	0.90	0.45	with Protein	1.60	Sugar 2.00
X	10 ounces in 20 has Fat.	3.50	3.00	2.50	2.00	1.50	1.00	0.50	with Protein	1.75	Sugar 2.25
XI	11 ounces in 20 has Fat.	3.80	3.30	2.75	2.20	1.65	1.10	0.55	with Protein	1.90	Sugar 2.45
XII	12 ounces in 20 has Fat.	.....	3.60	3.00	2.40	1.80	1.20	0.60	with Protein	2.10	Sugar 2.70
XIII	13 ounces in 20 has Fat.	.....	3.90	3.25	2.60	1.95	1.30	0.65	with Protein	2.25	Sugar 2.90
XIV	14 ounces in 20 has Fat.	.....	.....	3.50	2.80	2.10	1.40	0.70	with Protein	2.40	Sugar 3.15
XV	15 ounces in 20 has Fat.	.....	.....	.....	3.00	2.25	1.50	0.75	with Protein	2.60	Sugar 3.35

From 4 per cent. milk.............From 5 per cent. milk

To obtain 7 per cent. milk use upper 16 oz.............upper 20 oz.

To obtain 6 per cent. milk use upper 20 oz.............upper 24 oz.

To obtain 5 per cent. milk use upper 24 oz.............all

To obtain 4 per cent. milk use all.......................remainder after skimming off 2 oz.

To obtain 3 per cent. milk use remainder after skimming off 2 oz..remainder after skimming off 3 oz.

To obtain 2 per cent. milk use remainder after skimming off 4 oz..remainder after skimming off 5 oz.

To obtain 1 per cent. milk use remainder after skimming off 8 oz..remainder after skimming off 8 oz.

With Formulas I to V, enough sugar should be added to raise the amount to 5 per cent.

With Formulas VI to XV, enough sugar should be added to raise the amount to 6 per cent.

One ounce milk sugar by weight in 20-oz. mixture adds 5 per cent.

One ounce milk sugar by volume in 20-oz. mixture adds about 3 per cent.

One even tablespoonful   in 20 oz. mixture adds   1.75 per cent.

1 oz. 7 per cent. milk	27.5
1 oz. 6 per cent. milk	25.0
1 oz. 5 per cent. milk	22.5
1 oz. 4 per cent. milk	20.0
1 oz. 3 per cent. milk	17.5
1 oz. 2 per cent. milk	15.0
1 oz. 1 per cent. milk	12.5
1 oz. fat-free	10.0
1 oz. whey	10.0
1 oz. milk sugar by weight	116.0
1 oz. milk sugar by volume	72.0
1 even tablespoonful of milk sugar	44.0
1 oz. barley flour by weight	100.0
1 oz. barley water (1 tablespoonful to a pint)	2.0
1 oz. malt soup extract	80.0
1 oz. condensed milk	132.0
1 oz. olive oil by volume	245.0

Figure 2.1. Holt's method of calculating milk percentages. Source: L. Emmett Holt, "A new method of calculating milk percentages," *American Journal of Obstetrics and Diseases of Women and Children*, 64 (1911), 556

physicians used standard formulas without understanding the theory behind them, home-modified milk might be unsuccessful. Moreover, the charts were often "burdensome" and even "confusing." Physicians committed to the percentage method wanted practitioners to think in percentages and to have a simple method with which to translate these percentages "into terms of ordinary commercial articles."[19] Many so-called simple methods were proposed. Charles W. Townsend of the Harvard Medical School in 1899 formulated a series of rules based on Rotch's theory:

> Each ounce of 10-per-cent. cream in a twenty-ounce mixture represents .50 per cent. of fat, .20 per cent. of albuminoids and .20 per cent. of sugar; and each even tablespoon of sugar of milk represents 2 per cent.
>
> Thus if we order top milk four ounces, water fifteen ounces, lime-water one ounce, sugar of milk two tablespoonfuls, we are making a formula of fat 2 per cent., sugar 4.80, and albumenoids .80.[20]

Others presented their home-modification schemes in the form of algebraic equations. In 1898 Baner proposed one of the more popular sets of mathematical formulae, which continued to appear in print at least as late as 1923.[21]

Although Rotch preferred laboratory milk modifications above all other methods of artificial infant feeding, he too advocated a series of algebraic formulas for home use. Cognizant of the fact that many physicians found formulas inconvenient, "both because of the time required to make the computation and because of the difficulty which some minds experience in using algebraic formulae," he also recommended a card devised by Dr. Maynard Ladd of Harvard University (figure 2.2). This chart provided physicians with thirty possible combinations of fat, sugar, and proteids, compounded from cream, fat-free milk, lime-water, boiled water, and milk sugar.[22] Ladd's card and Holt's table graphically illustrate how complicated the percentage method had become. In addition, they suggest the major difficulty in the production of home-modified milk: the need to know the fat content of the cream used.

In reaction to the complexities of the percentage method, other theories based on European research were being proposed by the turn of the century. Within a decade, two feeding systems had emerged in the United States. One was Rotch's percentage, or American, method. Because most its adherents continued to cluster around Boston and the Harvard Medical School, proponents of this method became known as the Boston school. In opposition to them were physicians who based their theories on new European research

TABLE 18.

No.	℞. 20-oz. Mixtures. Percentage of Fat.	Sugar.	Prot'd.	Alk.	Ounces of Cream. 10%	12%	16%	20%	Ozs. Fat Free Milk Used with Creams of 10%	12%	16%	20%	Ounces Lm. Wtr.	Bld. Wtr.	Milk Sugar. meas.	Sugar % without dry sugar
1	1.50	4.50	0.25	5	*	*	*	1½	*	*	*	0	1	17½	2	0.33
2	1.50	4.50	0.50	5	3	2½	2	1½	0	½	1	1½	1	16	2	0.61
3	2.00	5.00	0.25	5	*	*	*	2	*	*	*	0	1	17	2¼	0.75
4	2.00	5.00	0.50	5	*	3¼	2½	2	*	0	½	1	1	15¾	2¼	0.73
5	2.00	5.00	0.75	5	4	3¼	2½	2	¾	1½	2¼	2¾	1	14½	2	1.01
6	2.00	5.50	1.00	5	4	3¼	2½	2	1¾	2½	3¼	3¾	1	13¼	2¼	1.30
7	2.50	5.00	0.50	5	*	*	3¼	2½	*	*	0	¾	1	15¾	2¼	0.78
8	2.50	5.50	0.75	5	*	4¼	3¼	2½	*	¼	1¼	2	1	14½	2¼	1.01
9	2.50	6.00	1.00	5	5	4¼	3¼	2½	1	1¾	2¾	3½	1	13½	2½	1.23
10	3.00	6.00	0.50	5	*	*	3¾	3	*	*	0	¾	1	15¼	2½	0.84
11	3.00	6.00	0.75	5	*	5	3¾	3	*	0	1¼	2	1	14	2½	1.12
12	3.00	6.00	1.00	5	6	5	3¾	3	0	1	2¼	3	1	13	2¼	1.35
13	3.00	6.00	1.25	5	6	5	3¾	3	1¼	2¼	3½	4¼	1	11¾	2¼	1.35
14	3.00	6.50	1.50	5	6	5	3¾	3	2½	3½	4¾	5½	1	10½	2¼	1.91
15	3.00	6.50	2.00	5	6	5	3¾	3	5½	6½	7¾	8½	1	7½	2	2.68
16	3.50	6.00	0.50	5	*	*	*	3½	*	*	*	0	1	15½	2½	0.78
17	3.50	6.00	0.75	5	*	*	4½	3½	*	*	0	1	1	14½	2½	1.01
18	3.50	6.50	1.00	5	*	5¾	4½	3½	*	0	1¼	2¼	1	13¼	2½	1.26
19	3.50	6.50	1.25	5	7	5¾	4½	3½	½	1¾	3	4	1	11½	2½	1.68
20	3.50	6.50	1.50	5	7	5¾	4½	3½	2	3¼	4½	5½	1	10	2¼	2.02
21	4.00	6.00	0.60	5	*	*	*	4	*	*	*	0	1	15	2½	0.78
22	4.00	6.00	0 75	5	*	*	5	4	*	*	0	1	1	14	2½	1.12
23	4.00	7.00	1.00	5	*	*	5	4	*	*	1	2	1	13	2¾	1.35
24	4.00	7.00	1.25	5	*	6¾	5	4	*	¾	2½	3½	1	11½	2½	1.68
25	4.00	7.00	1.50	5	8	6¾	5	4	1	2¼	4	5	1	10	2½	2.02
26	4.00	7.00	2.00	5	8	0¾	5	4	3½	4¾	6½	7½	1	7½	2¼	2.56
27	4.00	7.00	2.50	5	8	6¾	5	4	6¼	7½	9¼	10¼	1	4¾	2	3.20
28	4.00	7.00	3.00	5	8	6¾	5	4	9¼	10½	12¼	13¼	1	1¾	1½	3.88
29	4.00	6.00	3.00	5	8	6¾	5	4	9¼	10¼	12¼	13¼	1	1¾	1	3.88
30	4.00	5.50	3.00	5	8	6¾	5	4	9¼	10½	12¼	13¼	1	1¾	¾	3.88

For 25-oz. mixtures multiply amount of each ingredient by 1¼
For 30-oz. mixtures multiply amount of each ingredient by 1½
For 35-oz. mixtures multiply amount of each ingredient by 1¾
For 40-oz. mixtures multiply amount of each ingredient by 2
For 45-oz. mixtures multiply amount of each ingredient by 2¼
* Combination impossible with strength of cream indicated.

Figure 2.2. Dr. Maynard's card for calculating formulas. Source: Thomas Morgan Rotch, "The essential principles of infant feeding and the modern methods of applying them," *JAMA*, *41* (1903), 419

and used the so-called German, or caloric, method. Many of the most prolific and vocal proponents of this school, such as Dr. Joseph Brennemann and Dr. Isaac A. Abt, were located in Chicago; their method of simpler dilutions of milk, sugar, and water was sometimes called the Chicago method.[23]

Both schools investigated the digestibility, or indigestibility, of cow's milk in infant formulas. The Boston school named casein the culprit. They claimed that digestive and gastrointestinal disorders and dyspepsia all had their source in the firm, tough curds that cow's milk casein produced in the infant's digestive tract. Other researchers, most notably those influenced by German research, focused on the problem of fat digestion.[24] To these physicians, the indigestibility of fat, not protein, signaled that the percentage method was "erroneous." Furthermore, they argued that Rotch's method led to an "overfeeding" of fat, while the feeding of percentages left "undetermined the amount of food the baby gets"—that is, the caloric value of the food. This logic convinced physicians like Brennemann that the percentage method was "inadequate."[25]

Some investigators attempted to combine Rotch's method with the theories of fat indigestibility. Henry Dwight Chapin's rationale was typical. Though the caloric theory specified the amount of heat units, or calories, needed for an infant's growth and development, it did not specify which food was required. He therefore considered the caloric measure a necessary, but not sufficient, factor in infant feeding.[26] Dr. Frank Spooner Churchill, a professor at Rush Medical College, even claimed that the subject of infant feeding

> has now been crystallized into a study of the fats, sugars, and proteids, and the effects of feeding definite amounts of these elements. Obviously, such study has been made possible only by the method of percentage feeding, which has been gradually evolved and brought to its present high state of perfection by Rotch.[27]

Churchill and members of the Boston school praised the percentage method for its "elasticity," for "the power it places in the hands of the physician of exactly regulating the dosage of the various milk constituents," even the proportion of fat.[28]

Clearly, new data had forced changes in the percentage method. By 1906 even Rotch accepted a caloric measure as "of value to check percentage feeding," though he warned that "the number of calories, like the percentages of the ingredients, varies according to the pathological conditions present."[29] But a new debate was to undercut the theoretical foundations of the Boston method. Soon sugar came under investigation.

Rotch had always insisted that the only carbohydrate used in infant feeding be milk sugar (lactose). Though others preferred cane sugar (sucrose), which was less expensive and more readily available, Rotch had argued from analogy that since milk sugar was "always found in the milk of all mammals, it would be natural to suppose that this form of sugar had been put there for some good purpose." He rejected feeding an infant any "foreign" ingredient not found in human milk.[30] On the other hand, Abraham Jacobi, a leading pediatrician, preferred cane sugar because he worried about the change from milk sugar to lactic acid. "Some lactic acid was necessary for proper digestion," he believed, but "an over quantity produced hyperacidity and indigestion." Rotch dismissed this argument as "much exaggerated."[31] Throughout the 1890s and into the twentieth century, investigators continued to discuss the differences between various sugars. Holt concluded that milk sugar was best because it "supplies what exists in woman's milk." However, like other physicians of the time, he used cane sugar when good milk sugar was not available.[32]

By the end of the first decade of this century, American researchers had followed up some of the data German investigators had developed on the effects of different sugars. Brennemann applauded the use of maltose, recommended by some German pediatricians in cases of infant indigestion. Americans, he felt, were "handicapped in not having a desirable maltose . . . in this country." He had been forced to use an unnamed patent food "that is composed largely of maltose, with excellent results."[33] Rotch and John Lovett Morse, in their column in the *Boston Medical and Surgical Journal,* described some differences between various carbohydrates and, in doing so, also acknowledged the efficacy of some patent foods. If physicians found "unexplained success from the use of a food of which maltose [was] the principal ingredient," Rotch and Morse advised, then they should prescribe a milk mixture in which the lactose was replaced by maltose.[34]

Controversies among medical researchers affected infant-food manufacturers also. Mellin's produced a booklet that provided physicians with detailed instructions on using Mellin's Food in percentage feeding. The company included a table for preparing creams and top-milks from milks containing various percentages of fat.[35] Of course, the product could still be mixed and fed as it had been before the development of the percentage method. Smith, Kline & French added comments about fat digestion to its advertisements for Eskay's Food (figure 2.3).

> In modifying cow's milk for infant use, it is just as important to modify the
> fat as the casein, because the fat of cow's milk is much more indigestible
> than the fat of human milk, just as the casein of cow's milk is much more
> indigestible than the casein of human milk.[36]

With these and similar promotions, infant-food companies endeavored to convince physicians that their products represented the current state of infant-feeding research. When German-trained physicians returned to the United States imbued with the new caloric theories, the industry did more than alter advertising.

Jerome S. Leopold of the Post-Graduate Hospital and Medical School of New York City had studied medicine in Germany. In 1910, Leopold, who combined research with an urban practice, wrote of his European studies: "There is considerable difference in the influence on the organism of the different sugars. I have shown . . . that a combination of dextrin and maltose causes the least disturbance in infant feeding, and that lactose should not be used in milk dilutions."[37] But as Brennemann had pointed out several years earlier, the desired carbohydrate was not readily available in the United States. A short time later, in 1911, Joe Quilligan, senior sales representative of the Mead Johnson Company, called on Leopold, who was at that time in charge of the milk station of the New York Milk Committee. Leopold explained that he could not find a manufacturer willing to produce the maltose-dextrin. Quilligan suggested to E. Mead Johnson that their company could produce the desired sugar. Johnson agreed.[38]

At the time Johnson's son Lambert was studying chemistry at Cornell. He

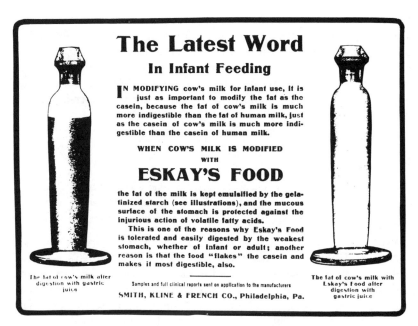

The Latest Word

In Infant Feeding

IN MODIFYING cow's milk for infant use, it is just as important to modify the fat as the casein, because the fat of cow's milk is much more indigestible than the fat of human milk, just as the casein of cow's milk is much more indigestible than the casein of human milk.

WHEN COW'S MILK IS MODIFIED
WITH

ESKAY'S FOOD

the fat of the milk is kept emulsified by the gelatinized starch (see illustrations), and the mucous surface of the stomach is protected against the injurious action of volatile fatty acids.

This is one of the reasons why Eskay's Food is tolerated and easily digested by the weakest stomach, whether of infant or adult; another reason is that the food "flakes" the casein and makes it most digestible, also.

The fat of cow's milk after digestion with gastric juice

Samples and full clinical reports sent on application to the manufacturers

SMITH, KLINE & FRENCH CO., Philadelphia, Pa.

The fat of cow's milk with Eskay's Food after digestion with gastric juice

Figure 2.3. Eskay's advertisement. Source: *JAMA*, *55* (4) (1910), adv. 52. Courtesy of the Archive, American Medical Association

was called home to work out the production problems and in a month developed a process that converted potato starch into dextrin and maltose. The product, Dextri-Maltose, was tested at the Babies' Ward of the New York Post-Graduate Hospital. When the company introduced Dextri-Maltose to the medical profession at the 1912 meeting of the American Medical Association, it was a singular product. Not only was it the first infant-food product developed in the United States by a commercial manufacturer at the instigation of a pediatric researcher, but it was advertised only to physicians, and its packaging contained no instructions for home use.[39]

The percentage method of infant feeding had dominated American pediatric thought for many years. By the 1910s, however, it has been generally discarded, except at Harvard, where, under the direction of Rotch's "staunch, loyal supporter and disciple," John Lovett Morse, the percentage method continued to be taught. Apparently, despite their disenchantment with the Boston method and the fact that few used it in their work, the staff felt that they had to instruct medical students in Rotch's method or lose their positions.[40] For most other researchers and teachers, investigations into infant digestion and metabolism had demonstrated the mistaken assumptions underlying Rotch's theory. The indigestibility of proteins did not explain all infantile indigestions; any one or all of the basic elements of fat, sugar, and protein could be responsible. For growth and development infants needed more than the correct percentages of ingredients; they also required a certain number of calories. But as Brennemann recalled many years later, in order to satisfy all the criteria, percentage feeding

> became increasingly more complicated and involved, as ever new and so-called "simpler" methods of calculation appeared until finally some of the articles seemed terrifyingly like treatises on mathematics or higher astronomy. . . . It all gradually became a headache to most of us. . . . The whole edifice finally collapsed because the superstructure was top heavy and the foundations weak, and because really simpler ideas came into play.[41]

Even proponents of the Boston method recognized problems with the percentage method.[42] By the 1910s they claimed that Rotch's scientific feeding of infants was not a particular formula or set of formulas, but rather a method of recording that established a common terminology for the various methods of infant feeding and a basis for comparing these methods. The percentage method, for them, was not a theory but a form of calculation, a convenient way of expressing the quantities of each food element and "a means of obtaining relative accuracy in the preparation of infant foods." They did retain one important aspect of Rotch's theoretical structure: the need to individualize cow's-milk formulas for artificially fed infants. The digestion and metabolism of each baby was unique; therefore, it was impossible to have one food for all babies. Rotch's followers believed that with a modified percentage method they had a flexible system for feeding all infants.[43] Other physicians, however, sought simpler feeding methods applicable to most, if not all, babies.

The legacy of the percentage method goes beyond any mere enumeration of its successes and failures. Rotch, by his work and writings, directly encouraged more that one generation of researchers to concentrate on the problem of infant feeding. As the next chapter will document, though his method fell into disfavor, his concern for infant nutrition continued to influence pediatric research.

III

"A Rational Means of Feeding the Baby"
1915–1950

Though the percentage method declined, infant feeding continued to attract the attention of researchers. Even physicians who proposed often radically different theories of infant feeding generally agreed on the importance of nutrition in pediatrics. Lewis Webb Hill, for example, advocated the Boston method; Jesse Robert Gerstley preferred the Chicago method. Yet when these two physicians contributed to the 1917 book *Clinical lectures on infant feeding,* both placed nutrition at the center of pediatrics. Hill began his first lecture:

> Pediatrics, or the study of diseases of children, is naturally divided into a number of sections, of which the most important is the feeding of infants and the treatment of the diarrheal diseases of infancy.

Gerstley's opening remarks were even more pointed:

> one almost might say that if we have mastered infant feeding, in addition to a little hygiene, there would be *no sick* babies. Don't take this statement too literally. But I make it boldly, and repeat it, to show how much emphasis I lay upon the subject.[1]

Numerous physicians expressed similar sentiments in the 1910s and 1920s.[2] Over the next several decades, however, the problems of infant feeding and nutrition receded from the forefront of pediatric research. Infant feeding was no longer a primary subject of investigation because the theory had become simplified, rationalized, and successful, as evidenced by the "remarkably reduced infant mortality."[3] Pediatric researchers published statistical studies that demonstrated that bottle-fed infants—"properly fed" with "supervised modern feeding"—compared favorably with breast-fed infants in terms of weight gain, growth, and morbidity. Indeed, some investigators found that bottle-fed infants sometimes did better than a breast-fed control group. Because for many years the specialty was synonymous with infant nutrition, success in infant feeding assured pediatrics a valued place in the profession.[4]

With the development of healthful artificial foods, researchers did not dismiss the use of breast milk; most considered mother's milk best for infants. Unfortunately, physicians alleged, many women did not have enough breast milk to feed their infants successfully until the recommended weaning age of seven or eight months, and some mothers could not produce enough milk even in their infants' early life. Indeed, human milk would be satisfactory only if the mother's diet was well-balanced and adequate. Even then, dietary supplements were needed. To prevent rickets, either the mother should be irradiated with ultraviolet light for a short time to increase the antirachitic potency of her milk, or the infant should be fed cod-liver oil; breast milk was not sufficiently antirachitic. To prevent scurvy, even breast-fed infants should receive daily doses of orange juice or tomato juice.[5] Many physicians expressed concern over the length of time it might take for newborns to regain their birth weight. They viewed any delay in the mother's lactation with alarm and often recommended offering the infant artificial food from the first day to obviate the initial weight loss.[6] These physicians and other researchers were quick to propose artificial feeding because they felt that infants brought up on the bottle generally would be as healthy as breast-fed babies. So convinced of the efficacy of bottle feeding was Dr. Abraham Tow that in 1934 he advised the meeting of the Clinical Section of the New York Polyclinic Medical School and Hospital to recommend the bottle whenever the baby failed to gain, when nursing was painful for the mother, or "when, for economic or other reasons, it [was] distasteful to the mother." He did not deny that breast milk was good, but he was ambivalent about its superiority and felt it "unnecessary to make undue sacrifices in continuing its use."[7]

Various factors contributed to this growing confidence in bottle feeding. Statistical studies demonstrating the healthfulness of artificial feeding encouraged this view; so too did advances in pediatric and nutritional research and the development of simple-to-use formulas. Dr. Manuel M. Glazier, an instructor at Tufts College Medical School, analyzed a group of 217 infants who attended well-baby clinics in Boston and compared their records with vital statistics from the Boston Health Department on 1,556 nonclinic infants who were followed for one year. He concluded in an oft-cited paper originally published in 1930:

I. Infant mortality and frequency of infection have a definite relationship to poor economic and hygienic conditions. In group studies, "breast" or "bottle" feeding alone are not the determining factors in frequency of infection and infant mortality.

II. Infants in a district with poor economic and hygienic conditions have more frequency of infections, deficiency diseases, and greater infant mortality, irrespective of breast or bottle feeding.

III. In districts where economic and hygienic conditions are fairly good, the average bottle-fed infant does as well as the average breast-fed infant.

IV. Clinic infants have a mortality of one-half that of nonclinic infants in the same district.

Clinic infants—that is, infants "under proper medical and nursing care"—were healthier than nonclinic infants, regardless of the mode of feeding. Another study published in the same year by Joseph Garland, M.D., and Mabel Rich, R.N., extended Glazier's work and stated definitely that given medical supervision, "actually the social status, the intelligence and the environment of the mother are more important factors in assuring the health and well-being of the child than is the type of feeding.[8]

Nutritional research in the 1910s and 1920s further encouraged the routine use of simple milk mixtures. Previously, a major obstacle to successful artificial infant feeding was the supposed indigestibility of the casein or protein element in cow's milk, though German scientists early in the century had reported that this was not a problem. Dr. Joseph Brennemann, of Northwestern University, investigated why the large, tough curds (considered undigested protein curds) often found in the stools of American bottle-fed infants were not familiar to the German researchers.

During postgraduate study in Germany in 1910, Brennemann had noted that the Germans almost invariably fed their infants boiled milk. He hypothesized that boiling somehow altered the casein and produced a more digestible protein. In 1911, to determine whether heating did affect the curd, he fed four healthy infants alternately with raw and boiled cow's milk and found that he could produce or eliminate the tough curds at will. "We have never seen a hard curd unless a considerable amount of raw milk casein was given," concluded Brennemann, "and we have never seen them persist or occur when boiled milk, no matter what amount, was given." He produced similar results *in vitro* and observed that the more the milk was boiled or diluted, the slower the coagulation and the less firm the coagulum.[9] Brennemann sought to go beyond *in vitro* experiments and clinical tests to study what actually happened in the stomach. In 1913 he discovered a young man with normal digestion "who could promptly, with little effort and a minimum of trauma to the curds, empty the stomach by the simple method of passing the finger into the throat." Brennemann had intended to conduct only two experiments, "but the process was so free from serious discomfort, the disclosures so interesting, and the subject so willing," that he and his subject undertook many more.

During the next several years, Brennemann and this young man conducted nearly a hundred experiments using raw milk; boiled milk; evaporated milk; condensed milk; milk modified with lime-water, sodium citrate, sodium bicarbonate, barley flour, Mellin's Food, Dextri-Maltose, cane sugar, and maltose; and also patent foods such as Nestlé's Milk Food and Horlick's Malted Milk. The results demonstrated that "the size of the curd varies inversely as the dilution, or directly as the amount of casein." Furthermore, smaller, softer curds were produced from milk that had been boiled and also from most milks that had undergone a manufacturing process such as condensation or drying. Thus evaporated milk, condensed milk, and patent foods like Nestlé's and Horlick's were more digestible than raw milk. So too was milk modified by the addition of lime-water, sodium citrate, sodium bicarbonate, or starch. The addition of sugar had little effect on the curds (figure 3.1). Though Brennemann avoided any explicit recommendations, he pointedly observed that there was no evidence that boiled milk was less nutritious than raw, that no one claimed that boiled milk resulted in rickets, and that scurvy was less common in Germany and France, where infants regularly received boiled milk, than in the United States.[11] At this time Brennemann downplayed the indigestibility of protein but recommended that should the infant exhibit symptoms that suggested an intolerance for protein, the milk should be boiled or an alkali such as sodium citrate or lime-water added. Other researchers gave similar advice.[12]

While Brennemann investigated the digestibility of the protein element, a group at the Babies' Dispensary and Hospital and Western Reserve University in Cleveland, Ohio, focused their research on the fat component of cow's milk. These researchers, under the direction of Dr. H. J. Gerstenberger, followed up on German studies that had examined the qualitative differences between cow's-milk fat and breast-milk fat. They produced a homogenized mixture of several animal and vegetable fats that was "nearly identical with the fat of human milk." This emulsion they then mixed with cow's milk from which the fat had been removed. The group presented the resultant food, named "G-R," to the 1915 meeting of the American Pediatric Society. Continued research modified the food slightly, and by 1919 Gerstenberger reported that he had successfully tested what was now known as "S.M.A."

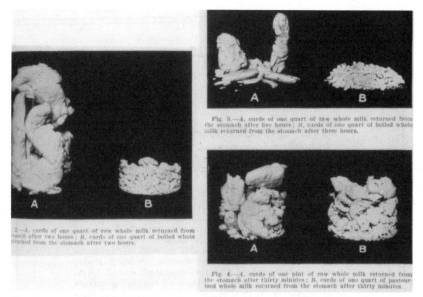

Fig. 3.—A, curds of one quart of raw whole milk returned from the stomach after five hours; B, curds of one quart of boiled whole milk returned from the stomach after three hours.

2.—A, curds of one quart of raw whole milk returned from stomach after two hours; B, curds of one quart of boiled whole returned from the stomach after two hours.

Fig. 4.—A, curds of one pint of raw whole milk returned from the stomach after thirty minutes; B, curds of one quart of pasteurized whole milk returned from the stomach after thirty minutes.

Figure 3.1. Curds analyzed in Brennemann's experiments. Source: Joseph Brennemann, "Boiled versus raw milk: An experimental study of milk coagulation in stomach, together with clinical observations on the use of raw and boiled milk," *JAMA*, 60 (1913), 575–582.

(Synthetic Milk Adapted) with 311 infants at the Babies' Dispensary. As with Dextri-Maltose, the impetus for this new infant food originated with the medical profession, which clinically tested it. The Laboratory Products Company marketed S.M.A. to the medical profession in the early 1920s, and several leading pediatric researchers cautiously, but enthusiastically, wrote of its value in infant feeding. In Gerstenberger's view, "the feeding of artificially-fed infants in the greatest per cent of cases can be, and in the future will be, successfully carried out in the simplest manner imaginable, both for family physician and parent, by the use of complete foods prepared on a large scale."[13] S.M.A. was not only simple to use, but "in certain details" it was superior to breast milk because it was antirachitic. Therefore, the company stressed, the value of S.M.A. lay not only in its superior fat content, but also because it contained cod-liver oil as a prophylactic against rickets[14] (figure 3.2).

In the late nineteenth and early twentieth centuries, the etiology of rickets was unclear. Causes cited included premature weaning, protracted lactation, the use of improper food, adverse living conditions such as dirty, damp, dark, and poorly ventilated apartments, and the lack of fresh air and sunshine. A

Figure 3.2. S.M.A. advertisement. Source: *JAMA*, 80 (26) (1923), adv. 11

connection between poor diet and the incidence of rickets was noted, though no one had a satisfactory explanation for breast-fed infants who became rachitic. Nutritional studies in the second and third decades of this century clarified the issue. The disease resulted from a deficiency of vitamin D. When this necessary element is lacking, it can be supplied by a dietary supplement, such as cod-liver oil. Moreover, when exposed to the sun or to ultraviolet light, the body can produce its own vitamin D.[15]

Though some physicians, even in the 1920s, resisted the widespread use of cod-liver oil, most others considered it a cure for rickets[16] and a preventative against it. Not surprisingly, then, the Laboratory Products Company advertised S.M.A. as "markedly anti-rachitic" and claimed that the product prevented rickets. Similarly, the Nestlé's Milk Food Company fortified its Milk Food with "the vitamin-content of cod-liver oil" and described the improved Milk Food as "an anti-rachitic polycarbohydrate milk modifier" (figure 3.3). Furthermore, uncertainty about the antirachitic potency of mother's milk led some physicians to advise cod-liver oil as a preventative even for breast-fed patients.

By the 1930s few disagreed with the proposition that bottle-fed infants needed some regular source of vitamin D for healthy growth and development. The popularity of cod-liver oil continued, but other forms of vitamin D appeared. In 1924, Alfred Hess of New York and Harry Steenbock of the University of Wisconsin independently reported that foods that were of no value in the prevention of rickets, such as cottonseed oil and linseed oil, could gain antirachitic properties by being exposed to ultraviolet light. In the years following, investigators irradiated other foods. Researchers produced vitamin D milk by irradiating whole milk, evaporated milk, and dried milk. These forms of vitamin D milk and that obtained by feeding cows irradiated yeast were both successful in curing and preventing rickets. The availability of these sources of vitamin D led to a marked decline in the incidence of rickets by mid-century.[17]

Twentieth-century researchers grappled with other problems that had plagued their predecessors. Before Brennemann examined heated milks from a physiologic point of view, other investigators had discussed the milk's bacteriological condition. In the late nineteenth century, physicians generally preferred raw milk for infant feeding, unless there was some doubt about the bacterial quality of the milk supply, in which case milk should be heated. By the turn of the century, physicians feared that high heat destroyed some of the nutritive factors in milk, and they therefore recommended pasteurization rather than sterilization. As Dr. Maurice Ostheimer, an instructor of pediatrics at the University of Pennsylvania, colorfully explained:

The Improved
NESTLÉ'S MILK FOOD
An anti-rachitic polycarbohydrate milk modifier

1. The Improved Nestlé's Milk Food, prepared with equal parts of fresh cow's milk and water, provides an ideal feeding for the normal infant—properly balanced in fat, protein, carbohydrate and mineral salts—and of excellent digestibility. The carbohydrate—being a *mixture* of lactose, saccharose, maltose, dextrin and starch—modifies the milk ideally.

2. The milk content of the Improved Nestlé's Milk Food has been made adequate for the infant's milk needs even when the Food is prepared with water only. It is, therefore, especially valuable (1) when infants do not tolerate fresh cow's milk, (2) when the milk supply is of doubtful purity, or (3) when it is advisable to give a feeding relatively low in fat and protein and high in carbohydrate.

3. Prepared with water only, it is an excellent aid in correcting constipation.

4. Small proportion of starch in it aids digestion and helps pave the way for introduction of cereals into diet later.

5. Mineral contents have been reinforced, especially in the needed calcium and phosphate.

6. It is an excellent supplementary food for breast-fed infants because of its nourishing qualities and digestibility.

7. It PROTECTS AGAINST RICKETS, because there has been added to it the vitamin-content of cod-liver oil without the disagreeable taste and odor.

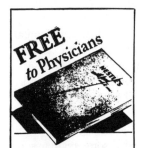

Helen L. Fales, formerly research chemist and nutritional worker at the Babies' Hospital, under the direction of Dr. L. Emmett Holt, has prepared an interesting and helpful booklet on the composition, properties and uses of the Improved Nestlé's Milk Food. If you have not yet received your copy, mail coupon below.

For samples of the Improved Nestlé's Milk Food, booklet and celluloid feeding table calculator, mail coupon below to Nestlé's Food Co., Inc., 2 Lafayette St., New York City.

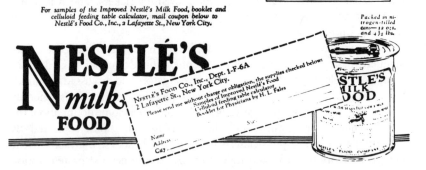

Figure 3.3. Nestlé's Milk Food advertisement. Source: *JAMA*, 90 (26) (1928), adv. 8. Courtesy of the Archive, American Medical Association

How much better off would the community be, were we able to furnish a clean milk to all, so that neither pasteurization nor sterilization need even be thought of! Sterilization causes decided changes, those which occur whenever milk is boiled, and should never be employed; while pasteurization, always an iniquity, though occasionally a necessary iniquity, can also be dispensed with when clean milk and cream are used.[18]

Dissatisfied with the commercial pasteurization of milk, which they feared was an imperfect process "used for the purpose of keeping dirty milk sweet until it can reach the consumer," researchers recommended home pasteurization. Dr. Clifford G. Grulee, of Rush Medical Collge, advised heating milk to a temperature of 140 or 150 degrees Fahrenheit and holding it there for 30 minutes. If no thermometer was available, he suggested heating the milk "until a scum forms on it, and maintaining it at that temperature for the time mentioned."[19] To pasteurize milk correctly at home was no easy procedure. A less complicated method of home heating, of course, was to boil milk. Following Brennemann's demonstration that boiled milk produced softer, smaller curds and also research that suggested that boiling did not significantly harm the nutritive value of milk, physicians such as Grulee began to recommend that milk used in infant feeding be sterilized at home by boiling it from five to twenty minutes.[20]

Researchers often discussed the place of heated milk, either pasteurized or sterilized, in the infant's diet. Almost invariably, whether they believed that raw milk was best or not, they opted for the safety of heated milk.[21] To correct any possible damage to the nutritive quality of heated milk, researchers began recommending regular dietary supplements. Furthermore, even in raw milk "the anti-scorbutic value of milk depends almost entirely upon the fodder of the cow," so physicians advised feeding an antiscorbutic such as orange juice whether raw, pasteurized, or boiled milk was used. A 1923 editorial in the *Boston Medical and Surgical Journal* summarized the opinion of a majority of the pediatric researchers of the day:

A boiled *fresh* milk, a milk that does not already contain the toxic products of bacterial growth, is the only entirely safe milk that can be fed to infants; it is a more digestible form of milk than either raw or pasteurized milk, and the slight disadvantage of lessened accessory product content is easily remedied.

To compensate for any possible vitamin loss, the editorial writer suggested "the addition of orange juice or orange juice and cod liver oil to the diet."[22]

Manufacturers were not unaware of the advisability of marketing an anti-scorbutic product. Gerstenberger helped the Laboratory Products Company develop a spray-dried orange juice–lactose combination that, added to S.M.A., served as a preventative against scurvy.[23]

Though Dr. Williams McKim Marriott, of Washington University, St. Louis, recognized that heating destroyed the vitamin C content of milk, he too promoted boiled milk for infant feeding because it was safe from a bacterial standpoint and more digestible than raw or pasteurized milk. Marriott approached pediatric research from a biochemical rather than a clinical background.[24] He not only supported the use of heated milk and antiscorbutics, but he also contributed to two other significant shifts in infant-feeding research. First, he introduced a new carbohydrate. Nine-teenth-century researchers had debated the use of milk sugar (lactose) and cane sugar (sucrose). Physicians in the early twentieth century could choose from among lactose, sucrose, maltose, dextrose, and also combinations of these and other carbohydrates, which pediatric investigators noted were superior to any single sugar.[25] Still, many physicians, especially those at infant welfare stations, continued to use cane sugar because it was readily available and cheap, though they resorted to proprietary combinations such as Dextri-Maltose for infants with digestive problems. In the early 1920s, when St. Louis was expanding its infant-care facilities, cane sugar became for a time scarce and quite expensive. Marriott recommended the substitution of Karo Syrup (corn syrup) for cane sugar. Karo Syrup was inexpensive and plentiful; it contained 50 percent dextrin, 30 percent maltose, and 10 percent each dextrose and sucrose, a combination similar to that found in many more expensive carbohydrate mixtures. Karo Syrup became the carbohydrate of choice for many physicians, especially during the Depression.[26]

Dextri-Maltose and S.M.A. were typical examples of infant foods pro-duced by manufacturers responding to the needs and wants of physicians. Marriott's other major contribution to artificial feeding reversed this sequence and was one of the first instances of a manufacturer approaching pediatric researchers. In the late 1920s the Evaporated Milk Association funded Marriott's research into the use of evaporated milk in infant feeding.[27]

The idea of feeding infants canned milk was not new. Gail Borden had developed and marketed Eagle Brand Condensed Milk in the United States during the mid-nineteenth century, at least in part, as an infant food. But since Borden preserved this milk by adding a significant quantity of sugar, most nineteenth-century physicians had decried its use for infant feeding. Unsweetened evaporated milk was not produced in the United States until the 1880s, when the Helvetia Milk Condensing Company of Highland, Illinois (later the Pet Milk Company), established a factory under the direction of John Meyenberg, a Swiss and a former employee of a European firm called the Anglo-Swiss Condensed Milk Company. Within a few years Helvetia was sending its sales personnel throughout the country and advertising its product for infant feeding. One of the retailers who bought some Highland Brand Evaporated Milk was E. A. Stuart of El Paso, Texas. In 1887 his young infant son was not thriving, and Stuart decided to try feeding him the canned milk. To the Stuarts' delight, the baby improved, and the retailer ordered more Highland Brand for his store. In 1899 Stuart bought a bankrupt condensery in Los Angeles and, with the help of Meyenberg, who had left Helvetia, established the Pacific Condensed Milk Company (later the Carnation Company). Both Pet and Carnation marketed their products for infant use, but because unsweetened evaporated milk was often confused with sweetened condensed milk, they and other, smaller evaporated milk companies had difficulty getting physicians to accept their product. The Evaporated Milk Association, an organization of manufacturers, aimed to demonstrate that evaporated milk was successful in infant feeding.[28]

Marriott had previously recommended evaporated milk for patients who lived in areas with doubtful milk supplies or who were traveling. Then, because evaporated milk was sterile, inexpensive, and generally available, he extended its use to "the poorer and more ignorant dispensary class of patients where it was felt that the mothers were not sufficiently intelligent to be trusted to sterilize formulas properly or did not have the facilities for the refrigeration of bottle milk." Even under such adverse circumstances, the results were "so generally satisfactory" that Marriott conducted a clinical study of evaporated milk feeding for "well and sick babies of all classes." From the summer of 1927 through the fall of 1928, he observed 752 infants, of whom 570 were newborns, 107 from dispensary and private practices, and 75 sick infants (including 11 premature babies) in a hospital. The study also included a control group of 670 infants who received breast milk or artifical feedings prepared from bottled milk. All infants in both groups received supplements of cod-liver oil and orange juice. Marriott reported that newborns fed on evaporated milk formulas regained their birth weight sooner than those fed exclusively at the breast or with supplementary bottled cow's-milk formulas. All the well infants, regardless of the form of feeding, showed the same average daily weight gain. Sick infants, especially the premature babies, did better on the evaporated milk formulas. Marriott concluded: "The known qualities of unsweetened evaporated milk—its sterility, its ready digestibility and uniformity of composition—are distinct advantages which recommend it for general use as milk for infants."[29]

Though Marriott had not been the first to recommend evaporated milk formulas, after the publication of his study in 1929 his enthusiasm for the product fired the interest of other researchers. By 1930 investigators had completed and reported on six other studies. Throughout the 1930s many other researchers undertook clinical tests to verify time and again that evaporated milk was superior to bottled cow's milk and even, in some cases, to breast milk.[30] The canned fluid was sterile, digestible, uniform; it was also easier to prepare (thus there was less likelihood of error or contamination), and, like Karo Syrup, it was readily available and economical.[31] An added advantage appeared in 1934 when Pet, Carnation, and several other brands used an irradiation process developed by Steenbock to market antirachitic vitamin D–enriched milks.[32] Dried milks too were found to be excellent for infant feeding—a readily digestible, sterile, and uniform product.[33]

By the 1930s and 1940s, pediatric theory had progressed to the stage where researchers were confident that, if they controlled the feeding, a bottle-fed baby could grow and develop as healthily as a breast-fed one, if not better. With their more detailed understanding of digestion and nutrition, many researchers accepted a general theory of infant feeding remarkably similar to the one originally outlined in 1915 by Roger H. Dennett of the Department of Pediatrics of the New York Post-Graduate Medical School and Hospital. Any successful infant food required three basic attributes: it must contain the proper elements; it must be digestible; and it must be given in the proper quantity as determined by its caloric value. Dennett believed that previous infant-feeding methods had failed because they "have been dependent upon one rather than upon all three of these equally important requirements. . . . Simple mixtures of cow's milk, water and sugar usually fulfill these requirements for an infant's food, and it is seldom necessary to use anything else."[34]

Dennett's plea for simplified infant feeding had been a direct reaction against his training in the percentage method. Rather than teach medical students and practitioners the complicated Boston method, he preferred to present them with one simple method of infant feeding and then to outline conditions under which special foods must be used for ill babies with digestive disturbances. In other words, most babies would receive a generalized or routine formula, not an individualized one.[35] Compared with Rotch's method, Dennett's system was sheer simplicity.

> The average infant having no digestive disturbances requires in twenty-four hours twice as many ounces of milk as he weighs in pounds, provided he can take 1½ ounces of sugar. This rule is a rough one only. Thin or emaciated infants need more. Fat infants need less.

As a check on this formula, Dennett recommended that the physician compare the calories per day required by the infant with the number of calories produced by the mixture. The caloric requirement he set at 40–45 calories per pound of body weight per day for fat infants over four months of age; 50–55 calories for infants under four months or thin infants of any age; and 60–65 calories for emaciated infants. If a more exact formula was needed, the physician determined the total number of calories required per day and subtracted the number of calories supplied by the chosen carbohydrate. The result was divided by 20 (the number of calories in an ounce of milk) to calculate the quantity of milk needed. This number was subtracted from the total ounces recommended for a twenty-four period to arrive at the quantity of water required in the final mixture.[36]

Not all researchers in the 1910s and 1920s praised Dennett's simpler methods. John Lovett Morse, Rotch's protégé, continued to advocate the percentage method, and most of the opposition to Dennett's procedures came from members of the Boston school. But by 1927 even Maynard Ladd, one of Rotch's most enthusiastic students, was recommending feeding infants by the caloric method, using whole milk with sugar and water added.[37] Other academicians utilized Dennett's method or their own variants of it in their teaching. For example, Dr. Ralph Scobey, of Syracuse University, taught his students simply that infants should have three ounces of fluid per pound of body weight, two grams of protein per pound (an ounce of milk contains one gram of protein), and one and a half ounces of sugar per day. By the 1930s and 1940s most researchers and teachers had proposed similar formulations.[38] To enhance the digestibility of the cow's milk, this ingredient was either boiled, evaporated, or dried. Various carbohydrates could be used to achieve the correct caloric value, depending on the health of the infant and the economic circumstances of the family.

The general acceptance of simple infant formulas was one major difference between early twentieth-century physicians and those of the 1930s and 1940s. Another significant distinction is evident in their approach to manufactured or patent foods. By the latter period, researchers themselves had initiated several commercial foods, notably Dextri-Maltose and S.M.A., and they had begun to examine other proprietary foods more closely. Published analyses usually rationalized that if doctors used them at all, they should know what they contained.[39] As combination sugars, like maltose-dextrin became more popular, researchers looked again at infant foods like Mellin's and Horlick's and found them satisfactory carbohydrates for infant feeding. Marriott noted, "A number of food mixtures have been devised for the feeding of normal infants and many of these are entirely satisfactory in practice, provided the fundamental nutritional requirements are met." He specifically named carbohydrates such as Mellin's and Horlick's and called S.M.A. the "most scientific" of the complete infant foods.[40]

Other researchers conducted clinical tests to ascertain the efficacy of at least one of S.M.A.'s competitors, Nestlé's Lactogen (figure 3.4). Comparing breast-fed infants and infants fed on Lactogen, Dr. Ralph Shapiro, of the Newark Department of Health, concluded, "On the whole, the results obtained show plainly that Lactogen when fed in proper amounts will not only produce a normal weight gain but also correct underweight conditions." Another study found that Lactogen "meets the nutritional requirements of the normal infant. . . . This food is easily digested by the normal infant." Whether Nestlé's funded these research projects is unknown, but other concerns, such as Borden's, Mead Johnson, and the Wisconsin Alumni Research Foundation, which held Steenbock's irradiation patent, regularly supplied researchers with money and materials to test their products.[41]

Though patent foods "used intelligently" could be healthful, some physicians objected to them because "their claims are exaggerated," and "their use tends to develop slipshod methods of feeding." There was another unfortunate drawback to these foods: "being led by the advertisements of the manufacturers of these foods to believe that the artificial feeding of infants is a very simple matter, parents attempt to feed their own babies on such foods instead of employing a physician to prescribe the feeding."[42] As will be seen in Chapter 5, the American Medical Association in the 1930s undertook to eliminate this difficulty by insisting that infant-food companies provide directions for use only to the medical profession.

By the middle decades of this century, pediatric researchers generally had arrived at a consensus; simplified, routinized forms of infant feeding replaced the controversial and complicated methods recommended previously. "Breast milk, when it is good, is the best food that we can give an infant," agreed most physicians at mid-century, but "still when the need arises, one must not hesitate to wean an infant."[43] Some researchers were so impressed with the advances of modern infant feeding that they suggested that the infant, not the food, was the cause of feeding problems: "Failure of a baby to gain on a well-balanced formula does not necessarily imply that the formula per se is at fault, and it certainly should not be considered an indication to change to something else—as it too frequently is. . . . The formula is rarely guilty."[44]

As the dangers and difficulties seemed to shrink, the artificial feeding of infants, which for many decades had commanded the attention of

Figure 3.4. Lactogen advertisement. Source: *JAMA, 100* (24) (1933), adv. 8

researchers, ceased to be a major component of pediatric investigations.
How the debates over infant feeding theories and the researchers' ultimate
faith in the efficacy of artificial feeding affected medical practice will be
discussed in the next section.

PART TWO

Infant Feeding in Medical Practice

IV

"For Humanity's Sake"
1890–1910

"It is a wonderfully mistaken idea that has been stalking abroad," one Auburn, Indiana, physician chided his colleagues in 1884, "that 'anybody' is competent to treat infants." In fact,

> no part of work requires so much care, science and judgment as our labors with the children; and no part will give such prompt and good results, such satisfaction and success, as a rational and scientific treatment of the little ones. . . . All [physicians] are invited to enter and assist in cultivating its soil and removing rank growth of error, skepticism, and failure, which we find preoccupying its surface.

Physicians had previously "surrendered" the children, and especially the babies, to the care of "'old women' and uneducated nurses," but this, he admonished, should no longer be; the treatment of children belonged to the family physician. "Come," he urged, "let us redeem it for humanity's sake and in the interests of the dear children."[1] Over the next several decades his vision flourished; by 1908, according to one estimate, pediatrics represented one-half of the practice of the typical family physician.[2]

Since medical practitioners of the late nineteenth and twentieth centuries believed that the greater proportion of infant morbidity and mortality resulted directly from poor diet, they focused much of their attention on improper feeding practices. "Every person who has the care of an infant," insisted one St. Louis doctor in 1896, "should be required to obtain medical advice as to its diet." He maintained that physician-directed infant feeding "indeed is as important to the life and health of the coming generation as that infants, when sick, should receive medical attention." Concerned that contemporary mothers, whether breast feeding or bottle feeding, did not know how best to nourish their babies, physicians made infant feeding the very foundation of pediatric practice.[3]

Medical researchers claimed that their theories and methods should shape medical practice. Nonetheless, while acknowledging the benefits of medical science, practitioners did not slavishly follow the precepts of scientific infant feeding. On the contrary, they were just as likely to recommend a formula that contradicted accepted theory, or even a commercial infant food, for their bottle-fed patients, when they were convinced that such a food was beneficial. Moreover, practitioners were less concerned than many of the medical researchers with the status of the new specialty of pediatrics. Rather, general practitioners recognized the growing economic importance of infant feeding in general medical practice. These physicians did not ignore the question of prestige, but they sought to elevate the role played by the family physician, not the specialist, in medically directed infant feeding, and to convince the public and the manufacturers of infant foods that infant feeding was a medical function.

Also, unlike researchers and educators such as Rotch and Leopold, who combined theory-building and practice, the practitioners discussed in this chapter and the next were physicians whose primary medical activity was practice.[4] They were not a homogeneous group. About the only characteristic they shared was that at some point, or points, in their careers they all used a public forum to address the problems of infant feeding in everyday practice. Most of these practitioners attended medical schools in the United States, though a few were educated in Europe. Those whose practices are discussed in this chapter received their education by and large in the 1870s and 1880s, though a few graduated before 1870 or after 1890; those discussed in Chapter 5 typically graduated in the twentieth century. Some of these physicians combined private practice with positions in urban institutions such as the New York Infant Asylum or the West End Dispensary in Boston or with lectureships. As late as the turn of the century, only a handful limited their practices to pediatrics or obstetrics and gynecology. Almost one-half of the practitioners discussed in this chapter were rural physicians; those in Chapter 5 were less likely to be rural, but few maintained extensive urban practices.

The biography of a given physician is no predictor of that individual's views or practices. Urban physicians, as a group, did not contrast sharply with rural physicians. Practitioners in the North and South often expressed similar opinions. Even sex was no predictor. In the area of infant feeding, female practitioners demonstrated the same styles of practice as male practitioners. Furthermore, infant-feeding practices recommended by so-called regular, or allopathic, physicians did not differ significantly from those advocated by "sectarian" physicians such as homeopaths and hydropaths. For example, a popular infant formula was whole cow's milk diluted with plain water. It was the preferred food of John Binnie, an 1875 graduate of Rush Medical College, who practiced in rural Poynette, Wisconsin; of W. A. Edmonds, a homeopath in St. Louis, Missouri, who graduated from the University of Louisville in 1846; and of Cuvier R. Marshall, an 1885 graduate of Bellevue Hospital Medical College, who spent a year as house physician of the City Hospital of Newark, New Jersey, and then practiced in Philadelphia. Though this heterogeneous group of physicians may have differed on the details of infant feeding in everyday practice, the extent of their agreement is striking.

The desire to alleviate the high rates of infant mortality and morbidity they saw each day in their practices and to replace the influence of "old women" and "uneducated nurses" with "rational and scientific treatment"—that is to say, humanitarian concerns—spurred practitioners' involvement in pediatrics in general and infant feeding in particular. And so too did economics. "It frequently falls to the lot of the general practitioner," one Stoughton, Wisconsin, physician reminded fellow members of the Medical Society of Wisconsin in 1900, "to lay out the diet-list for infants."[5] Several years later the health officer of Gallatin, Tennessee, explained the importance of pediatric work for general practitioners, particularly those residing in rural communities:

> For the young man beginning his professional career a knowledge of
> pediatric work will create a reputation and give a foothold in establishing a
> practice as soon as anything I know. For one woman whose baby's life he
> has saved will give him more advertisements in the community than a full
> page ad in his county paper.

For him, infant feeding represented a significant aspect of pediatric work.[6] John M. Keating, a medical lecturer, called infant feeding the "bread and butter" of the practice of the average doctor.[7] Though not always so explicitly articulated, the economic importance of infant feeding underlay many of the practitioners' discussions.

Like researchers, practitioners began with the assumption that "among the different causes of infantile disease and therefore infantile mortality none perhaps figures more prominently than improper feeding."[8] Also like their more theoretically minded counterparts, practicing physicians did not limit the definition of poor nutrition to bottle feeding. Mothers who ate overly rich food, who lacked exercise, or who were nervous or easily excited produced poor, possibly poisonous milk.[9] To avoid such calamity, practitioners took it upon themselves to teach mothers the rules of healthy living and thus ensure a nutritious milk supply.[10]

Recognizing that despite their educational efforts suitable mother's milk was not always available, practitioners wanted a reasonable substitute for infants deprived of a mother's breast. An obvious alternative was the milk of other women. However, turn-of-the-century physicians despaired as had their predecessors, emphasizing the almost insurmountable difficulties involved in finding and keeping a suitable wet-nurse. On a practical level, if faced with a choice between artificial feeding and the uncertain and undesirable side-effects of wet-nursing, medical practitioners preferred the bottle.[11]

Physicians proudly announced that bottle feeding under the direction of a doctor was a healthful alternative to mother's milk. At first glance, this attitude seems curious, since analyses of infant mortality showed that a significantly greater proportion of bottle-fed than breast-fed infants died from digestive disturbances. However, statistical studies that looked beyond the mode of feeding and took into account environmental and economic factors convinced practitioners that under favorable circumstances artificially fed infants thrived. Perhaps even more important, physicians found bottle feeding successful in their own practices. As early as 1884, one Brooklyn physician felt so confident of his ability to direct the artificial feeding of infants that he ardently claimed, "It is not one of the greatest evils that a mother can not nurse her child."[12] Furthermore, rather than worry about the changeable nature of mother's milk, several practitioners preferred bottle feeding because "it is easier to control cows than women" or because with an artificial food one could be certain of what the infant was receiving.[13]

Not surprisingly then, late nineteenth- and early twentieth-century practitioners began to stress the benefits of artificial infant feeding. They most particularly recommended mixed feeding—that is, a combination of breast and bottle feeding. If a mother's milk supply decreased in the early months of nursing—and doctors reported seeing more and more cases of this—then the physician would recommend supplementary bottles. In this way the child would continue to receive the advantages of maternal nursing and would not be weaned prematurely. Such combination feeding could even enhance a woman's ability to lactate. A relief bottle would give the mother respite "from the very confining duties of nursing." Freed for exercise and recreation, she would be more relaxed and thus would produce more milk. Similarly, practitioners hoped that this "freedom" might encourage some women, especially those who were otherwise disinclined to nurse because it might interfere with their social life, to breast feed at least partially.[14] In any case, all these practitioners assumed that women needed doctors to tell them how to bottle feed.

Given the economic importance of infant feeding to their practices, physicians needed an efficacious method of artificial infant feeding. To some extent their answers to the question "how shall I feed the baby?" reflected and were conditioned by contemporary medical hypotheses and research. Ultimately, though, practitioners believed that "*experience* must be the final arbiter as to the fitness and value of any material as an article of diet."[15] In other words, they stressed clinical practice, not theory, in their discussions and descriptions of bottle feeding.

In practice, as in theory, healthful artificial infant feeding started with the readily available cow's milk. Unfortunately, the milk delivered to the home often was not safe and pure; it could, practitioners feared, contain harmful bacteria. Boiling, sterilizing, pasteurizing, could kill germs, but did they also, as researchers claimed, affect the nutritional qualities or the digestibility of the milk? Although practitioners did not deny the possibility that heated milk might not be as nutritious as raw milk, they considered heated milk safer and preferable. Heating milk, they stressed, eliminated germs—"one of the greatest dangers of artificial feeding."[16] Some practitioners recommended boiling the milk. By the 1880s and 1890s, several physicians had developed home sterilizers, what Brennemann in later years characterized as "a sort of family altar on which a daily ritual of food preparation for the baby was performed."[17] Consumers could purchase devices that pasteurized, devices that sterilized, and devices that did both (figure 4.1). Though practitioners did not agree on the best method for destroying disease-carrying microorganisms in home-delivered milk, they did advocate the safety of heated milk over raw.

Heating, however, would not improve unwholesome milk. In order to remedy the problem of contaminated milk, doctors from rural and urban areas took it upon themselves to educate the public on the importance of improving local milk supplies. At the turn of the century, physicians cited statistics from New York, Brooklyn, Chicago, and Milwaukee proving that death rates from diarrheal diseases decreased as the local milk supply improved.[18] In numerous articles addressed to nonmedical audiences, as well as in medical society discussions, physicians stressed the benefits of the regulation of milk production, handling, and transport.[19]

By the 1890s some individuals dissatisfied with the level of municipal control attempted to establish other means for providing pure milk to

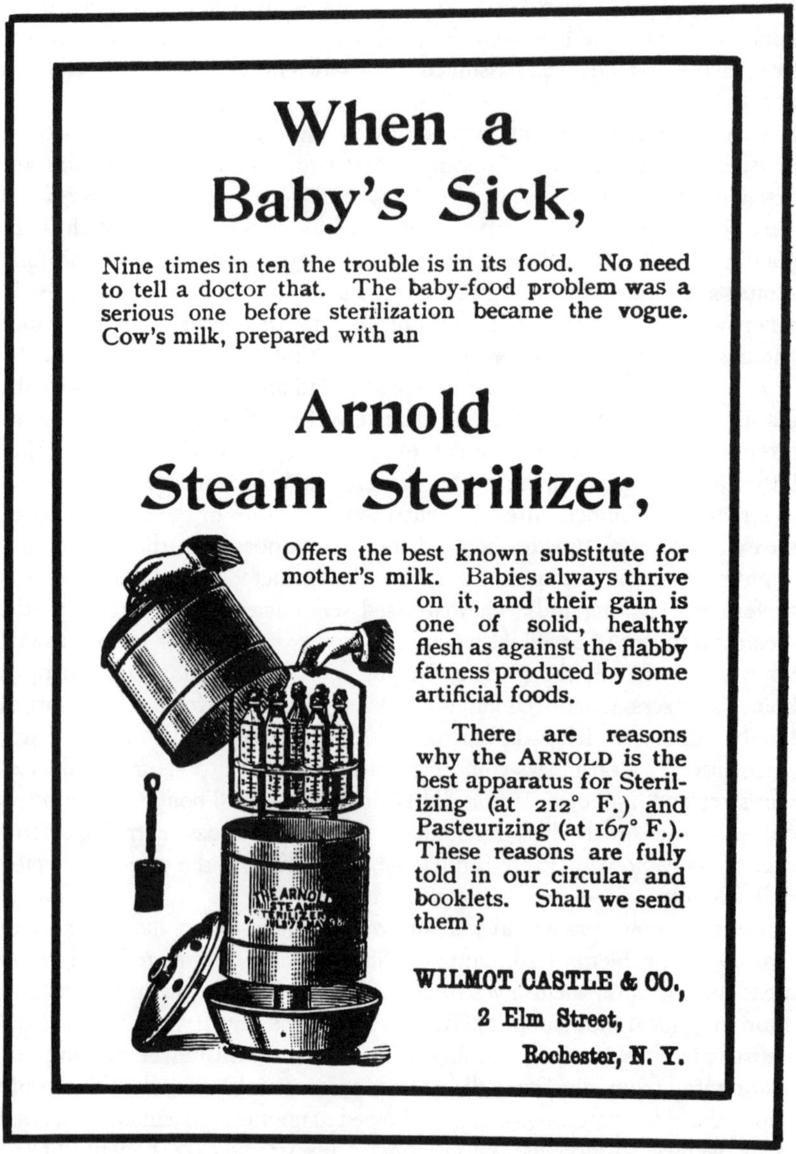

Figure 4.1. Arnold Steam Sterilizer advertisemment. Source: *New York Medical Journal, 61* (22 June 1895), adv. 10

bottle-fed infants. The most famous of such organizations in the last decade of the nineteenth century and the early years of the twentieth was the milk station or milk depot. Though Dr. Henry Koplik established the first such distribution center in the United States in 1889 on the Lower East Side of New York City, the name usually associated with these depots was Nathan Straus, the New York philanthropist. In 1893 Straus directed and financially supported the construction of several pasteurizing plants that distributed both pure pasteurized milk and six-ounce bottles of prepared milk formulas through stations set up in various areas of New York. Within a decade he had donated plants to Philadelphia and Chicago so that infants of those cities too might enjoy the benefits of pasteurized milk. Public-health-oriented physicians in other cities spearheaded drives to establish milk stations for their infants. Straus and his supporters pointed with pride to statistics that documented declines in infant death rates following the establishment of pasteurizing plants and distribution centers.[20]

In general, then, physicians favored the safety of heated milk and applauded the efforts of Straus-type milk depots. Some, however, were more interested in the production and transportation of milk. One such practitioner, E. F. Brush of Mount Vernon, New York, established his own dairy. According to Brush, milk from unhealthy or incorrectly fed cows and milk that had been improperly handled contributed to the failure of artificial infant feeding. Using recent discoveries in bacteriology and the nutritional sciences, he designed a plan for the proper care and feeding of dairy cows, which he published in JAMA in 1889. Brush put his ideas into practice as early as 1889, and advertisements for this dairy appeared in national magazines at least as late as 1902.[21]

Brush's effort foreshadowed a more influential movement to provide pure raw milk: the push for certification. Henry L. Coit, a Newark, New Jersey, physician, introduced his plan for producing milk of "uniform nutritive value, reliable keeping qualities, and [free] from pathogenic bacteria" in an 1893 paper.[22] He saw the production of this certified milk as requiring close cooperation between medical commissions and dairy farmers. A commission would establish the feeding and living standards for the herd and the procedures by which the milk producer would collect and handle the product. The dairy farmer would agree to abide by all such regulations. Responsibility for the inspection of the dairy stock and for the chemical and bacteriological examination of the herd and the product would rest with the members of the commission, physicians serving without financial compensation. The product ultimately sent to the consumer would be a raw, unheated, unprocessed milk that could contain no more than a set level of bacterial activity.

Coit and other New Jersey practitioners established the first medical milk commission in 1893; and the doctor received the first bottle of certified milk from the Fairfield Dairy Company in May 1894. By 1907 commissions from all over the country had banded together to form the American Association of Medical Milk Commissions. Because of the stringent production requirements and economic considerations, the milk often cost twice as much as ordinary milk. It is not surprising, then, that certified milk represented less than 1 percent of the total milk supply of large cities. By the end of the first decade of this century, the push for certified milk had abated. Fraudulent use of the certified label had promoted public distrust of this milk. Moreover, statistical data, such as the figures collected for the Straus milk-depot experiments, demonstrated the value of pasteurized milk in reducing infant mortality; and pasteurized milk was less expensive than certified milk. Cities like Chicago passed ordinances requiring the pasteurization of milk sold within their boundaries.

Clearly, in the care and handling of cow's milk, practitioners were pragmatic. That raw milk was, in theory, best for infant feeding they freely admitted; however, they also recognized the dangers inherent in all but the best raw milk and the expenses involved in procuring a safe unheated product. Rather than worry about such difficulties and uncertainties, practitioners opted for the safety of heated milk.

Of course even pure, clean cow's milk needed modification. Many theoretical solutions to the problem of "humanizing" cow's milk were being proposed by researchers and teachers, but practitioners were less concerned with the theoretical correctness of any given formula and more concerned with its clinical efficacy. "I have tried the following mixture as a substitute for mother's milk, in a number of cases, and it has always proved very successful; so much so that I felt encouraged to advise its use"—so physicians typically began their reports of artificial infant feeding. They did not ignore theory, but they put more trust in their own observations. Thus, they "strongly favor[ed] common-sense success against theoretical procedures."[23]

Though the differences between the various formulations loomed large to contemporaries, from today's perspective practitioners can be said to have used three basic cow's-milk mixtures. A popular one, consisting of diluted cream, was described by a Seneca Falls physician in a letter to the editor of the *Medical Record* in 1890. Strain fresh cow's milk into a pan that has a small hole closed with a cork, he advised. After waiting for the cream to rise, remove the cork and allow one-half of the milk to run out. Dilute and sweeten the remaining milk. He claimed that his mixture, which he had successfully employed for five years, was "a food for infants second in value to nothing, save good wholesome mother's milk, which is, at the present day, exceedingly difficult to obtain."[24] An Omaha, Nebraska, physician told the 1898 AMA meeting of a flexible cream-milk-water mixture he had recommended in eighteen cases. He had directed mothers to mix three ounces of cream, two ounces of milk, one ounce of milk sugar, and ten ounces of water; all the infants were "well developed." Under certain conditions he eliminated the milk and used only cream and water; in other cases he prescribed only one-eighth part cream and seven-eighths water, but "then after a few days I increased the amount of cream until I got about the normal proportions," he reported.[25] Some physicians who recommended similar cream-milk-water mixtures discussed the theoretical rationale behind their formulations, but more usually they favored formulas based on their own clinical experience.[26]

Another common cow's-milk formula, described by a rural Wisconsin physician in 1883, called for the dilution of whole milk with barley- or oatmeal-water. An ounce of pearl barley was added to one pint of boiling water; after the mixture had cooled, it was strained. He then mixed one-third of a pint of this barley-water with two-thirds of a pint of cow's milk and one teaspoon of milk sugar. Several years later he wrote a more detailed report of his procedure, recommending that the proportions of barley-water and milk be adjusted according to the age of the infant and that in "diseased conditions" the barley-water be replaced with oatmeal- or rice-water. Stressing his experience, he concluded: "After four years use of this food in a country practice, where I have had every chance to know when it agreed or when disagreed, and how, enables me to urge you to give it a thorough and impartial trial. I have never found it to fail."[27] A Boston physician concurred, warning that this formula "needs care in its preparation and in its administration." But, he added, "it will do as well in cities as the majority of those who use breast milk," because, especially in urban areas, mothers have many causes of excitement and fright "which the animal is free from."[28]

Practitioners also fed infants cow's milk diluted with plain water, altering the ingredients and proportions as conditions warranted. Writing in the *Medical Record* in 1884, one physician claimed that on the basis of his "extensive" practice, he "truly believed that many a mother's milk is not so good as proper artificial feeding." For a small infant, he preferred mixing three or four parts warm water with one part milk, adding "a little fine white sugar." By the time the child was four months old, the mixture should contain equal amounts of milk and water, but circumstances must be the guide for adjusting the formula, this doctor insisted. If the infant appeared undernourished, increase the milk more rapidly or dilute it with barley-water, a formula also recommended in cases of diarrhea.[29] In the late nineteenth century, other rural and urban physicians in private practice, as well as some associated with urban institutions such as the Out-door Department of Bellevue Hospital, New York, claimed success with similar diluted milk mixtures.[30]

Here again, practice took precedence over theory. Many practitioners advocated the use of milks or creams diluted with cereal-waters, despite the fact that theoretically infants were incapable of digesting starch. As Dr. Henry Dwight Chapin explained, "while proper theorizing is desirable in practice, the ultimate and final decision upon a therapeutic question must rest upon clinical experience." Theoretically, cereals adversely affected the digestive systems of infants, but as experience had shown that "infants are able to utilize them then their use is rational"—that is, clinically correct.[31]

By the 1890s another variation of cow's-milk formulations had attracted the attention of some practitioners—Rotch's percentage method. Yet despite its supposed scientific validity, the theory never dominated practical infant feeding, because physicians recognized the difficulties it posed for the general practitioner. The percentage method was criticized for its "complexity and elaborateness," which made the theory so difficult to comprehend that "discouragement [was] apt to follow." Some professors admired Rotch's "scientific study of feeding," but preferred to "teach the practitioner practical methods." Even Holt's "ingenious" table (see figure 2.1) was too complicated for physician-teachers, who recommended "simpler dilutions of milk" to make "the subject easier for the general practitioner and medical student." Some physicians feared that the proliferation of so-called simpler methods, many in conflict with one another, was causing practitioners to give up infant feeding "in despair" and driving them "to the use of patent baby foods as the easiest way out of the difficulty."[32] Practitioners frequently praised Rotch's work, but preferred to use a few fixed formulas.[33]

Leaving aside the complicated mathematics, practitioners faced other problems when they attempted to employ the percentage method in their everyday practices. The fat percentage of cream proved to be particularly troublesome. Some formula proponents simply assumed that the top quarter of milk that had stood for three or four hours contained 10 percent cream: that is, cream with 10 percent fat.[34] But soon this procedure seemed too imprecise, because a variation of 1 or 2 percent could make a significant difference in compounding an infant's formula. Westcott published the records of four of his own cases in which he claimed that variations as small as 0.1 or 0.2 percent could affect the baby's health.[35] In 1901 Holt wrote that most milk used for infant feeding contained 4 percent fat, and that after standing for several hours the upper third of this milk contained 10 percent fat and the upper half 7 percent fat. He therefore established formulas calling for 10 percent or 7 percent cream. In 1911, however, he admitted that since the fat percentage of the milk depended on the breed of cow, one could not assume how much fat the cream contained unless one knew from what variety of cow the milk had come. For this reason he constructed the table illustrated in figure 2.1, which allowed the physician to order formulas using whichever cream was available. During a 1901 lecture at the New York Post Graduate Medical School, Dr. Henry Dwight Chapin lamented "the extremely fine alterations of percentages" demanded by Rotch's method; then he too produced a detailed picture of the various percentages of fat in different layers of the cream from 4 percent milk and pointed out how much milks could vary in their fat content (figure 4.2).[36] In addition, the accuracy of the formula depended on how intelligently and conscientiously a person followed the physicians' mixing instructions. Even when mixed with cream and milk of known composition, the formula could differ significantly from the prescription if compounded carelessly.[37] Supposedly, laboratories, such as the Walker-Gordon Laboratory founded by Rotch in Boston in 1891, could overcome these obstacles.

Once the doctor had calculated which percentages to prescribe, it was a simple matter to fill out a prescription blank and pass it on to the Walker-Gordon Laboratory. The milk used to make up the formula came from a special farm under the direction of the laboratory, which ensured that the milk was as pure and as clean as possible. The laboratory processed the milk in a centrifugal separator and produced a cream with a stable percentage of fat. A laboratory employee, a "modifying clerk," compounded the physician's prescription with this cream, milk, and a standard 20 percent sugar solution, diluting it with lime-water, if necessary, and plain water. The clerk then divided the formula into tubes designed as nursing bottles and placed the tubes in a wicker basket for delivery (figures 4.3 and 4.4). Before the baskets left the laboratory, they were sent through a sterilizer and quickly cooled. The laboratory delivered the baskets to the homes of the consumers, and the basket and tubes from the previous day were returned for washing and sterilizing.[38]

After postgraduate study in Boston and New York, Dr. Tunstall R. Taylor returned to Baltimore determined that his city should enjoy the advantages of a milk laboratory. To create a demand that would persuade the Walker-Gordon Company to establish a branch in Baltimore, he told other city physicians that

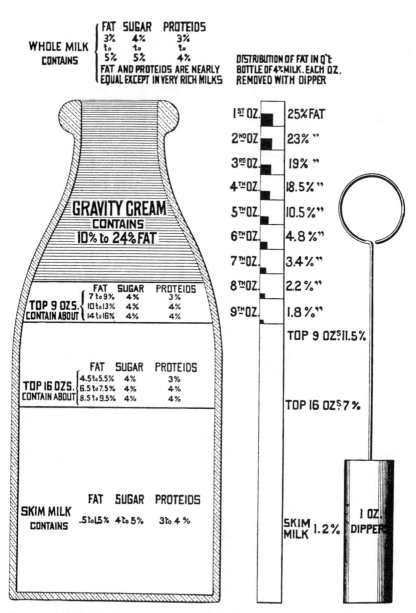

Figure 4.2. Fat content of cow's milk. Source: Henry Dwight Chapin, "Infant feeding: A clinical lecture delivered at the New York Post Graduate Medical School and Hospital," *American Journal of Obstetrics and Diseases of Women and Children*, 43 (1901), 602

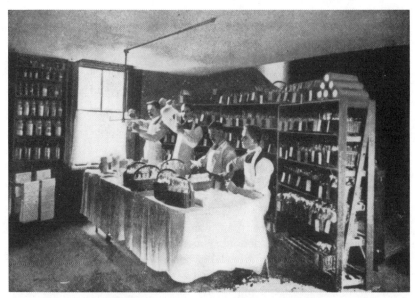

Figure 4.3. Modifying room, Walker-Gordon Milk Laboratory.

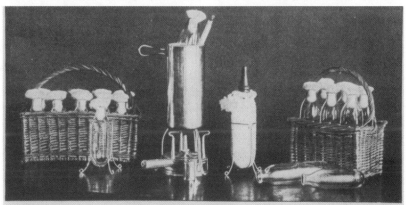

In the left of the picture is a basket holding eight tubes of a capacity of six ounces each. In front of this basket is a four-ounce tube in a wire stand. In the middle of the picture is a tin apparatus for warming the milk at the time of feeding. An alcohol lamp is shown beneath the warmer, and a tube of milk and a thermometer for testing the temperature of the milk are in the tin-warmer. Next to and to the right of the tin-warmer is a tube with a capacity of eight ounces. It is enclosed in a white worsted cozy, has the rubber nipple in place, and is supported in a wire stand. In the right of the picture is a basket containing six tubes with a capacity of eight ounces each. In front of this basket are an eight-ounce tube and a four-ounce tube.

Figure 4.4. Equipment used at the Walker-Gordon Milk Laboratory.

Source for figures 4.3 and 4.4: Thomas Morgan Rotch, *Pediatrics: The hygienic and medical treatment of children* (Philadelphia: J. B. Lippincott, 1895), p. 249 (fig. 4.3) and p. 262 (fig. 4.4)

> One has but to see the little crates of bottled "modified milk" daily left at
> the houses, ready for almost immediate use, to appreciate not only the
> convenience to the mothers, but the relief experienced by the physicians as
> expressed by them of "knowing that the milk is as it should be."

Apparently Taylor was effective, because a year later the city had a milk
laboratory. By 1907 there were Walker-Gordon Laboratories in twenty cities
in the United States and Canada, and numerous physicians across the country had reported their pleasure in using laboratory milk.[39]

At the same time, however, many more practitioners, both opponents and
proponents of the percentage method, were very dissatisfied with the milk
laboratories. Some praised milk laboratories for demonstrating that good,
clean milk could be produced commercially but claimed that it was this milk,
not the formula, that made laboratory-modified milk so efficacious.[40] Other
physicians claimed that infants fed laboratory milk over a long period of time
were not as healthy as those brought up on home-modified milk.[41] Supporters of the Walker-Gordon Company replied that physicians who lacked the
"knowledge of the percentages required by various conditions to use this
valuable agent intelligently" had probably caused these failures.[42] If they
understood the theory of the percentage method and frequently changed
their prescriptions, physicians could employ milk laboratories and avoid the
problems characteristic of home modification: namely, the uncertain nature
of the milk and the errors often encountered when untrained people compounded the formulas.

While promoting the percentage method, some physicians lambasted the
Walker-Gordon Company, asserting that the milk laboratories did not always
live up to the company's ideals of accuracy and cleanliness. Two Michigan
doctors described a visit to the Boston branch:

> The laboratory is pictured as perfect in its appointments and immaculate in
> its cleanliness. What greeted the eye, however, was not even the cleanliness
> of a down town butcher shop, nor could we be impressed that it was
> sterilized uncleanliness. The man at the rack was juggling prescriptions, it
> seemed to us, at the rate of 50 per minute. Occasionally a little milk slopped
> over. It did not seem to us that the care of a drug store prescription clerk
> was given to the combining of the various constituents of the milk
> modification.[43]

In 1902 Dr. A. H. Wentworth, working at the Pharmacological Laboratory of Harvard Medical School, analyzed samples of "modifications of milk
procured from an establishment that devotes especial attention to the prepa-

ration of milk for infant feeding" and found that the bottles delivered to the patients were incorrect: that is, they did not agree with the formula ordered by the physician. On the basis of his analyses and clinical observations, he determined that "within certain limits, accurate percentages of the constituents of modifications of milk are not essential in a large proportion of cases."[44] His results seemingly disproved the claims of researchers like Rotch and Westcott, who held that minute changes in the percentages of various ingredients had a significant effect on the health of infants. Yet Wentworth did not use this research to repudiate Rotch's theory; in fact, his article called for more accurate modifications of milk both in the laboratory and at home.

There were other practical objections to the laboratories. At least one physician preferred not to use laboratory milk because he feared that the family could become dependent on it; then, "if some accident should happen to prevent the making of the food for one, two or three days, we would be in an unfortunate predicament."[45] Geography further limited the use of laboratory milk; laboratories existed only in large cities and did not distribute their milk beyond a 100-mile radius.[46]

Practitioners frequently cited financial drawbacks as well. Laboratory-modified milk was too expensive; it was artificial feeding only for the well-to-do. Estimates of the cost of one day's feeding (approximately one quart) ranged from 30 to 90 cents, though the cost could drop to 20 cents a quart when the laboratory produced formula "in bulk." (This, however, would seem to negate a major tenet of the percentage method: namely, that each infant presented a unique case whose formula had to be individualized.)[47] Rotch's connection with the Walker-Gordon Company was also questioned. Rotch explained that he had consciously sought to disassociate himself from the commercial aspects of the milk laboratories because he felt that "to have proper influence in persuading both physicians and laity," he should "have no connection with the commercial side of its development." But not all practitioners accepted the sincerity of his disclaimer.[48]

For many reasons, then, by the second decade of the century milk laboratories had almost totally disappeared.[49] In practice the laboratories did not measure up to their own standards of cleanliness and accuracy, and they were inconvenient to use because of both expense and limited geographic distribution. Careful home preparation of infant food was as successful as laboratory production, if not more so. And, of course, practitioners who did not appreciate the percentage method found the laboratories unnecessary. Significant also was the growing disillusionment with Rotch's method as more and more practitioners recognized from their own clinical experience that the absolute accuracy of formulations demanded by the theory was not needed.

In medical journals and at society meetings, many of these physicians called for simplicity, not complexity, in infant feeding.[50]

Obviously, practitioners agreed on little. Many medical observers worried that this lack of consensus would be interpreted as a sign that physicians were not knowledgeable experts on infant feeding. Viewing the situation from Atlanta, Georgia, one practitioner asked, "Is it any wonder the layman [sic] has begun to look on us with suspicion" when a mother might see five different physicians and have each one order a different food?[51] Physicians also feared that their colleagues would "shrink from the task of puzzling over" confusing and otherwise contradictory formulations and turn instead to the easier to prepare and prescribe patent foods.[52] Manufacturers of infant foods cultivated this dissatisfaction with contemporary infant-feeding techniques among general practitioners, while at the same time using the latest theoretical advances to add a veneer of scientific respectability to their products. Though these foods were not prescription items, companies directed much of their advertising to practitioners and attempted to convince them that patent infant foods answered the practical problems of artificial infant feeding.

According to each infant-food company, its product was unique; only its food represented the best way to feed the infant. Yet the companies were quite similar, at least in their approaches to the medical profession. They all advertised extensively in medical journals. Most companies exhibited their products at medical conventions. They all distributed free samples and reprinted testimonials and endorsements. And, most important, they all provided practitioners with a host of helpful aids, usually in the form of booklets, to simplify infant feeding. The company that produced Horlick's Malted Milk offered to send physicians "A Practical Modification of Milk" and "How to Ensure Pure Milk for the Infant During the Hot Summer Months," pamphlets that described its food in terms of contemporary scientific knowledge and gave detailed instructions for infant feeding. The manufacturer of Mellin's published "The Mellin's Food Method of Percentage Feeding," 183 pages that gave doctors nearly 500 combinations of Mellin's, milk, cream, and water to construct formulas with specific percentages of proteids, fats, and carbohydrates (figure 4.5).[53]

How many practitioners regularly recommended these products is impossible to assess. The products' longevity and the extensiveness of the infant-food companies' promotional campaigns, however, indicate that the manufacturers were prosperous. And evidence in the medical literature confirms

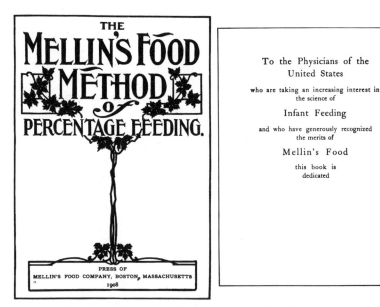

Figure 4.5. Title page and dedication of *Mellin's Food Method of Percentage Feeding* (Boston: Mellin's Food Company, 1908)

that many individual practitioners were quite impressed with these proprietary foods.

In some instances doctors recommended specific patent foods. Charles Warrington Earle, a leading Chicago physician, told the 1888 AMA meeting that Mellin's Food "certainly has stood the test, and at the bedside has been found of great value in the practice of those who are studying [infant feeding] and whose opinions are worthy of respect." The manufacturer was quick to reprint this statement in an advertisement, of course neglecting to inform readers that Earle had also praised other foods, such as Nestlé's, in the same address. In 1898 a Philadelphia practitioner wrote in the *Journal of the American Medical Association (JAMA)* that Mellin's was widely used in his city; his rationale for its popularity echoed the claims of the manufacturer: the product was simple to use and flexible.[54] Physicians praised complete infant foods such as Nestlé's specifically for their ease of preparation: "nothing is left to the discretion or whim of nurses, who, when not too disposed to spoil the child's food by excess of sugar, are so often careless in preparing it." Even "in the hands of the most ignorant," such food "may be safely used."[55]

Many practitioners appreciated the availability of manufactured infant foods, reporting cases in which they had successfully employed specific patent foods. Even those who used cow's-milk formulas found reason to praise commercial infant foods. A Boston physician who worked at the West End Dispensary and also had a private practice found a variety of foods helpful. When the living conditions were good, he recommended malted foods or milk and barley; however, "where the hygiene is poor, I am strongly led by my personal experience to rely on condensed milk."[56] Another doctor, in Minneapolis, complained that physicians were "compelled to commercial foods" because "the great trouble with us in the West here is the milk supply."[57] Physicians lauded "the services to mankind, and our profession, rendered by honest infant-food manufacturers," and spoke of a "debt of gratitude" due these companies.[58] One can also gauge the extent to which physicians employed patent foods from statements by writers opposed to such products. One 1910 estimate claimed that 40 percent of the medical profession ordered some manufactured food for their bottle-fed patients.[59]

At national medical conventions and state and local meetings, in medical journals and textbooks, practitioners heard arguments against patent foods. Theoretical shortcomings were pointed out: these products did not contain the proper nutrients in the correct proportions for healthful infant feeding. Those who used commercial infant foods dismissed these alleged drawbacks by pointing to cases in which they had recommended proprietary products and their patients flourished. More telling objections to patent foods involved the question of control: who would direct the feeding of the infant?

Many practitioners opposed to patent foods protested that such products denied doctors their rightful position as scientific advisors on infant feeding. For one thing, many manufacturers did not publish the formulas of their products. Without this information, physicians were forced to experiment to find the correct food for an infant. If doctors knew the constituents of the various foods, then they could decide for themselves which foods to use in what circumstances rather than having to follow the suggestions of the manufacturers. But the crux of the problem was printed directions appearing on the packages of commercial infant foods. Instructions supplied by the manufacturer made a product easier to use for both the physician and the mother, but they also, in effect, eliminated the need for medical advice on infant feeding. A physician confused about how to feed an infant could advise a mother to buy a certain product and follow the instructions provided. The mother was apt to take this as a general sanction for that particular food, and this could lead to its indiscriminate use and abuse.[60]

Plainly, by 1910 practitioners had reached no consensus on the topic of infant feeding. True, pediatrics—and most particularly infant nutrition—had become an important area of general medical practice, but still the question of how to feed the infant appeared to have many, often contradictory, answers. During the next several decades, practitioners would eliminate much of the confusion, and a generally accepted mode of infant feeding would evolve.

V

"Under the Supervision of the Physician"
1910–1950

By the mid-twentieth century, practitioners had moved from a belief that bottle feeding could healthfully augment or replace breast feeding to a conviction that artificial feeding generally had positive benefits for infant health. Investigations demonstrated possible nutritional deficiencies in human milk. Studies documented that carefully supervised bottle feeding was as healthful as breast feeding, if not healthier. Mothers, according to urban and rural practitioners alike, more and more frequently requested bottle-feeding advice. Artificial infant feeding became less complex and confusing as physicians refined and simplified formulations and as infant-food products gained acceptance. Consequently, practitioners focused less on the advantages or shortcomings of breast feeding and placed more stress on the ease and healthfulness of medically directed bottle feeding.

Not all artificial feeding situations, however, were considered safe and nutritious. Since the late nineteenth century, some doctors had argued that all instructions on infant feeding must originate with the medical profession in order to ensure the health of the infant and physicians' economic self-interest. In the twentieth century, the profession fought for and gained control over the dissemination of infant-feeding information. Through organizational efforts physicians were able to limit the sources of artificial-feeding directions to practitioners.

Twentieth-century scientific and clinical investigations more clearly delineated the limitations of breast milk suggested by earlier research. For example, increasingly detailed analyses disclosed that the vitamin content of mother's milk varied among women and even changed in the same woman with different diets. To avoid the possibility of scurvy or rickets, practitioners advised that all infants receive dietary supplements of vitamins C and D. In the opinion of at least one rural Wisconsin physician, the most important change that occurred in infant feeding in the second quarter of this century was the regular employment of cod-liver oil and orange juice in the diets of even breast-fed babies.[1]

Practitioners did not worry only about possible qualitative deficiencies of breast milk. Concerned that mothers produced insufficient amounts of breast milk, doctors turned to the problem of weight loss that they often observed in newborns. For the first several days after birth, mothers secrete colostrum, a fluid that differs from the later breast milk. Physicians, fearing that infants received little or no nourishment from colostrum, advised that newborns be given supplemental bottles until the mothers were lactating adequately. Some practitioners viewed such supplemental feeding as tampering with nature; many others, however, considered the initial weight loss itself unnatural. "The Lord . . . had in mind a less highly developed nervous system than [we] are dealing with today," remarked one Seattle, Washington, physician at the 1921 meeting of the American Medical Association.[2] Civilized women, these practitioners suspected, lived under a strain that upset their systems. Though "primitive" women did not require assistance, modern mothers did. Physicians opposed to this supplemental feeding pointed out that such artificial feeding often signaled the first step toward weaning. Yet given physicians' faith in bottle feeding, this was not a serious drawback. A Sioux City physician writing to the editor of *JAMA* in 1925 expressed a commonly held opinion: "A large number of infants need something to burn before it is provided by the mother. The gratifying results one sees when fluids, sugar solutions, or milk dilutions are given to dehydrated infants more than offsets any danger there may be of the baby later refusing the breast." Other practitioners wrote glowingly about how they minimized the problem of weight loss by following insufficient breast-milk feedings with complementary bottles.[3]

Aware of studies such as those of Glazier and Garland and Rich (see Chapter 3), physicians viewed artificial feeding not merely as a corrective for negative aspects of breast feeding, but also as a healthful, positive form of infant nutrition. Many practitioners continued to advocate maternal nursing as the best form of infant feeding, but they steadily tempered this stand. In the late 1910s one finds many comments to the effect that after the first three or six months of life babies will do as well, if not better, on bottle formulas. Physicians in the 1920s frequently wrote that there was little difference between breast milk and artificial food, and that few infants would not thrive on carefully prepared cow's milk mixtures. By mid-century most practitioners believed that if a mother did not wish to breast feed her infant, then the doctor should accept her decision, since most babies, even newborns, did well with bottle feeding that was medically directed.[4]

74

Not that physicians rejected breast feeding; some, particularly in the 1910s and 1920s, encouraged maternal nursing under medical supervision. Dr. J. P. Sedgwick led a highly publicized campaign for breast feeding in Minneapolis in the late 1910s. Drawing on an analogy from dairy farming, the doctor attributed unsuccessful lactation to the nurslings' failure to stimulate the breast by emptying it completely. To compensate for this, he trained mothers to express manually any milk that remained after the infant had nursed. Sedgwick was proud of the results of this program: at one month of age, over 97 percent of the infants whom he followed were fed at the breast; at three months, over 93 percent; and at seven months, over 83 percent. A few other proponents of maternal nursing imitated Sedgwick's methods. One practitioner hired a registered nurse to visit the homes of his patients in the "upper or well to do class" and instruct them in correct breast-feeding techniques. The nurse reported success in teaching these women to express their milk.[5]

In other cases, though, mothers and physicians who were confident about the healthfulness of bottle feeding lacked the motivation to implement Sedgwick's procedures. This point is clearly illustrated in the story of one doctor who trained under Sedgwick in 1921 at Minneapolis General Hospital. When he then interned under Gerstenberger at Cleveland City Hospital, he recalled, he was unable to implement Sedgwick's ideas for two reasons. The mothers there refused to be treated like animals; one reportedly told him, "[You] ain't gonna make no cow out of me." Also, the hospital had been a testing site for S.M.A. Convinced that "S.M.A. pretty well solved the problem" of insufficient mother's milk, the staff was not committed to breast feeding.[6]

Even practitioners committed to maternal nursing did not reject artificial infant feeding. In the statistics that Sedgwick and his imitators cited to document the effectiveness of their programs, an unspecified proportion of their breast-fed infants actually received some bottle feeding to complement their mothers' milk. Twentieth-century physicians recommended supplementary bottles to ameliorate nutritional problems and to facilitate breast feeding, as did their predecessors who had advised a bottle or two a day to augment the infant's diet or to relieve the mother of a tied-down feeling. Now practitioners touted additional advantages for the "happy combination." They stressed that weaning should be a gradual process. Unfortunately, unless the baby had previous experience with a bottle, weaning could be difficult, for the child might obstinately refuse any form of feeding other than the breast. Such circumstances "may necessitate starving the infant into submission." On the other hand, if one had used the bottle each day, then the baby, being accustomed to it, could easily be weaned. Furthermore, practitioners feared that some emergency might separate the mother and child or cause the mother's milk to dry up; in this century physicians frequently noted that mothers lost their milk in the third or fourth month. For babies who had already received some artificial food, a sudden loss of mother's milk would not be a major problem because the infant was accustomed to the bottle. Thus doctors logically considered supplemental feeding "a good idea" and regularly recommended one bottle a day for their breast-fed patients.[7]

Several other, nonmedical, factors influenced the general practitioners' positive opinions about artificial feeding. Physicians correlated the very growth of pediatrics in general medical practice with the inability or unwillingness of modern mothers to nurse their babies. All but equating pediatric practice with feeding problems, by the late 1920s and early 1930s they estimated that 25 percent or more of the case loads of general practitioners consisted in directing the routine feeding of infants. They also complained that mothers demanded that doctors supply them with formulas. And as one St. Louis practitioner mourned, "We have to, for if we did not the other doctor across the street would."[8] Artificial feeding, then, continued to have economic importance for the general practitioner.

Moreover, physicians heard, read, and learned much more about bottle feeding than breast feeding. According to doctors, the hours in medical school devoted to artificial feeding "stand out in striking contrast to the casual attitude which is so frequently taken in discussing with students the advantages of maternal nursing."[9] Consequently, if a mother had any difficulty in breast feeding, the average practitioner was ill-equipped to advise her and preferred instead to wean the infant to a bottle. One doctor defensively queried in *American Medicine* in 1928, "If one's medical course and postgraduate teaching have not emphasized breast feeding . . . can he be held entirely blameworthy for not using it?"[10] Textbooks of the period typically presented a few pages on breast feeding and many more pages on the intricacies of artificial feeding. And most articles on infant feeding merely mentioned breast feeding in passing before going on to discuss in detail "the accepted modes of infant feeding"—that is, bottle feeding.[11]

Just as a combination of theoretical and practical factors convinced practitioners that artificial feeding was a necessary and important element in their practices, a similar mixture of science and clinical experience answered the question of what to put in the bottle. In the early years of this century, physicians had faced a confusing array of infant-feeding formulas and patent infant foods. During the following decades physicians utilized new advances in nutrition research, modified by practical experience, to develop simpler methods of infant feeding. For instance, Dr. S. Josephine Baker, director of the Bureau of Child Hygiene in New York City, found that complicated methods were not practical for the city's baby health stations. Despite objections from more theoretically minded physicians, she directed practitioners at the stations to prescribe simple whole-milk mixtures, which were successful.[12] She and other physicians reported that minute fractional changes in the percentages of various food elements were not necessary; the feeding of the average infant did not have to be complicated. Moreover, mothers—even the more educated, and thus supposedly more capable, private patients—need not fret and puzzle over complex formulas. Since simple mixtures were easier for mothers to prepare, and since most children thrived on these formulas, infants should be fed ordinary milk dilutions with some additional carbohydrate—under medical supervision, of course. As one practitioner told the American Association for the Study and Prevention of Infant Mortality in 1913, "Simplicity and efficiency is the keynote."[13]

Consensus over the simpler form of cow's-milk formulas did not develop immediately. Medical-school pediatric departments and most textbooks continued to present their readers with a multitude of infant-feeding formulas. However, they increasingly emphasized that most babies—some said 90 percent or more—would do well on simple whole-milk mixtures; other formulations were reserved for the difficult or sick infant. Even proponents of the percentage method began in the 1910s to modify their method and simplify the procedures they recommended for formula construction. While extolling the virtues of this "scientific modification of milk," these practitioners often admitted that the large majority of infants could be successfully fed on relatively simple formulas.[14]

Growing numbers of physicians across the country employed simple-to-make formulas. Based on the protein and caloric needs of the infant, the formula usually consisted of 1.5 to 2.0 ounces of cow's milk per pound of body weight per day with an eighth of an ounce of sugar per pound per day and enough water to provide a total of three ounces of fluid volume per pound per day. The milk used was either boiled whole milk or evaporated or powdered milk.[15] This method of infant feeding was simple for the physician to calculate (as one 1935 medical school graduate put it, "Feeding was sort of routine") and easy for the mother to use.[16] By the fourth decade of this century, practitioners made little mention of the complicated methods of formula construction, except to say that they were no longer necessary. The use of simple milk dilutions with the addition of carbohydrates was "the most common and rational procedure" for infant feeding.[17]

Physicians continued to admit that human milk was, in theory, best, but among their private patients and mothers who attended carefully supervised clinics, they saw little difference between maternal nursing and bottle feeding. Some mothers reported that doctors told them it was better to bottle feed than to nurse because "with the bottle you always know how much you have, with the breast you don't." Not only was the quantity unknown, but the quality also. If an infant reacted poorly to a bottle formula, one could easily modify the mixture. It was much more difficult to modify mother's milk.[18]

Seeing little difference between the two modes of infant feeding, practitioners usually did not insist that women nurse their babies. One Madison, Wisconsin, pediatrician, H. Kent Tenney, recalled: "I always told these young mothers, the best thing you can do is feed this baby yourself. . . . But if you can't, I will. I'll fix you up with a formula that will be satisfactory."[19] Since he believed that worry could ruin a mother's milk supply and that women rejected nursing because they feared being "tied down," Tenney often advised mixed feeding to relieve anxiety. He recommended that a lactating mother periodically substitute a bottle for a breast feeding, even as early as the first month, so that the infant would learn to recognize the bottle as "a friend when the time comes for him to have a bottle fairly regularly." Complementary feedings were also necessary, in his opinion, for the large number of women "who need help after about two months"; only a few mothers could "supply full rations for many months." Tenney told mothers that "if simplicity is anything in your life, I would say that the simplest of all feedings is diluted evaporated milk to which sugar is added." According to Tenney, the simplicity of evaporated milk mixtures was one of the most significant developments in infant feeding in the twentieth century. Thus, though breast milk with the addition of cod-liver oil and orange juice was best for an infant, Tenney was comfortable and confident directing his patients in bottle feeding.

Aware of practitioners' concerns, manufacturers of infant foods emphasized that their products were nutritionally satisfactory and could simplify infant feeding. The Mead Johnson Company was most aggressive in its pursuit of physicians. From the beginning, when the company unveiled Dextri-Maltose at the 1912 AMA convention, Mead Johnson advertised almost exclusively to the medical profession, appearing regularly at the AMA and other medical society meetings, advertising extensively in medical journals, and also providing physicians with free samples and with booklets that described the scientific basis of Dextri-Maltose. The company prepared a sales manual for its detailmen that supplied likely questions from general practitioners and outlined answers explaining the superiority of Mead Johnson products. Thus trained, these sales representatives visited doctors' offices all over the country, discussing the products and distributing free samples and various devices to simplify infant feeding and to make it "easier for the general practitioner to obtain better cooperation from mothers." With a feeding calculator, the physician could dial the infant's age and weight and see at a glance the correct amounts of milk, water, and Dextri-Maltose needed for a day's formula (figure 5.1). Formula blanks imprinted with the doctor's name and address instructed the mother how to mix the formula and feed it to her child; each blank also reminded her to bring the baby back to the physician for a checkup and a new Dextri-Maltose formula on a specified date. Directing the mothers to doctors for infant-feeding advice was a constant theme in Mead Johnson's promotional campaigns.[20]

Mead Johnson marketed Dextri-Maltose as a nonprescription but "ethical" product (figure 5.2). The company proudly proclaimed that

> MEAD'S Infant Diet Materials are advertised only to physicians. No feeding directions accompany trade packages. Information in regard to feeding is supplied to the mother by written instructions from her doctor, who changes the feedings from time to time to meet the nutritional requirements of the growing infant.

The few advertisements that appeared in national magazines like *Hygeia* gave no feeding instructions but rather pointed out to mothers the advantages of medical supervision. In the 1930s Mead Johnson produced a film, "The Preparation of Modified Milk Formulas," to teach women the correct procedures for bottle feeding; the viewer repeatedly heard that artificial feeding should be "prescribed by physician" and that infant feeding should be under "physicians' direction." The company often told physicians that with this policy doctors controlled infant feeding. Unlike products that a mother could buy off the shelf, with instructions printed on the package, prescription of Dextri-Maltose directed the mother back to the physician. Not only did this protect the infant's nutritional status and growth, but it also added to the physician's practice. As L. S. Johnson, an official of the company, remarked in an informal company history many years later, one of the points emphasized in the early advertising campaigns directed to physicians was that the use of Dextri-Maltose "added to their practices and put money in their pockets."[21] In this way the Mead Johnson Company astutely played upon the fears and desires of general practitioners in order to sell its products. The company described its relationship with the medical profession in terms of "enlightened self-interest and co-operation": both manufacturer and the medical profession would profit under Mead Johnson's advertising policy.[22]

The manufacturer of S.M.A., another twentieth-century product, also

BABY'S AGE 6 MONTHS
WEIGHT 15 POUNDS

BABY'S AGE 7 MONTHS
WEIGHT 17 POUNDS

TURN DIAL

1-6 MONTHS | 7-12 MONTHS

ALWAYS SPECIFY A
STANDARD TABLE-
SPOON. (1½ FLUID
OUNCE CAPACITY)

FEEDING CALCULATOR
FOR AVERAGE BABIES
MIXTURES OF COW'S MILK, WATER AND
DEXTRI-MALTOSE

MILK 26 OZ.	MILK 30 OZ.
WATER 9 OZ.	WATER 10 OZ.
DEXTRI-MALTOSE 6 LEVEL TABLESPOONFULS	DEXTRI-MALTOSE 6 LEVEL TABLESPOONFULS
7 OZ. EACH FEEDING	8 OZ. EACH FEEDING
5 FEEDINGS IN 24 HRS.	5 FEEDINGS IN 24 HRS.

1½ TIMES AS MANY TABLESPOONFULS ARE REQUIRED WHEN "DEXTRI-MALTOSE
WITH VITAMINS B AND G" IS USED, THAN WITH DEXTRI-MALTOSE NOS. 1, 2 OR 3.

Preparation --- Heat milk and water until nearly boiling. Add the Dextri-Maltose, measured from a standard tablespoon and leveled with a table knife, and stir into solution with a fork. Then boil the mixture for 3 minutes. (If desired, the Dextri-Maltose may be added after the milk and water have been boiled, while still hot.) Add enough boiled water to bring mixture up to original volume.

HOW TO USE THE CALCULATOR: Turn dial until the baby's age and weight appear in the upper window. The feeding formula will then appear in the window below. The left-hand dial is for babies 1 to 6 mos. old, the right-hand dial is for babies 7 to 12 mos. old.

For average babies use Dextri-Maltose No. 1

For constipated babies use Dextri-Maltose No. 3

When first starting a baby on artificial feeding, use one half the amount of Dextri-Maltose shown on the formulas. Then, after 2 or 3 days, gradually increase to the full amount.

Evaporated Milk, diluted to normal strength, also may be used in these formulae.

ORANGE JUICE: After the baby is two months old, begin giving between meals one teaspoonful strained orange juice daily. Gradually increase the quantity one teaspoonful at a time until, at six months of age, the baby is getting the juice of a whole orange daily.

COD LIVER OIL: As a preventive of rickets the baby should receive a highly potent cod liver oil, such as Mead's Standardized and Biologically Assayed Cod Liver Oil. Dose: Up to 1 month, ½ teaspoonful daily. 1 to 2 months, 1 teaspoonful twice daily. 2 months on, 1 teaspoonful three times daily.

Mead's Powdered Whole Milk, reliquified to normal strength also, may be used in these formulae.

24 HOUR FORMULAS FOR AVERAGE BABIES UNDER ONE MONTH

Baby's Age Days	Oz. Milk	Oz. Water	Level Tablespoonfuls Dextri-Maltose	No. Feedings in 24 hours
4	4	12	1	7
8	5	12	2	7
14	7	11	2	7
21	9	12	3	7
28	13	11	3	7

For babies of this age the milk and water should be boiled together for three minutes.

LITERATURE AVAILABLE ON REQUEST

Dextri-Maltose with Casec in Loose Green Stools	No. 109
Dextri-Maltose with Protein Milk	" 122
Dextri-Maltose with Lactic Acid Milk	" 169

Copyright 1935, Mead Johnson & Co., Evansville, Ind., U. S. A.

Figure 5.1. Front and back sides of Dextri-Maltose feeding calculator, 1935

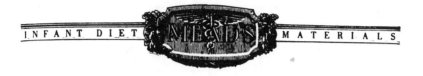

HEALTHY BABIES

The Nation Marches Forward on the Feet of Little Children

The future health of our Nation largely depends on the health of the babies of *today*.

Proper food, supervised by physicians, is one of the most important factors to keep the baby *well*.

A FOOD worthy of consideration is
Fresh Cow's Milk, Water and
MEAD'S DEXTRI-MALTOSE
(Dextrins and Maltose)

The Mead Johnson Policy

MEAD'S Infant Diet Materials are advertised only to physicians. No feeding directions accompany trade packages. Information in regard to feeding is supplied to the mother by written instructions from her doctor, who changes the feedings from time to time to meet the nutritional requirements of the growing infant. Literature furnished only to physicians.

MEAD JOHNSON & COMPANY
Evansville, Ind., U. S. A.

Figure 5.2. Mead Johnson advertisement with ethical policy. Source: *JAMA, 84* (12) (1925), adv. 45. Courtesy of the Archive, American Medical Association

exhibited at medical meetings and advertised extensively in medical journals. Advertisements appearing in nonmedical journals provided no feeding directions but told readers that S.M.A. was "to be used only on the order of a physician." Advertisements and booklets for practitioners stressed that S.M.A. was scientifically constructed and simple to use (figure 5.3). Because of this simplicity, "the physician is relieved of exacting detail" in prescribing it, and the patient "can prepare it properly" with little chance of error. In addition to distributing feeding calculators, free samples, and literature, the company encouraged physicians to advise it on possible new products and at one time allowed doctors to put their own labels on standard S.M.A. products.[23]

Nineteenth-century infant-food manufacturers updated their promotional campaigns in the twentieth century. The Mellin's Company continued to exhibit at AMA meetings and to advertise in medical and nonmedical journals. As the percentage method declined, however, and simpler methods gained in popularity, the company dropped its booklet about percentage feeding. Instead, advertisements stressed that Mellin's was simple to use and that a mixture of Mellin's, water, and milk provided the recommended quantities of food elements needed by most babies (figure 5.4). The company offered a formula card that presented in tabular form the simple milk mixtures preferred by contemporary physicians (figure 5.5).[24]

As the Horlick's Company and the Nestlé's Company developed additional products in the 1920s, they imitated Mead Johnson's advertising techniques and policy. Horlick's promoted its new Maltose and Dextrin Milk Modifier to physicians with free samples, feeding calculators, and formula pads, informing doctors that "directions for its use are to be furnished to physicians only. No feeding directions accompany the package, but each wrapper will bear the statement: 'The proportions for the modification of milk should be directed by a physician, in order to suit the needs of the individual case.'" Similarly, Nestlé's distributed no feeding instructions with its new product, Lactogen, and instead directed mothers to physicians. However, the companies continued to supply directions for use on packages of Horlick's Malted Milk and Nestlé's Milk Food.[25]

Canned-milk companies employed promotional techniques similar to those of the Mellin's Food Company, advertising their products as safe and inexpensive forms of infant feeding and offering both mothers and doctors free literature. Manufacturers such as the Pet Milk Company, Carnation Milk, and Borden's and trade organizations like the Evaporated Milk Association exhibited at medical society meetings from the 1920s on. To ease the physician's work, the association and individual manufacturers provided

S.M.A. The Only Antirachitic Breast Milk Adaptation

SO SIMPLE

that even Mrs. _____* can prepare it properly.

SO SIMPLE

that Mrs._____ ‡ will thank you for sparing her much worry and trouble.

(* ‡ No doubt you can supply names from your practice.)

ANYONE CAN FOLLOW THESE SIMPLE INSTRUCTIONS

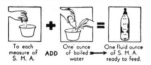

To each measure of S. M. A. **ADD** One ounce of boiled water ➡ One fluid ounce of S. M. A. ready to feed.

This proportion remains unchanged. As the infant grows older you merely increase the quantity as with breast milk. (See table below.)

SUGGESTED FEEDING TABLE

Infant	Total Quantity In 24 Hours In Ounces *	No. of Feedings •	Quantity per Feeding In Ounces *
2 days	1 to 2½	2 to 3	½ to 1
3 days	2½ to 5	3 to 4	½ to 1½
4 days	5 to 7½	4 to 5	1 to 1½
5 days	7½ to 10	5 to 7	1 to 2
6 days	10 to 12½	5 to 7	1½ to 2½
7 days	12½ to 15	5 to 7	2 to 3
2 weeks	15 to 17½	5 to 7	2 to 3½
4 weeks	17½ to 20	5 to 7	2½ to 4
6 weeks	20 to 22½	5 to 7	3 to 4½
2 months	22½ to 25	5 to 6	3½ to 5
2½ months	25 to 27½	5 to 6	4 to 5½
3 months	27½ to 30	5	5½ to 6
3½ months	30 to 32½	5	6 to 6½
4 months	32½ to 35	5	6½ to 7
5 months	32½ to 37½	5	6½ to 7½
6 months to 1 year	32½ to 40	5 to 4	6½ to 10

6 to 7 Mos.. At this age it is customary to add soups and vegetables to the diet, especially spinach.

* These quantities refer to fluid ounces of S. M. A. diluted according to directions.

TIME SCHEDULE

7 feedings: 6, 9, 12, 3, 6, 9 and once during night.
6 feedings: 6, 9, 12, 3, 6 and 9 or later.
6 feedings: 6, 10, 2, 6, 10 and 2.
5 feedings: 6, 10, 2, 6 and 10 or later.
5 feedings: 6, 9, 12, 3 and 6 or later.

NUMBER OF FEEDINGS IN 24 HOURS.

The number of feedings in 24 hours should likewise be the same as those allowed breast-fed infants; generally stated not more than seven and not less than five. However, when the infant reaches the age of 6 to 7 months, it is customary to replace one of the feedings with an 8 ounce meal of farina broth soup.

SAVES PHYSICIAN'S TIME, TOO

S M A. is simple to prescribe. The busy physician is relieved of exacting detail because he has only to increase the *amount* of S.M.A. (as with breast milk) when in his judgment it becomes necessary. The accompanying chart suggests average amounts.

The physician's time is also saved because the chances are good for excellent results under his skilled supervision. S.M.A. was proved clinically before it was offered to physicians generally in 1921, and has demonstrated its worth over and over again.

S.M.A. RESEMBLES BREAST MILK

S.M.A. is a food for infants — derived from tuberculin tested cows' milk, the fat of which is replaced by animal and vegetable fats including biologically-tested cod liver oil; with the addition of milk sugar, potassium chloride, and salts; altogether forming *an antirachitic food*. When diluted according to directions, it is *essentially similar to human milk* in percentages of protein, fat, carbohydrates and ash, in chemical constants of the fat and in physical properties.

If you have not already availed yourself of these advantages, prescribe S.M.A. for your next feeding case. The results will please you. If you wish a complimentary pocket celluloid feeding chart, containing the information illustrated above, and S.M.A. physician's booklet, simply mail us a letter or postcard referring to this offer. S.M.A. Corporation, Cleveland, Ohio.

ETHICAL OF COURSE

•

If babies were all alike, it might not be quite so necessary to have a physician plan and supervise feedings. However, from the very beginning every package of S. M. A. has carried these instructions prominently on the label: *"Use only on order and under supervision of a licensed physician. He will give you instructions."*

S.M.A. PRODUCES RESULTS - MORE SIMPLY, MORE QUICKLY

Figure 5.3. S.M.A. advertisement. Source: *JAMA, 101* (14) (1933), adv. 12

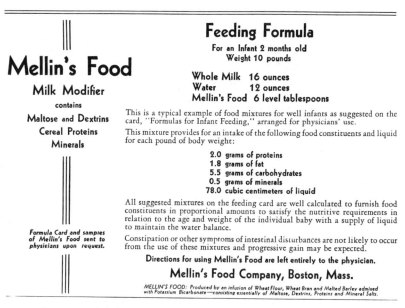

Figure 5.4. Mellin's advertisement. Source: *JAMA, 107* (26) (1936), adv. 37

booklets and feeding schedules.[26] In the 1930s, after Marriott had published his studies on the efficacy of canned unsweetened milk in infant feeding, Pet Milk hired him to show Q. J. Papineau, head of its medical relations department, the right and wrong ways to contact a doctor. Papineau also studied clinical and hospital procedures and learned the technical aspects of infant feeding. In order to get past the receptionist of a doctor's office, he had cards printed that identified him as "Q. J. Papineau, Research Division, Pet Milk Company." In the 1930s the staff of this "research division" grew from a few dozen sales representatives to fifty-five employees. As was typical of infant-food manufacturers, the Pet Milk Company offered physicians literature, free samples, and prescription blanks. To encourage hospitals to use the product, the company produced films, trained nurses in formula preparation, and, most important, adopted a policy of supplying free goods to hospitals for nursery use.[27] Like other manufacturers of infant-food items, evaporated milk producers emphasized the simplicity and safety of formulas composed of their products.

These promotional campaigns apparently struck a responsive chord in many practitioners. Especially in the 1910s, observers discovered that many physicians thought cow's-milk formulas were too complex and preferred the easier-to-use manufactured foods. One 1914 study at the Vanderbilt Clinic

These formulas, which are arranged for normal infants of average weight, meet the generally accepted requirement for protein, fat, carbohydrate and liquid per pound of body weight — *with a liberal supply of mineral salts.*

In beginning bottle feedings it is best to use a little less milk than called for in the formulas, adding enough water to keep the measure. It is rarely advisable to use less Mellin's Food than suggested, but not infrequently an increase is desirable, particularly if the baby is underweight or if constipation is an annoying symptom.

Formulas are readily changed to satisfy the needs of babies other than normal. Variations in weight, size or condition may be met by properly adjusting the formula.

The underlying principle of this workable method makes possible an unlimited range of adaptation and opens the way to *fitting the food to the baby* — the correct approach to bottle feeding.

Analysis of Mellin's Food

Fat	0.2 %
Protein	10.3 %
Reducing Sugars as Maltose	58.9 %
Dextrins (by difference)	20.7 %
Ash	3.9 %
Moisture	5.6 %

Six level tablespoonfuls of Mellin's Food — the minimum amount added to a full day's feeding — enhances the value of milk in the suggested formulas by contributing the following food constituents in approximate amounts as stated:

Maltose	24 grams
Dextrins	8 "
Cereal Proteins	4 "
Mineral Elements	
Phosphorus	130 milligrams
Magnesium	36 "
Sodium	32 "
Calcium	8 "
Iron	2 "
Copper	0.36 "
Manganese	0.12 "

The above constituents are derived from wheat flour, wheat bran and malted barley from which Mellin's Food is made. There is also contributed to the mixture seven-tenths of a gram of potassium, due to the addition of potassium bicarbonate in the process of manufacture.

Mellin's Food Company, Boston, Mass.

Formulas furnished to Physicians Only

Fresh Milk Formulas for Infant Feeding

Age Months	Weight Pounds	Whole Milk Ounces	Mellin's Food Level Table-spoons	Water Ounces	Ounces per Feeding	Feedings in 24 Hours	Calories per Pound
One	8	13	6	15	4	7	52
Two	10	16	6	12	4	7	48
Three	12	19	7	13	4½	7	48
Four	14	23	7	12	5	7	47
Five	15	24	8	12	6	6	47
Six	16	27	8	9	6	6	47
Seven	17	30	8	9	6½	6	48
Eight	18	32	8	8	8	5	48
Nine	19	32	8	8	8	5	45
Ten	20	32	8	8	8	5	43
Eleven	20½	32	8	8	8	5	42
Twelve	21	32	8	8	8	5	41

Evaporated Milk Formulas for Infant Feeding

Age Months	Weight Pounds	Evaporated Milk Ounces	Mellin's Food Level Table-spoons	Water Ounces	Ounces per Feeding	Feedings in 24 Hours	Calories per Pound
One	8	7	6	21	4	7	55
Two	10	9	6	19	4	7	52
Three	12	11	7	21	4½	7	53
Four	14	12	7	23	5	7	48
Five	15	13	8	23	6	6	49
Six	16	14	8	22	6	6	49
Seven	17	15	8	24	6½	6	48
Eight	18	16	8	24	8	5	48
Nine	19	16	8	24	8	5	45
Ten	20	16	8	24	8	5	43
Eleven	20½	16	8	24	8	5	42
Twelve	21	16	8	24	8	5	41

All formulas provide for an amount of mixture sufficient for twenty-four hours. To prepare: Dissolve the Mellin's Food in the water (previously boiled, then cooled), and then add the milk. Let the mixture stand in the refrigerator for about two hours before using the first feeding.

Orange juice should be given daily after 2nd or 3rd month.

Figure 5.5. Front and back sides of Mellin's feeding card

disclosed that out of 200 feeding cases previously on a food prescribed by a doctor, only 19 percent were on a milk formula; the other 81 percent were fed some patent food. This very small, select sample suggests that practitioners were resorting to manufactured foods to avoid complex formulas.[28] In large measure physicians blamed the use of patent foods, if not the rise of bottle feeding itself, not only on the complexity of milk formulations but, more specifically, on the extensive advertising of proprietary infant foods to physicians.[29] How valid was this charge? True, physicians received much of their information from advertising, booklets, and sales representatives of infant-food companies. But they also learned about products in medical school and postgraduate courses, and they certainly read about them in articles in medical journals and textbooks.[30] These medical sources usually did not denounce all proprietary foods; rather, they cautioned that any physician who used these products should be knowledgeable about their composition and cognizant of the circumstances for which they were suitable.

The growing popularity of evaporated milk formulations in the late 1920s and 1930s demonstrates the difficulty one encounters in attempting to evaluate the relative influences of advertising and medical expertise on modes of infant feeding. In this case, at approximately the same time, medical researchers published studies that showed the effectiveness of evaporated milk, textbooks discussed in positive tones infant formulas mixed with evaporated milk, and evaporated milk producers stepped up their advertising campaigns. No one factor clearly dominated.

Influenced by this combination of medical research, advertising, and personal experience, the majority of practitioners no longer condemned manufactured infant foods. Though a few continued to rail against their use, preferring instead simple whole-milk mixtures with carbohydrate added,[31] doctors generally accepted that commercial products could provide satisfactory nutrition for infants. In 1933 an Upper Darby, Pennsylvania, practitioner counted seventeen advertisements for baby food in one issue of *JAMA* and wrote that most of these were "quite satisfactory foods." In the same year, another practitioner declared in the *Archives of Pediatrics* that "the ever increasing use of commercial milk products designed for infant feeding has been one of the outstanding features of pediatrics in the last decade." Practitioners accepted these foods because of the "scientific methods" of their production, the cleanliness and safety of the products, and the simplicity of their use.[32] Tenney employed manufactured infant foods, having learned of them from sales representatives whom he regarded as "nice men," because he considered these products nutritionally satisfactory and simple to use: "all you had to do was dilute and feed." Other doctors were similarly impressed.[33]

Practitioners feared, however, that even with simpler methods of bottle feeding, most mothers generally lacked the knowledge necessary "to carry the child through infancy and childhood in such a manner that he may reach adult life sound in body and mind." A woman might have a keen sense of duty toward her child, but left to trust instinct alone, she would not "bring up the baby in a model fashion."[34] Earlier physicians had recognized that the surest way of reducing infant mortality was through the education of the mother. As the *Archives of Pediatrics* editorialized in 1912, "the purest milk in the world, alone, will not solve the problem of infant mortality. Ignorance kills more babies than bad milk."[35] In the ensuing decades practitioners often claimed that the declining infant death rate was a direct result of better-educated mothers, in particular stressing the mothers' increased knowledge of nutrition and milk modification for infant feeding.[36] A significant component of this knowledge was that mothers had learned to turn more frequently to medical advisors for information on child care. Studies such as those from the Vanderbilt Clinic, Glazier, and Garland and Rich had shown the importance of medical supervision and education. Moreover, as one member of the American Academy of Pediatrics put it in 1938, educating the mother gave her "a lasting impression of the advantages of modern obstetrics and pediatrics for herself and her baby."[37]

It is difficult to evaluate how much this judgment reflected physicians' humanitarian concerns about the well-being of children and how much their financial interest in attracting patients. But whether for health or economic reasons, physicians increasingly insisted that mothers go to private physicians or well-baby clinics for advice on child care in general and infant feeding in particular. By the 1910s milk stations and depots laid greater stress on medical instruction than on distributing pure milk.[38] Practitioners emphasized that even educated mothers needed the careful supervision of a medical attendant to ensure success in infant feeding.[39] Mothers should not only call upon a physician when their children were ill but should take even healthy children to a doctor regularly. Child-care manuals, such as *Simplifying Motherhood,* described this as "a 'keep-well' system, in which all responsibility rests, not on the mother, but on the shoulders of the doctor who is directing the baby's whole regime." Especially in the realm of bottle feeding, responsibility for selection of the infant's food rested with the physician.[40] Infant-care books written by practitioners and containing sample bottle formulas urged women "on no account to use them without medical advice."[41] Mothers also received infant-care advice from governmental agencies, philanthropic and private health organizations, and hospitals as well as from columns in women's magazines. By the 1940s these sources too stressed the necessity of regular visits to the doctor, regardless of whether the infant was nursed or bottle-fed (see Chapter 7). Since information about infant feeding also came from the manufacturers of infant foods, one of the goals of these educational campaigns was that women would rely on the advice of physicians and ignore the advertisements for proprietary foods.[42]

A few physicians discovered some unexpected deleterious side-effects of all this maternal education. The widespread dissemination of child-care information gave some mothers, in physicians' views, a false sense of security that resulted in physicians' seeing infants less frequently. For this reason, one California physician estimated in 1936 that the routine care of babies under two years of age had decreased by 50 percent in his state.[43] On the other hand, when educated mothers did seek the assistance of doctors, the practitioner could have problems also. Dr. Joseph Brennemann lamented:

> That lay education is desirable may be granted as an axiom. . . . [But] In
> actual practice the young mother with a nutritionally untutored mind who

frankly states that she knows nothing about babies and leaves the instruction to me is a treasure; the mother who has perhaps specialized in dietetics while in college, or who approached the subject with a McCollum in one hand and a Gesell in the other is sometimes more of a problem than is her baby.[44]

Basically practitioners saw the situation as one of control. A woman educated enough to be aware of the important advances in science and medicine was more open to her physician's direction. Unfortunately, too much education led her to think that she knew as much as or more than her doctor. Physicians wanted mothers to understand that they needed to visit doctors and to follow the physician's instructions but not to possess so much information that they could ignore or interfere with the physician's advice. If practitioners were to have responsibility for infant feeding, then they must be the sole dispensers of information about artificial feeding.[45]

With the publication of the Children's Bureau pamphlet *Infant Care* in 1914, national medical associations became involved in the controversy over the role of medical practitioners in child care. Julia Lathrop, bureau chief, had appointed Mary Mills West, a mother of five and graduate of the University of Minnesota, to write the booklet. West complemented the works of leading physicians with her own practical experience. This combination of scientific knowledge and common sense reflected the bureau's view that child health was not strictly a medical problem. Nevertheless, West warned her readers that *Infant Care* was not meant to replace the physician. Following the publication of *Infant Care,* the medical profession pressured Lathrop to appoint an Advisory Medical Committee, composed of representatives of the American Pediatric Society, the Pediatrics Section of the AMA, and the American Child Hygiene Association, to review all bureau publications dealing with the techniques of child care. In a letter dated 9 October 1919, the committee told Lathrop that the pamphlet was "merely a compilation; therefore it should not have an author's name given." West, understanding Lathrop's situation, in a 1920 letter accepted the decision to delete her name as author. In the 1921 revision of *Infant Care,* West no longer appeared as author, though Lathrop did acknowledge her assistance, along with that of Dr. Dorothy Reed Mendenhall, in a letter of transmittal printed at the beginning of the booklet. By the late 1920s all the compilers of *Infant Care* were physicians. The bureau increasingly characterized child health as a medical problem, and in both pamphlets and correspondence the bureau's leaders recommended that women see their physicians regularly and bring their questions to a medical adviser.[46]

Practitioners also feared that manufacturers of infant foods threatened their role as child-care advisors. Advertising campaigns to nonmedical audiences presented bottle feeding as safe and simple without medical supervision. And because mothers could follow the directions on the package and read about infant care in booklets provided free by the manufacturer, the companies' actions seemingly eliminated the need to take the child to a physician. In a 1933 article cogently entitled "The Importance of Infant Feeding to the General Practitioner," one physician argued that doctors who recommended such products to their patients tacitly encouraged the assumption that bottle-fed infants did not need medical supervision, and in so doing they permitted "a lucrative practice" to slip through their fingers. He warned that once a physician instructed a mother to feed her baby according to the directions on the container, she would buy the same product for subsequent children and would recommend the food to her friends. "Thus, not one but several patients are lost by the practitioner through his endorsement of the baby food," and babies would be fed without medical oversight.[47]

In opposing the use of manufactured infant foods, practitioners less often discussed the nutritional deficiencies of the products themselves and more frequently objected that doctors lacked control over their use. In 1915 a group of physicians presented the AMA's Section on Diseases of Children with a resolution attacking the advertising techniques of infant-food companies. A few years later the section appointed a committee to investigate the general question of advertising proprietary infant foods.[48]

Basing its 1925 report on a questionnaire answered by 628 physicians from across the country, the committee found that many practitioners considered these products at the very least "convenient, helpful and serv[ing] a purpose," if not "essential," in their own infant-feeding cases. When asked if it was possible or advisable to "dispense entirely with proprietary foods in the feeding of infants in your practice," a majority admitted that these foods, especially canned milks, were vital in their work. Respondents expressed dissatisfaction not with the nutritional value of proprietary foods but with their advertising:

> The opinion is almost unanimous that the means of advertisement must be
> limited to medical journals and literature and personal contact with the
> physician. Such a method will permit the physician to discriminate between
> foods that are offered and to judge these foods on the basis of their
> composition and the material which they contain in its relation to the
> nutritional requirements of the infant.

In other words, patent infant foods were useful, but their dissemination must be controlled. Not surprisingly, given these responses, the committee concluded that "it is impracticable at the present time to dispense entirely with all proprietary foods." The committee recognized the importance of formulating "a definite program for control of the method of advertising in all medical journals and in all periodicals," but it did not propose any specific regulations.

At the end of the report, the AMA committee commended unnamed manufacturers of proprietary foods for cooperating with the medical profession and its medical journals. The writers were probably referring to the producers of products like Dextri-Maltose and S.M.A., both of which had developed their advertising campaigns around the theme of medically directed infant feeding. These companies appear to have decided from the first that their success lay in persuading the medical profession to use their products; product recognition among the general public was secondary. Dextri-Maltose and S.M.A. were obviously profitable. By the 1920s other companies had noted their success and also recognized the growing involvement of the medical profession in directing infant feeding. When Nestlé's introduced Lactogen and Horlick's its Milk Modifier, these companies too directed their advertising almost exclusively to physicians and supplied no feeding directions on their packages. Though the AMA committee applauded this technique, many other products, such as canned milk, Mellin's, Nestlé's Milk Food, and Horlick's Malted Milk, continued to provide feeding instructions to nonmedical users like mothers.

Why all this interest in advertising coalesced into organizational action in the mid-1920s is unclear. Two facts, however, are most significant: the manufacture of infant food had grown into a large, profitable industry, and artificial infant feeding had become widely accepted among medical practitioners and the general public. Physicians who recognized the importance of infant feeding in their practices were undoubtedly upset with foods that made their advice unnecessary. A mother might not take her child to the doctor if she could read about various products in magazines, decide for herself which one was best, and then walk into a drugstore, buy it, and use it according to the directions printed on the label. Similarly, if a doctor recommended a food that included preprinted instructions, the mother did not have to return to the physician for additional information. No matter which way the mother learned about such a product, the result could be the same: a doctor was not needed to supervise the feeding of the infant. Such a situation could be physically unhealthful for the infant and economically harmful to the physician. Whatever the reasons that prodded the profession into examining the advertising of infant foods, the 1925 investigation disclosed how important these products were to the practitioner.

Four years later the AMA became more directly involved with the establishment of a Committee on Foods within the Council on Pharmacy and Chemistry to approve the content claims and advertising of proprietary food products.[49] Though the committee was not specifically concerned with infant foods, many manufacturers of such items presented their products for AMA approval. In its acceptance notice for one of the first infant-food products approved, Borden's Evaporated Milk, the committee commended the company's policy of advertising the infant-feeding potential of its canned milk to the medical profession only; Borden's advertisements to nonmedical audiences discussed general household uses. Despite the fact that other products such as Mellin's and Horlick's Malted Milk printed feeding instructions on their packages, they too won the seal of approval.[50] At this time the committee was more concerned with erroneous content lists and unwarranted advertising claims than with control of feeding directions. In 1931 one committee member remarked, "It is most encouraging to find that most of the baby food manufacturers have agreed to eliminate extravagant claims."[51]

Feeling that more was needed, the executive council of the American Pediatric Society in 1932 suggested to the Committee on Foods that it "withhold its acceptance and approval of infant foods formulae for which are advertised directly to the laity." Shortly thereafter the committee issued specific regulations dealing with infant foods. First stating that "the breast fed and doubly so the artificially fed should be under the supervision of the physician who is experienced and skilled in the care and feeding of infants," the committee went on to explain its concern:

> The feeding of an infant by routine feeding formulas and instructions
> distributed by food manufacturers, or according to directions, printed
> material, or advice of any person other than the attending physician who
> can personally observe the condition of the baby, may seriously endanger the
> health of the infant.

For this reason, "the promulgation of feeding formulas in advertising to the laity is considered to be in conflict with the best experience, authoritative judgment, and basic principles in infant feeding and is not permissible."[52] Basically the new rule accepted in principle the use of manufactured infant foods while simultaneously seeking to restrain companies from publishing formulas or distributing them to nonmedical personnel.

The Mellin's Food Company quickly changed its labels to comply with the committee's new rule. At medical meetings the company reminded physicians that it limited distribution of feeding instructions to medical practitioners, and its advertisements pointed up this change (figure 5.6).[53] Mellin's halted its advertisements in nonmedical journals and limited itself

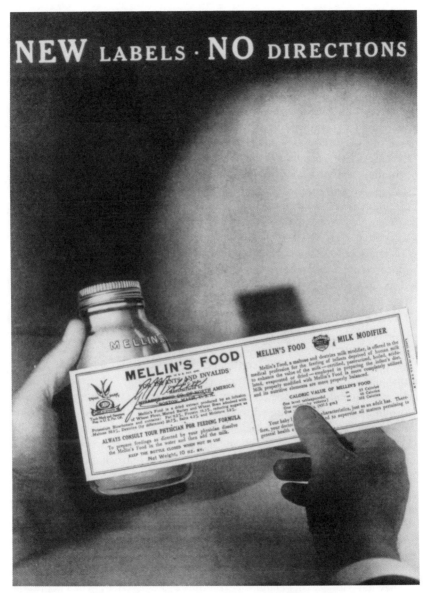

Figure 5.6. Mellin's advertisement with new labels. Source: *JAMA*, 99 (27) (1932), adv. 8

strictly to medical publications. Nestlé's did not have to change its Lactogen promotional campaigns, but it did stop advertising Nestlé's Milk Food, now called Nestlé's Food, to the general public and distributed feeding directions to physicians only (figure 5.7). Other companies followed suit.

Companies made such changes because they understood the importance of the AMA's seal of approval. The appearance of the seal on promotional material suggested that the medical profession had confidence in the product. And, more important, its absence made it more difficult for a company to attract the attention of practitioners; without the approval of the Committee on Foods, a product could not be advertised in AMA publications or exhibited at AMA meetings. In addition, many major medical publications, such as the *New England Journal of Medicine,* received advertising contracts through the AMA's Cooperative Medical Advertising Bureau. This bureau would approve copy only for "drugs, therapeutic agents and foods which are acceptable to the respective approving committees of the American Medical Association." Similarly, regional medical societies would allow only approved products to be exhibited at their meetings. Some textbooks, such as Marriott's *Infant Nutrition,* discontinued listing specific infant foods and instead directed readers to the AMA's approved list.[54] Thus denial of the seal limited the company's promotional sphere.

Despite the importance of the Seal, not all manufacturers were amenable to the requirement of the Committee on Foods. The labels and advertising for Horlick's Malted Milk continued to "present explicit infant feeding formulas for infants aged from one week to 12 months." When the committee recommended that the company alter its copy and "remove the feeding formulas from advertising addressed to the public," Horlick's refused and lost the right to display the seal.[55] Over a decade later Frank E. Hartman, Horlick's executive vice-president, blamed the medical profession for the company's declining sales. He contended that pediatricians did not want infant foods designed for fixed-feeding formulas; rather, they demanded products with more flexibility. Using items such as Dextri-Maltose and evaporated milks, medical practitioners could manipulate the composition of the infant's food, and, Hartman claimed, physicians felt that they needed such adaptable products "if the profession was to extend its activities to a profitable point." Horlick's Malted Milk was not suitable for this purpose. (The fact that the AMA accepted relatively inflexible products like S.M.A. somewhat vitiates this claim.) Furthermore, he asserted, when reputable medical journals denied Horlick's advertising space as a result of the decision of the Committee on Foods, they eliminated a vital link between the firm and doctors.[56]

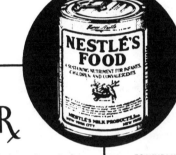

℞

FOR INFANTS who cannot thrive on formulas which simulate human milk in percentage composition—

℞

FOR INFANTS who have suffered digestive disturbances due to previous diet, overfeeding, infection or improper formulas—

℞

FOR INFANTS who have a limited tolerance for cow's milk, whether fresh or processed —

℞

FOR INFANTS who are markedly below normal weight due to excessive activity or previous illness—

(Malted whole wheat, malt, dry milk, sucrose, wheat flour, salt, dicalcium and tricalcium phosphate, iron citrate and cod liver oil extract. Contains vitamins A, B and D.)

Nestlé's Food is ideally indicated in such cases and has attained an enviable reputation among physicians who have had experience with it.

Nestlé's Food has been accepted by the Committee on Foods of the American Medical Association.

●   ●   ●

No feeding directions given except to physicians. No laity advertising. For free samples and literature, please send your professional blank to:

NESTLÉ'S MILK PRODUCTS · Inc.

2 Lafayette Street   •   Dept. 1N3   •   New York City

Figure 5.7. Nestlé's Food advertisement with new advertising policy. Source: *JAMA* 100 (11) (1933), adv. 10

Though the demise of the Horlick's company in the United States is more complex than Hartman's analysis would suggest, undoubtedly the action of the Committee on Foods significantly lessened the use of Horlick's products in infant feeding. Companies that allowed the committee to approve their promotional material fared much better financially. The Mead Johnson Company succinctly summarized how this symbiotic bond functioned:

> When mothers in America feed their babies by lay advice, the control of your pediatric cases passes out of your hands, Doctor. Our interest in this important phase of medical economics springs not from any motives of altruism, philanthropy or paternalism, but rather from a spirit of enlightened self interest and co-operation because [our] infant diet materials are advertised only to you, never to the public.[57]

Theoretical considerations, clinically proven, simple cow's-milk formulas, pliant manufacturers of infant foods, and economic self-interest interacted to influence the activities of medical practitioners in the area of infant feeding. Throughout the first half of the twentieth century, practitioners' growing involvement in the area of infant feeding was, in part, an acknowledgment of the scientific and medical advances that made artificial feeding a safe and healthful alternative to maternal nursing. It was also a response to the perception that increasing numbers of women were unable or unwilling to nurse their infants. Practitioners saw that to enhance their economic position and to protect the nutrition of infants they had to direct infant feeding. By mid-century American women commonly bottle fed their infants under medical supervision.

PART THREE

Scientific Motherhood

VI

"The Noblest Profession" 1890–1920

While physicians debated the virtues of bottle feeding, the variety of artificial foods, and the doctor's role in infant feeding, while manufacturers proclaimed the advantages of one product over another, mothers faced the question: "How shall I feed my baby?" Medical discussions and pronouncements shaped the options available, infant-food advertisements suggested new alternatives, but they were not the only factors influencing women's choices. In order to understand how women decided between breast feeding and bottle feeding, how they selected the foods they fed their infants, we must also examine the significant transformation in women's idealized maternal role from the cult of domesticity to scientific motherhood.

In the late nineteenth and early twentieth centuries, scientific motherhood appeared as a coherent ideology but not usually an organized movement. Scientific motherhood, like the "cult of domesticity," defined women in terms of their maternal role centered in the domestic sphere. At the same time, however, it increasingly emphasized the importance of scientific and medical expertise to the development of proper childrearing techniques. Thus the ideology of scientific motherhood shared with various Progressive reform movements of the time a faith in science and an appreciation of expert knowledge. Women retained the responsibility for child care, but, according to proponents of scientific motherhood, they needed expert advice in order to perform their duties successfully.[1]

The definition of woman developed under the ideology of scientific motherhood did not constitute a sharp break with the past. As had the proponents of the cult of true womenhood, commentators on women's place in society maintained the centrality of home and family in women's lives. An 1886 article in the popular childcare magazine *Babyhood* paints a poignant picture of woman as mother:

> For motherhood is the crown and glory of a woman's life. It comes
> sometimes as a thorny crown, but it is worth all its costs. The bliss of
> motherhood, which is like nothing else on earth, is placed in compensation
> over against all the pain and care which so often seem to be woman's
> peculiar burden. And it compensates.

Motherhood was both "the highest honor and noblest profession possible to woman" and "a privilege to be gratefully appreciated."[2]

This abstract, idealized vision of woman as mother remained fairly constant through the period, but various changes in American society affected the substance of the maternal role. By the 1880s and 1890s, increasing numbers of women were employed as teachers, social workers, and nurses. The professions of law and medicine attracted others, and many women found employment in factories or as pieceworkers. Even more significant in drawing large numbers of women out of the home were the host of organizations established in the last quarter of the nineteenth century, groups such as the Women's Christian Temperance Union (WCTU), the Daughters of the American Revolution, the Congress of Mothers (later the National Parent and Teachers Association), and the General Federation of Women's Clubs.

Though women's groups frequently began as lecture and discussion clubs, by the 1880s and 1890s they had gradually become more involved in social reform efforts. For example, lectures on art might have stirred a local club's interest in beautifying the city, leading to a drive for public parks that in turn stimulated an investigation of local housing conditions and a push to improve tenement houses. Groups did not necessarily limit themselves to a single reform effort. Along with the prohibition of alcohol and stricter moral codes, for instance, the WCTU reported the benefits of exercise and dress reform for women's health; it pushed for the establishment of kindergartens, the employment of matrons to work in women's prisons, and passage of child labor legislation. The group also published a baby-care journal variously titled *Mother's Friend, New Crusade,* and *American Motherhood.* For many years its editor was Mary Wood-Allen, the national superintendent of the Purity Department of the WCTU, who was followed by Marion A. McBridge, WCTU's superintendent of Domestic Science and Sanitation.

The clubs both enlarged and confirmed women's domestic roles. True, such organizations did draw women outside the home, but the reform movements in which they most visibly participated were extensions of their domestic duties. Thus it was not surprising that women's groups were concerned with schooling, playgrounds and parks, and pure food and drugs, activities that would make society safer, cleaner, and healthier for families and children.

Despite the development of new options that took some women outside the domestic sphere, the overwhelming majority of women became wives and mothers, and popular imagery continued to equate praiseworthy womanhood and the maternal role. "Woman's labors and successes in the various fields and affairs of life, are calling daily for more and more attention," noted one woman physician in her 1901 medical manual for women. But, she cautioned, "while we admire her in her new role, with her efforts toward success in society, literature, science, politics and the arts, we must not lose sight of her most divine and sublime mission in life—womanhood and motherhood."[3] Around the turn of the century, even feminists as radical as Ellen Key, Emma Goldman, and Charlotte Perkins Gilman claimed that motherhood was woman's chief fulfillment in life.[4]

But the environment of that motherhood was changing as technological innovations within the home altered women's lives. Devices such as carpet sweepers, vacuum cleaners, refrigerators, and washing machines slowly became available to growing numbers of households. The introduction of new equipment had considerable consequences for women's domestic work. In the kitchen, for example, the move from coal or wood stoves to gas, oil, or electric models eliminated such chores as loading fuel and removing ashes. The new stoves themselves were easier to light, maintain, and regulate; and because coal dust was not regularly tracked through the room, the kitchen was easier to clean. Cookbooks became more "scientific," speaking of a tablespoon of compressed yeast rather than a walnut-sized piece. The emerging commercial food industry further modified American women's cooking tasks, as the variety of canned foods first available in the mid-nineteenth century expanded greatly by the second decade of this century. Lighting in the home moved from candles to kerosene-burning lamps to gaslights and eventually to electric lights. These changes did not reach all women at the same time, of course. Nonetheless, modern and expanding networks of communication and transportation, including such developments as rural free delivery, mail-order merchandising, mass-circulation magazines, the telephone, and transcontinental railroads, facilitated the movement of goods and services and transformed the domestic experiences of women.[5]

Regarded negatively, these changes could appear to devalue the importance of women's work in the home and could encourage women to seek an identity outside the domestic sphere. Concurrently, though, the ideology of scientific motherhood elevated the nurturing of children to the status of a profession. The expectation that science should shape domestic work dates from at least as early as the 1840s with the publication of Catharine Beecher's *Treatise on Domestic Economy.* Gathering together in one volume the whole spectrum of domestic tasks—household maintenance, childrearing, gardening, cooking, cleaning, and doctoring—Beecher defined a new role for women within the home. Scientific explanations provided the rationale for her advice. Beecher did not present herself as the expert in matters such as physiology and health, but instead acknowledged the medical sources she used and implied that anyone could easily learn from them. Beecher and her followers promoted the idea that housekeeping was a full-time scientific profession. Just as men studied and trained for their professions, women must educate themselves for their life's work, mothering. Women needed to "equip themselves for motherhood as thoughtfully, conscientiously, and zealously as any other scientist prepares himself for an exacting career."[6] The exact meaning of the term "science" remained extremely vague: in various contexts it suggested laboratory work and research, and in other circumstances it meant developing a set of more exacting measures. Though its definition remained elusive, the word "science" added a veneer of professionalism to a wide range of activities. In addition to scientific motherhood, there was, for example, domestic science in the kitchen, and women published books with titles such as *Household engineering: Scientific management in the home.*[7]

Scientific motherhood established science as the informing agent in child-rearing and health matters. Scientific discoveries would help mothers raise healthier children. Moreover, as the prestige of science grew in American society, the application of scientific advances in the domestic sphere could enhance the status of women's work. As one mother wrote in an 1899 issue of the *Ladies' Home Journal,* "Ideal motherhood, you see, is the work not of instinct, but of enlightened knowledge conscientiously acquired and carefully digested. If maternity is an instinct, motherhood is a profession." She claimed that four-fifths of the ill-health of children could be avoided with proper maternal training. Women, she insisted, needed to "cultivate a new way of looking at their children," a scientific way, like men. Although acknowledging that women always have fed their babies, this mother was convinced that "it is the men chemists and physicians who have given babies their dietary formulas, obtained through chemical analysis and conforming to physiological laws." "In point of fact," wrote another woman in 1913, "to feed a baby properly in this day of nostrums, germs and stomach destroyers requires education, the best that science can provide." "Instinct has equipped us only with the means to acquire that education," she believed, and only with training would motherhood "be regarded as the highest profession among us, and one for which every woman should have some fundamental preparation."[8] Scientific motherhood elevated science and denigrated instinct.

The themes of science and professionalism pervade the scientific motherhood literature throughout the late nineteenth and early twentieth centuries. Whether written by feminists like Gilman, doctors, home economists, mothers, or educational and governmental agencies, these materials insisted that scientific training was essential to motherhood. Gilman, for example, accepted that women were instinctually maternal, but the force of maternal love needed direction. Her prime example of this was "the futility of unaided maternal love and instinct in the simple act of feeding the child." Unfortunately, "this instinct has not taught her such habits of life as insure her ability to fulfill this natural function," nor to select a healthful substitute for mother's milk. Mothers' responsibility for the health of their families necessitated training in scientific motherhood. Similarly, a writer who signed herself simply "A trained mother" wrote in *Good Housekeeping* in 1911 that "maternal instinct is not knowledge. It is love, patience, and unselfishness. . . . [But] maternal instinct left alone succeeds in killing a large proportion of the babies born into this world."[9]

Trained mothers could reduce this mortality. A brochure distributed by Smith, Kline & French to promote Eskay's Food reminded women that motherhood was not an accident but a profession, not an incident but a supreme event. Mothers should not trust their childrearing responsibilities to Providence, but they should seek out and use the knowledge produced by science. These and other articles and books through the period increasingly stressed the awesome task a woman had in protecting her family's health and well-being: she dare not depend on instinct alone; she needed training and knowledge of the latest scientific and medical developments.[10]

The emphasis on scientific training transformed the values and codes of behavior for women. Evident at first primarily among the middle classes in the late nineteenth century, the ideal of trained motherhood gradually spread to all parts of the country through many channels of communication. Journals, such as the *Ladies' Home Journal* and *Good Housekeeping,* and other publications promoted the view that women were not innately equipped to handle their mothering tasks; they needed some instruction. Governmental and philanthropic agencies, too, established institutional forums to help educate working-class women.

The milk stations, which had begun in the 1890s, provided the nucleus for many of the well-baby clinics and baby health stations that developed in urban areas during the early twentieth century. Under the aegis of Dr. S. Josephine Baker of the city health department, New York used its milk depots not only to distribute milk to poor families but also to educate tenement mothers in scientific child care. Many other cities copied this pattern of clinics, sometimes instituted by public health departments and sometimes by charitable organizations. In Madison, Wisconsin, in the summer of 1915, a group of philanthropic women, called the Attic Angels, began a summertime child health center under the direction of Dr. Dorothy Reed Mendenhall. By February 1916 the Attic Angels had established a permanent center, and more were developed in the next several decades. These centers were typical of those created in many other parts of the country: physicians examined infants, mothers received advice on the feeding and care of children. These were well-baby clinics; ill babies were sent to outside physicians. The Attic Angels did not claim all the credit for Madison's declining infant mortality rate, but they pointed with pride to the role their centers played in its reduction.[11]

Baker was also instrumental in the development of another significant educational agency, Little Mothers' Clubs. Influenced by John Spargo's *Bitter Cry of the Children*[12] and her own experiences in New York City, Baker concluded that "little mothers"—that is, young, untrained girls who often had to take charge of their younger siblings while their mothers worked—were primary sources of infant mortality. The doctor accepted that "the little mother was an inevitable makeshift," one who "would be far less dangerous to her charges if she were intelligently trained."[13] Accordingly, Baker established seventy-one Little Mothers' Leagues in New York City in 1910. These girls' clubs would attack the problem of infant mortality and morbidity in the tenements in two ways. First, nurses would give the girls practical instruction in baby feeding, exercising, dressing, and other aspects of baby care. Second, the girls would instruct their mothers and neighborhood women in scientific motherhood. Baker called these girls "our most efficient missionaries." They persuaded their mothers and neighborhood women to attend baby health stations and told "every mother they met all about what they were learning." Within a year New York had 183 leagues and approximately 20,000 trained little mothers.[14]

The success of Baker's Little Mothers' Leagues prompted health departments across the country to initiate similar programs. Dr. E. T. Lobedan, chief of the Milwaukee City Health Board's Bureau of Child Welfare, introduced Little Mothers' Clubs in Wisconsin. By 1913 Milwaukee had fifteen classes instructing almost 2,000 girls. The Babies' Dispensary in Cleveland during 1911 and 1912 demonstrated the importance of teaching infant hygiene to young girls, and as a result child-care courses were introduced into the public school curriculum there. And the story was repeated over and over again throughout the nation as tens of thousands of students attended these courses over the next several decades.[15]

Baby health stations and Little Mothers' Leagues, however, reached only a limited, primarily urban population. Often the people who attended them were already involved in mothering. That is to say, the instruction often was an after-the-fact response to practical child-care problems. Therefore, although these institutions educated girls and women in scientific motherhood, their existence and even successes are not enough to explain how the general concept found its way into American life. Other educational forums attracted wider audiences.

Most women's colleges in the late nineteenth century supported the idea of educated motherhood. Schools such as Vassar were founded on the premise that women should have the same educational opportunities as men, should study the same curriculum. But they also gave instruction in domestic economy in order "to maintain a just appreciation of the dignity of woman's home sphere . . . to teach a correct *theory,* at least, of the household and its management." Collegiate instructors of home economics emphasized that their students would not reject woman's place in the home. Women so educated would perform their homemaking tasks more efficiently, would improve the quality of life for their charges, and thus would bring the benefits of science to their families. Rationalizing college chemistry courses for women, one writer in an 1871 issue of the domestic magazine *Hearth and Home* wrote:

> Why should chemistry be generally studied by our girls if they are not assisted by such knowledge to make better bread, to compound more wholesome dishes, and to preside with increased skill and scientific knowledge over the households of which they become mistresses?

Proponents of domestic science accepted the traditional role of women in the home, but these teachers wanted to use science education to improve women's domestic lives.[16]

Though home-economics courses, baby health stations, and Little Mothers' Leagues were widespread, their influence was somewhat restricted because they depended on face-to-face instruction. The ideals and techniques of scientific motherhood reached a broader audience through the growing number of pamphlets and books published on child care. State and local boards of health and bureaus of child hygiene distributed many of these publications. In 1911 the American Medical Association listed sixteen states that issued child-care pamphlets and estimated that in 1910 alone over 100,000 copies had been distributed. The AMA itself distributed booklets. Women did not have to seek out these publications; governmental agencies often sent them to prospective and new mothers.[17]

The child-care books that appeared in the late nineteenth and early twentieth centuries promoted, implicitly and explicitly, the ideology of scientific motherhood. They reiterated time and again that maternal instinct was not sufficient for the healthful rearing of children. "Whether or not a child shall become a healthy, happy, vigorous adult depends very largely on the care he may have received during the earliest months of life," explained the 1913 edition of *Our Baby Book*. Hospitals were crowded with "half starved, wrinkled, rachitic, miserable little scraps of humanity, mostly because of the inability or ignorance of mothers to give them intelligent care." Hence, the book claimed, "the necessity for instructing mothers in the hygiene of the child." Many of these child-care books were written by physicians for both their private patients and the general public. One of the most significant was *The Care and Feeding of Children*, by L. Emmett Holt. It began as a four-page catechism for nursery maids training at Babies' Hospital in New York City in the early 1890s. Students carried the booklet into the private homes in which they worked, and their employers soon asked for copies of their own. In 1894 Holt published the catechism as a sixty-six-page book. *Care and Feeding* went through seventy-five printings and twelve revisions by the mid-1920s and was translated into several foreign languages.[18]

Women's periodicals also fostered the ideal of scientific motherhood.[19] *Babyhood* emphasized that "there is a science in bringing up children and this magazine is the voice of that science."[20] Other magazines were less specific about their calling, but numerous child-care and health-related articles implied that successful mothering depended on scientific knowledge. Journals expressly designed for mothers and women's magazines concerned with the whole range of homemaking problems initiated columns on child-care topics and invited readers to write them for advice. They also distributed booklets to mothers.

For many years the *Ladies' Home Journal* published a column called "Mother's Corner," edited by Elizabeth Robinson Scovil, a trained nurse. Scovil noted that "among the questions that are poured into" the *Journal*, "there is none more often asked than 'How shall I feed my baby'?" In 1892, in response to these and other inquiries, she prepared "a little booklet called 'A Baby's Requirements,' giving practical advice as to the first wardrobe, the necessary toilet articles, the preparations needed for the mother's comfort, the food and the general care of a young baby."[21]

Eighteen years later Dr. Emelyn Lincoln Coolidge instituted a "Young Mother's Register" through her monthly column in the *Journal*. Within a year over 500 women had registered and sent to Coolidge monthly reports on their children's development. In return the doctor answered their questions about child care. Pleased with the growing number of registrants, in 1912 Coolidge reported, "The young mother is fast becoming educated, being no longer satisfied to follow the advice of well-meaning but inexperienced neighbors, but preferring to turn to a higher authority for help on solving nursery problems." By 1918 the number of registered babies had grown to over 60,000. The columns in the *Journal* were not unique. *Good Housekeeping* hired a physician, Josephine Hemenway Kenyon, to direct its "Health and Happiness Club," a column on child care. Other magazines instituted advice columns and entertained letters to the editor soliciting child-care information.[22]

Popular magazines also contained advertising that used the ideology of scientific motherhood to sell a wide range of products and services. Manufacturers expounded on the importance of science for mothers and then employed scientific evidence to demonstrate the superiority of their products. This was particularly true of infant-food advertisements. In their advertising copy, companies implied that mothers who wanted healthy children would appreciate the importance of the science of nutrition (figure 6.1). Two points must be remembered in ascertaining the impact of advertising on the reader. First, in the 1890s Edward W. Bok, editor of the *Ladies' Home Journal,* instituted the practice of mixing advertising matter among editorial pages. Formerly advertising material had appeared primarily in the front and back of magazines, isolated from the feature articles and editorials. When articles and advertisements appeared on the same page, the reader was more likely to notice the advertisements. Other magazines quickly adopted the new format. Second, in several instances journals specifically directed readers to advertising material. *American Motherhood*'s 1907 disclaimer of any responsibility for advertisements that appeared in its pages was unusual. The editorial staffs of other journals highlighted their advertising content.[23]

Housewives Magazine, organ of the Housewives League, considered advertising "an integral part" of the journal's function and an important means of educating intelligent consumers. The league endorsed products only after analyzing the "quality and value" of the item; the magazine printed advertisements only for endorsed products.[24] In 1912 *Good Housekeeping*

Advice to Mothers.

The swelling tide of infantile disease and mortality, resulting from injudicious feeding, the ignorant attempts to supply a substitute for human milk, can only be checked by enlightened parental care.

If possible, mothers should nurse their children, and every healthy mother should make the effort to perform this duty ; artificial food should never be substituted for the aliment which nature has provided in the healthy mother. But while it is undoubted that the healthy mother should esteem it her bounden duty, and for her good and that of her babe, that she should suckle him, constitutional incapacity, the claims of society, artificial surroundings, and other causes, have been potent in promoting the use, if not the necessity, of artificial food. We must endeavor to get a substitute for mothers' milk that approaches it as nearly as possible in its chemical constituents, in order to maintain the functional integrity and growing powers of a child.

Cows' milk immediately suggests itself as a probable substitute, and we find that it more nearly approximates to human milk than that of any other animal ; it is plentiful, readily obtained, and cheap, and has been commonly used as such substitute. But its use has always been attended with far from satisfactory results ; the excessively delicate digestive organs of the infant are generally thrown into derangement : while the irritability, fretfulness, and crying, followed, perhaps, by vomiting or diarrhœa, indicate in no uncertain manner that these organs are taxed beyond their powers, and that some modification of the diet is demanded, and must be made, or graver complications will surely ensue.

A compound suitable for the infant's diet must be alkaline in reaction ; must be rich in heat-producers, with a proper admixture of albuminoids of a readily digestible nature, together with the necessary salts and moisture. Men of the highest scientific attainments of modern times, both physiologists and chemists, have devoted themselves to careful investigation and experiment in devising a suitable substitute for human milk. The distinguished German, Baron Justus Von Liebig, chemist, physiologist, and philanthropist, made his name famous throughout the civilized world by nearly the last and the crowning work of his life, the publication of a formula for the preparation of a proper Infants' Food.

To prepare the food according to his directions, however, requires great care, much skill, and considerable time, and this difficulty of preparation was found almost to forbid its use in the family. Many variations of these directions were proposed, but all met with similar objections. It remained for Mr. Mellin, of London, England, to devise a process of manufacture that fitted it for introduction to general use.

Mellin's Food is entirely free from cane sugar and starch, the starch having been transformed into grape-sugar and dextrine by the diastase of the malt. Unlike cane-sugar, grape-sugar, upon being dissolved in water, is immediately taken into the circulation through the absorbent glands of the stomach and intestine.

An analysis of the Mellin's Food prepared with water and cows' milk, according to the directions, shows the closest approximation to analyses of human milk. It is the only Infants' Food prepared in accordance with known laws of physiology, and which fulfils the requirements of Liebig's principles.

We believe this food to be worthy the confidence of mothers ; that it is exactly suited to the ordinary powers of the babe's digestive organs, and that by its use and the exercise of proper care those diseases which work such frightful havoc among infants— diarrhœa, convulsions, the various wasting diseases, etc.—would be reduced to a minimum, and their fatal results be largely decreased.

This opinion is not based on theoretical assumption, but on observation and experience with the little ones whom I have attended, and with confidence born of this experience I heartily recommend its trial and use. The babe will thrive on cows' milk and Mellin's Food alone, and will need no addition to its diet till about twelve months of age, or until dentition is well advanced. . . . . Ever bear in mind that the young infant's organism is of the most delicate and sensitive construction ; from the first helpless to a degree, till gradually the stream of life acquires power, it commends itself to the utmost patience, vigilance, and care of the mother, and her unceasing love.—*From Advice to Mothers, by Dr. Hanaford.*

A copy of the book from which the above are extracts, also a valuable little work, " The Care and Feeding of Infants," may be had free by addressing

DOLIBER, GOODALE & CO.,

Figure 6.1. Mellin's advertisement. Source: *Babyhood*, *1* (4) (1885), v

hired Dr. Harvey Wiley to perform a similar service. Wiley had fought hard for the passage of the Pure Food and Drug Act of 1906 and then had led the United States Bureau of Chemistry, which was charged with implementing the legislation. The magazine gave Wiley absolute authority to reject advertising for drugs and cosmetics that did not meet his standards. Though Wiley recognized the need for artificial infant feeding in some instances, he believed that patent foods should never be recommended to mothers for general use. He allowed no manufacturer of infant foods to purchase advertising space in *Good Housekeeping,* although by the 1920s he did permit infant-feeding advertisements by evaporated milk companies.[25]

Many diverse aspects of women's magazines promoted and reinforced the ideology of scientific motherhood. Articles implied or boldly stated that maternal instinct alone would not produce healthy children. Echoing the sentiments expressed in home-economics courses and child-care books and pamphlets, the journals insisted that every woman needed instruction based on scientific principles and discoveries to rear her children successfully. Similarly, companies that advertised in these magazines used the rhetoric of scientific motherhood to sell their products. Editorial support for advertisements added to the visibility and respectability of the products. The relationship between the editorial content of the magazines and the advertising in them was important to the development of scientific motherhood. Both editorials and advertising, independently and in concert, fostered the assumption that a woman alone could not decide between different products; she needed to rely on the expertise of others to direct her choices.

The free booklets on child care offered by many companies also emphasized the importance of science. Mellin's produced "The Care and Feeding of Infants." Borden's furnished pamphlets entitled "Babies" and "Infant Health." Advertisements for KLIM, a dried milk, invited readers to send for the pamphlet "Child Health and Child Feeding."[26] These publications naturally publicized the infant-food product of the sponsoring company, but they also included instruction in general child care based on scientific principles. Other companies, including the Ivory Soap Company and the Metropolitan Life Insurance Company, provided mothers with similar infant-care information.[27]

Carnrick's "Our Baby's First and Second Years" combines scientific child-care advice and product advertising in a booklet written by Marion Harland, a popular author of novels and homemaking books. "Modern science has robbed the dentition period of many terrors by showing that since it is a normal process," Harland assured her readers, "the complications attendant upon it—particularly in hot weather—are to be governed by natural laws."

She pointed out that "heat, undue excitement, *change of food,* or perseverance in the use of an improper food, sudden check of perspiration—any one of a dozen imprudences—may derange digestion or bring on a fever, and the teeth get the full blame."[28] As to proper diet, "the healthy mother ought to nurse her child," but, unfortunately, few mothers could "supply enough milk for the entire nourishment of a hearty, growing infant of six or eight months old." Harland advised that "the conscientious mother," seeking out "that which will meet the increasing needs of her little one," should judge the value of the infant foods by observing "the analyses made by trustworthy chemists." Several pages later the reader finds a testimonial letter from Harland to the manufacturer praising Carnrick's Soluble Food.[29]

Proponents of scientific motherhood agreed that family nutrition was the responsibility and duty of mothers, and, they stressed, the good mother, the modern mother, would utilize the advances of science in the rearing of her children. Specifically, the discoveries of nutrition should inform her decisions on feeding. According to one speaker at a meeting of the Mothers' Union of Kansas City, Missouri, in 1899: "Child-building is an art, and the wise mother will put forth every effort to secure information as to how she can best bring her child into healthy and vigorous manhood or womanhood. And then she will look carefully into the dietary of those intrusted to her care." A few years later, a popular health-care manual explained the importance of applying theory to practice. Characterizing the usual methods of feeding as "hap-hazard," the book stated that "any mother who will study the nature of food products . . . will comprehend at once the value of dietetic knowledge in the selection and preparation of wholesome food for her family." Among the most consistent themes of scientific motherhood were the correlation between infant feeding and the health of the child, the mother's responsibility for her family's nourishment, and the assumption that science provided the answers for healthful nutrition.[30]

Scientific motherhood advocated the use of contemporary science to shape appropriate mothering practices; consequently, specific recommendations on infant feeding changed over time with new discoveries in the nutritional sciences. From the late nineteenth century to the early twentieth century, the insistence on breast feeding gradually became less adamant and bottle feeding more acceptable. Similarly, child-care advisors increasingly discussed the importance of the medical supervision of infant feeding.

Whether written by medical or nonmedical persons, the child-care literature of the period invariably began with the dictum that mothers should nurse their children. A few writers endowed maternal nursing with theological overtones. Harland pitied the woman who did not nurse her child: "The case comes under the solemn statute—'What God hath joined together let no man (or woman) put asunder.'" Writers reasoned that mother's milk was baby's "natural food." They frequently expressed the sentiment that "the law of Nature is, that a babe . . . shall be brought up by the breast; and Nature's laws cannot be broken with impunity." Mothers who did not nurse were irresponsible. Home medical manuals, articles in women's magazines and popular health journals, governmental brochures, home-economics textbooks, and booklets distributed by infant-food manufacturers—all the diverse forms of trained motherhood literature—advanced the claim that the mother's breast furnished "the natural and therefore the best means" of nourishing an infant. Even some advertisements for infant foods repeated this theme.[31]

Mother's milk might be the ideal form of infant feeding; however, alternatives to mother's milk were not only discussed but encouraged. The prescription "breast milk is best" was often followed with descriptions of breast milk insufficiency. Warning that breast milk could be or become deficient in quality or quantity, the home economist Anna Richardson concluded that "owing to illness or inability to nurse their children, thousands of mothers must feed their infants artificially." As early as 1902, an article in *Babyhood* remarked:

> Formerly if a child was at the breast, there was, so to speak, the end of it; he throve or not, according to the quantity or quality of his nourishment. Now it is not the end of it. . . . In those days many persons nursed who could not properly do it. Many now wisely aid their breast with additional food, or even totally wean their children, who would formerly have, with the best intent, half-starved their sucklings. This is not a plea for abandoning suckling. A good breast is a blessing, a poor one may be a "delusion, a mockery, and a snare."

In addition, even if a mother's supply appeared adequate, she was advised to feed her child at least one bottle a day. This supplemental feeding would give the mother "a little freedom" and make "weaning much easier."[32] Bottle feeding, of course, was not the same as breast feeding. However, explained the scientific-motherhood literature, by analyzing the differences in composition and digestibility between human and cow's milk, science had demonstrated how to "humanize" the bovine fluid. According to motherhood educators, especially in the early twentieth century, advances in nutritional sciences had rendered breast feeding no longer "an absolute necessity for a healthy baby."[33]

The contents of women's magazines document other, perhaps more subtle, influences on the growing acceptability of bottle feeding. The overwhelming preponderance of advice on infant feeding dealt with artificial feeding. Writing to Coolidge at the *Journal,* "a very young mother" complained that she could find little information about breast feeding:

> You speak often of diet-lists, etc., for bottle-babies and older children, but have you nothing of the kind for breast-fed babies? I nurse my three-months-old baby, and there are many little points as to length of time to nurse her, the hours, the number of meals in twenty-four hours, etc., that I would like to know about.

Coolidge had written some articles for nursing mothers, but most of her columns discussed either bottle feeding or mixed feeding.[34] Moreover, most of the infant-feeding correspondence from mothers pertained to artificial feeding. The wealth of editorial material and the high proportion of letters discussing bottle feeding taken together suggest that infant feeding by the early twentieth century was by no means synonymous with breast feeding. The imbalance between information on breast feeding and that on bottle feeding is also evident in child-care manuals and in the instruction women and girls received at well-baby clinics and Little Mothers' Clubs.

On the specifics of infant feeding, scientific motherhood literature mirrored the state of contemporary medical and scientific knowledge. For example, the first edition of Holt's *Care and Feeding* states categorically, "What is the best infant's food? Mother's milk."[35] However, many factors, including "extreme nervousness, fright, fatigue, grief or passion," might compromise a mother's ability to suckle her child. Even if there was no nursing problem, the infant should receive one bottle a day. Supplemental feeding would obviate difficulties at weaning time and would allow the mother a period of rest during the nursing period. Holt reiterated these sentiments in all subsequent editions.

When discussing bottle feeding, Holt, like writers of other child-care manuals, emphasized the scientific bases of good artificial feeding. He outlined the known differences between human and cow's milk and used these analyses to rationalize the formulas he proposed. In 1894 he recommended diluting cow's milk with water and adding top-milk and sugar. By the fourth edition (1906), Holt, a proponent of Rotch's theory, provided readers with a simplified form of the percentage method. Sixteen years later he advised using 1.5 ounces of whole milk per pound of body weight per day, 1.0 ounce of sugar per day, and water. As his formulas changed in the various editions of his book, so too did the scientific arguments he used to support them.

Science was also invoked to justify the use of patent infant foods. While extolling the virtues of mother's milk, companies detailed the scientific bases of their products in various publications sent to mothers and in advertisements in women's magazines. The 1891 edition of *Mellin's Food for Infants and Invalids* explained:

> It is universally admitted that a mother should, if she is able, nurse her child; if she cannot, or if for some good reasons it is not advisable either for herself or for the child, then the best alternative is the use of a proper artificial food. The substitute should correspond as closely as possible, both chemically and physiologically, to mother's milk, because nature's work can never be improved. . . . Mellin's food . . . is the only perfect substitute for mother's milk, being the only infant food corresponding chemically and physiologically to mother's milk.[36]

The manufacturer supplied charts comparing human and cow's milk and asserted that the addition of Mellin's Food to cow's milk produced "the perfect food for infants." The company's promotions almost invariably paid at least lip service to the superiority of breast milk and characterized Mellin's as the best substitute for mother's milk, but one to be used only when necessary. In at least one instance, though, the graphics of an advertisement for Mellin's belied the text (figure 6.2).

The books and advertisements of infant-food companies emphasized "scientific" infant feeding—the importance of using the latest scientific discoveries to evaluate modes of infant feeding. One very significant factor, however, differentiated most infant-food companies' materials from other scientific motherhood literature and instruction. On the one hand, Mellin's and other manufacturers implied that the mother should and would direct the feeding of her infant. In 1887 Harland advised the mother to decide which food to feed her infant—to "judge for herself" which product to use. "The duty," she reminded her readers, "is plain. If it is not easy, it is, nevertheless, duty and hers."[32] On the other hand, Holt's book, despite its detailed instructions on bottle feeding, assumed that a physician was supervising the infant's diet; he intended the information in *Care and Feeding* to help the mother to understand and carry out the directions of the doctor.

In the nineteenth century the ideology of scientific motherhood gave mothers broad decision-making powers; after the turn of the century, increasing numbers of trained motherhood publications insisted that a mother alone could not choose the appropriate food for her child. Books that

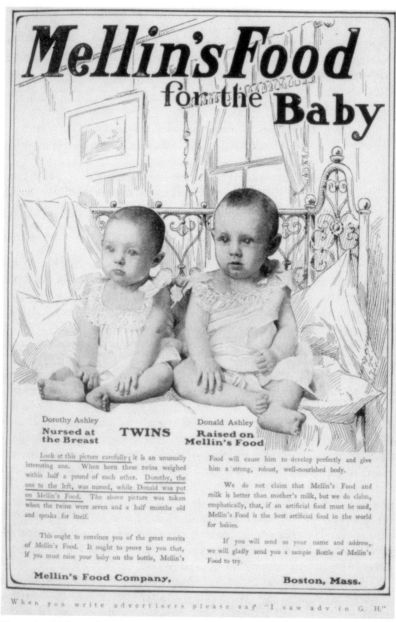

Figure 6.2. Mellin's advertisement. Source: *Good Housekeeping*, 44 (1907), advertisement section

supplied bottle formulas did so with the proviso that the recipes "may serve as a guide for mothers who for any reason cannot consult a physician. A mother should not attempt to decide the proper formula when she can get the advice of a physician."[38] Similarly, Coolidge admonished readers of her column to "get regular formulas from the doctor if possible; if not, write me, and I will gladly send them. . . . [H]ave *skilled* advice from the first."[39] By the second decade of this century, child-care columns in other popular magazines and domestic medical manuals, while providing detailed instructions on artificial feeding, became more insistent about the need for direct medical supervision.

The rise of the ideology of scientific motherhood coupled with developments in nutritional and medical sciences significantly affected views of infant feeding. In the nineteenth century the bottle-fed baby was an object of pity; by the twentieth century artificial feeding was widely discussed. Though breast milk was the best food for infants, now infant foods constructed by knowledgeable persons according to the most up-to-date scientific information were reasonable substitutes for mother's milk. Well-baby clinics and Little Mothers' Clubs, child-care manuals and columns in women's magazines, advertising campaigns of infant-food manufacturers, all promoted scientific infant feeding and scientific motherhood. All agreed that motherhood represented woman's proper and ideal role. All acknowledged the importance of scientific knowledge for correcting mothering practices. And all proclaimed that a mother alone could not decide which food was best for her infant. Disagreement arose over the question of who should select the food. The infant-food companies placed the decision in the hands of mothers. However, by the early twentieth century, other advocates of scientific motherhood insisted on the medical supervision of artificial infant feeding. Balancing a mother's responsibility for the health of her child with her dependence upon expert advice created a tension within the ideology of scientific motherhood. In attempting to resolve this tension, scientific-motherhood proponents in the twentieth century accorded physicians an increasingly significant role in infant feeding.

VII

"The Doctor Should Decide"
1920–1950

The ideology of scientific motherhood lost none of its potency in the twentieth century. Throughout the 1920s, 1930s, and 1940s, despite opportunities opening for women outside the home and the traumas of the Depression and World War II, traditional concepts continued to influence ideas about women's proper place in society. One mother of seven, in her 1935 book *Common Sense for Mothers,* described women's maternal role in terms only slightly more prosaic than her predecessors:

> I am convinced that what we do in the secrecy of our own four walls, as
> housewives and as mothers, still has the most profound and far-reaching
> effect on civilization; in other words, I believe that our most important work
> in the world is to run a good home and to bring up our children well. . . .
> Home must come first. That is not mere highsounding platitude; it is not
> merely an old-fashioned but honorable sentiment. It is sound, plain everyday
> sense.[1]

While continuing to define motherhood as women's primary role, scientific motherhood increasingly accentuated the inadequacy of maternal instinct and highlighted the positive necessity for mothercraft education. Mothers did not "just naturally" know how to care for infants and children; they needed instruction in proper childrearing techniques. Giving birth made a woman a mother in the physical, biological sense only; a good mother had to learn about mothering from authoritative sources. Ill-health, excessive crying, any negative characteristic of an infant, could be, and was, blamed on maternal ignorance. The scientific motherhood literature of the twentieth century consistently reiterated the importance of expert advice and oversight to successful childrearing and increasingly stressed the need for physician-directed instruction. Women were reminded again and again that no matter how much they studied, how much they read, they needed professionals, primarily physicians, to supervise their mothering practices. Throughout the first half of the twentieth century, these themes, the basic tenets of the ideology of scientific motherhood, attained wider circulation.

Motherhood education took many diverse forms. Increasing utilization of hospital maternity facilities created new situations in which thousands of women learned to appreciate the benefits of medical expertise in infant care. The value of sources that had informed previous generations shifted; women were encouraged to reject the assistance of female relatives, neighbors, and friends, whose reliability and validity as child-care experts were questioned; women's magazines even more pointedly instructed readers on the importance of science and expert advice in healthful, modern child rearing. Frequently these older instructional forms were modified to reach a broader audience. For instance, the success of Little Mothers' Clubs inspired the development of home-economics and child-care courses in the public schools.

Equating women's life role with homemaking and motherhood, public school home-economics courses pursued two goals. Educators feared that "the feminist movement with its insistence on equal rights for men and women" taught girls to consider a career first and motherhood second, if at all; teachers intended practical child-care classes "to create the proper attitude in girls" toward motherhood[2]—in other words, to make motherhood women's profession. Second, like the advocates of earlier Little Mothers' Clubs, course writers wanted to replace tradition, or folklore, with scientific child care as a way of combatting infant mortality and morbidity. Unlike their predecessors, however, home-economics classes were not designed primarily for immigrant "little mothers." Instituted in elementary and high schools across the country, they were aimed at the general female student population.

Domestic science courses, in the words of a Baltimore supervisor of Home Economics Education, sought "to establish standards of judgment and ideals of achievement" in homemaking. While teaching the technical aspects of the subject, these classes would also instruct students in right habits and attitudes about women's work in the domestic setting.[3] Justifying mandatory home-economics and child-care courses, instructors asserted:

> It is expected that every woman will have at some time in her life the care of babies and young children. It is not reasonable to expect that she should know how to care for them wisely without definite instruction and training in the skill and art of mothercraft.[4]

The syllabi and textbooks for these courses repeatedly stressed that motherhood was more than instinct, that good mothers needed to be educated in the science of mothering. For example, one popular 1929 high school text aimed

> to urge the importance of the right start in the rearing of children; to
> emphasize the close relationship between the physical and the mental health
> of children; and to teach by text, demonstration, and observation the
> essential principles involved in the physical, mental, emotional, and social
> development of the child in the first five years.

The course of study presented in this book included sections on "the need for child study" and "parental responsibility for the coming baby," as well as instruction in such practical matters as selecting a layette, laundering baby clothes, the diet and care of the nursing mother, the preparation and care of the baby's food, and artificial feeding.[5]

Courses developed under the auspices of state health departments and departments of education also reached out beyond schoolgirls to women in the community. To provide mothers with the benefits of science, Girls' High School in Reading, Pennsylvania, rewrote its popular high school course, "The care of infants," renamed it "Course for mothers," and offered it to adult women. By 1926 over 7,000 women had attended Minnesota's fifteen-lesson course, "Maternal and child hygiene." The Indiana State Department of Health created a prenatal and child-care course consisting of five classes taught by department physicians and nurses. More than 45,000 women had taken these classes by 1928.[6]

Collegiate programs also added more domestic science to their curricula, and the education at women's colleges further reinforced the image of women as wives and mothers. At the 1923 convention of the American Collegiate Association, a group of insurgents condemned women's schools for not preparing their students for their life-roles in homemaking and childrearing. In fact, these schools were moving to institute home economics on the college level. In the spring of 1924 the Vassar board of trustees created an inter-disciplinary School of Euthenics to study the development and care of the family, educating women for their domestic responsibilities and motherhood with courses such as Husband and Wife, Motherhood, and the Family as an Economic Unit. Considering lecture courses alone inadequate, Cornell's College of Home Economics after 1919 arranged for its students to undertake child-care training with "practice babies." Cornell rapidly became a center for domestic science, and state university domestic-science programs began to blossom in the 1920s.[7]

Brochures and pamphlets remained a common means of disseminating information about scientific motherhood and mothering practices. The American Medical Association distributed tens of thousands of pamphlets such as "Baby Welfare," "Save the Babies," and "Summer Care of the Baby." The boards of health of many states wrote and mailed out publications with prenatal information and child-care instructions, usually in the form of a series of letters or wall cards. Michigan alone mailed out over 117,000 letters in a five-year period from 1922 to 1927.[8] And the federal government produced the quintessential governmental publication, *Infant Care*.

First published in 1914 by the U.S. Children's Bureau, *Infant Care* rapidly became the most popular government publication ever. In many respects the advice dispensed through the various revisions of *Infant Care* represented contemporary middle-class values and opinions. As the historian Nancy Pottisham Weiss discovered, "the Children's Bureau advice on child care was a barometer of emergent middle-class opinion on the topic and helped to promulgate the idea motherhood was a scientific undertaking not a state of sanctification." However, the pamphlet was widely distributed by governmental agencies and congressional representatives, and its circulation reached beyond the middle class. By 1930 over 5 million copies had been distributed; by 1940, over 12 million; by 1955, after ten editions, over 34 million. The bureau's statistics suggest the tremendous popularity of *Infant Care*. Between the first issuance of the pamphlet and 1965, approximately 163 million children were born in the United States. Within the same time almost 52 million copies of *Infant Care* were distributed, and the bureau estimated that each copy was probably used for more than one child and sometimes by more than one family.[9]

Journals also continued to promote the tenets of scientific motherhood. Thousands of research scientists, doctors, dieticians, and nurses were trying to determine how to give children the best possible start in life, explained one home economist in *Parents' Magazine* in 1928. However, their endeavors would mean nothing "unless the mother picks up the work there and carries it wisely." The writer recommended to mothers that "as inspiration to support you in the daily grind of carrying out the details of feeding the baby, remember that you are laying the foundation for possibly three-score years of 'ease' or 'dis-ease' for the child." "Scientific care," meaning "right feeding," could reduce the already lowered infant death rate by one-half, declared another writer in the *Farmer's Wife* a year later. Many women's magazines enlarged their child-care advice columns. Dr. Josephine Hemenway Kenyon's column continued in *Good Housekeeping*. In 1922 she wrote two booklets, one on prenatal care and one on baby's first year. Within a year the magazine had received thousands of requests for the publications. Other journals, like *Modern Priscilla,* offered to send readers copies of Children's Bureau pamphlets.[10]

Magazines influenced the development and dissemination of scientific motherhood through their advertising as well. Some journals continued to direct readers specifically to advertisements, to promote the products and advertising copy published in their pages. *Hygeia,* the popular health journal published by the AMA, editorialized:

> If Hygeia advertisements merely shouted at you to do this or to do that "for health" I could not be so enthusiastic in recommending that you read each one carefully. But they are not empty generalities. They are packed with facts. Read the advertisements as you do the articles in the magazine.

At times its recommendations were even more specific. In 1934 the column "Among Hygeia Advertisers" singled out for praise an advertisement for Pet Milk because the irradiated product contained vitamin D. The article, however, failed to mention a similar advantage in irradiated Carnation Milk, also advertised in the same issue.[11]

The advertising content of journals affected the spread of scientific motherhood in a more subtle manner also. Various analysts of twentieth-century advertising have concluded that advertisements tend to reflect cultural, particularly middle-class, values (to do otherwise might offend consumers and repel potential buyers) and to reinforce these values by repeatedly presenting them before the public. Of course, neither reflection nor reinforcement means reality; advertisements do not necessarily portray the way people live, but they do depict society's idealized lifestyle.[12] Viewed in this light, the dominant trend in advertising copy aimed at mothers from the early to the mid-twentieth century supported and furthered the ideology of scientific motherhood. A good mother, a modern mother, is concerned with the scientific basis of products, with the vitamin content of foods, with the germ-killing power of cleansers. Women continually read in these magazines about the importance of expert advice in successful homemaking and childrearing.

Child-care manuals, too, continued to instruct women in scientific motherhood. While Holt's *Care and Feeding of Children* remained popular, other doctors entered the market with their own books. Herman Bundesen, a Chicago physician, first published his book, *Our Babies,* in 1925. Within fourteen years over nine million copies had been distributed. Mothers could, of course, buy Bundesen's book, but numerous copies were distributed free. For example, in 1933 the Infants' Wear Department of Baron Bros., Inc., a Madison, Wisconsin, department store, gave *Our Babies* to pregnant women visiting the store. In addition, the store promised that each month a woman returned to the department, she would be given another booklet written by Bundesen describing the monthly development and requirements of infants.[13]

As popular as Bundesen was, he has been overshadowed by one physician-author who preceded him and another who followed. Our foremothers spoke of raising a Holt baby; later generations debated the merits and failings of Spock babies. Benjamin Spock's *Common Sense Book of Baby and Child Care* first appeared in May 1946. Within two months it had sold over 500,000 copies in paperback and almost 6,500 copies in hardcover, numbers that rivaled the entire distribution of Holt's *Care and Feeding of Children*. Within three years paperback sales had reached one million copies a year. By 1985 Spock's book had gone through four editions and sold over 30 million copies in 38 languages. The book probably attained and maintained its popularity because of the author's writing style. He uses short words (often colloquialisms) in short sentences; his advice is basic, and, as his title promises, based on common sense as much as on medical theory. Spock claimed that he wanted a book that would increase parents' comfort, independence, and confidence, and thus their effectiveness. He considered earlier child-care books "condescending, scolding, or intimidating in tone," and he wrote as he did to "help the parent build self-confidence."[14] In Spock's words: "Bringing up your child won't be a complicated job if you take it easy, trust your instincts, and follow the directions that your doctor gives you."[15] Despite Spock's call to "trust your instincts," his book is a clear example of the mid-twentieth-century version of scientific motherhood. Mothering is not difficult *with expert advice,* if you follow directions.

By the 1920s, another influential institution, the hospital, had begun to teach increasing numbers of women the tenets of scientific motherhood, especially the need for medical oversight. Because of inexperience and lack of self-confidence, new mothers are often highly susceptible to suggestions about child-care techniques. The institutional environment of the hospital, cloaked in the aura of medical authority, provided a fertile ground for such education. Reports of hospital nurseries often described the training women received there.[16] "How to weigh, bathe and dress the baby, how to prepare a formula, how to care for his skin and hair and how to keep him healthy and happy are subjects which claim her closest attention in this hospital class," proclaimed an article in *Hygeia* in 1938 (figure 7.1).

In addition to explicit instruction, women were also undoubtedly influenced by hospital procedures—practices based on the fear that newborns in the hospital nursery might be exposed to infections. Outbreaks of diarrheal

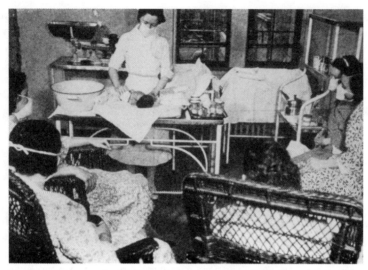

Figure 7.1. Photograph of a hospital class for new mothers. Source: *Hygeia, 16* (1938), 423

diseases were not uncommon, as one physician explained when describing the newborn nursery procedures instituted at the California Hospital, Los Angeles, in 1938: "One small cloud is never absent from the horizon of those responsible for the management of modern obstetric hospitals. . . . They [epidemics] form a constant threat to our peace of mind."[17]

To minimize this danger, babies were kept in virtual isolation, separated from their mothers immediately after birth and cared for in large, sterile nurseries by nurses typically wearing face-masks. Since contemporary pediatric thought gave at least lip-service to the benefits of maternal nursing, at certain times in the day infants had to be removed from this protected environment. Hospitals instituted various procedures to lessen the chance that infection might reach the infant from the mother. At the Maternity Hospital of Cleveland:

> The [mother's] breast is cleansed thoroughly each day with soap and water. Before the baby is brought to the mother, her hands are carefully washed with soap and water, and she is warned to touch nothing after that until her baby is at the breast. The binder is unpinned, with the mother resting on her side. The nurse, with scrubbed hands, lays a sterile receiver by the mother and the child is placed upon that. After the nursing, the nipple and aureola are sponged with 35 per cent alcohol, and a fresh sterile binder is applied.[18]

Most hospitals instituted similar, sometimes more stringent, procedures to avoid the danger of the mother contaminating the child, or of carrying contamination back to the nursery. At minimum these routines reinforced the idea that hospitals, and by extension medical experts, could care for babies better than mothers could and that babies needed protection from their own mothers.

Manufacturers recognized the significance of the hospital environment for the future behavior of new mothers. The Pet Milk Company consciously used the hospital milieu to develop consumer interest in its product (figure 7.2). Martin L. Bell, historian of the company, described Pet's rationale:

> The expectant mother may first hear about PET milk when learning about formula preparation in the hospital orientation class. She and her husband may select the baby's name from a list supplied by a company medical relations representative [sales representative]. The name card on her baby's crib in the hospital might bear the PET insignia. Most important, her baby's first bottle of formula may very well be made with PET brand evaporated milk. These "little things" add up to a convincing acceptance of the PET brand.[19]

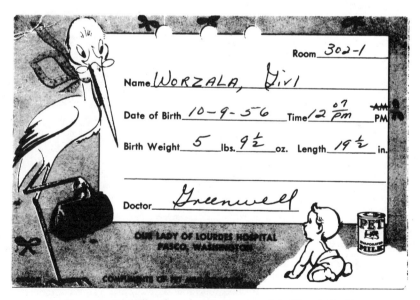

Figure 7.2. Pet Milk crib card, 1956. Courtesy of the Worzala family

The Carnation Milk Company similarly made its presence felt in American hospitals (figure 7.3). Women viewed hospitals as modern, scientific institutions, and scientific mothers would attempt to emulate hospital procedures at home (figure 7.4).[20]

Thus trends begun in the nineteenth century gained strength in the twentieth as domestic-science and home-economics courses, child-care pamphlets and books, hospital classes and routines, all fostered and reinforced the basic tenets of scientific motherhood. Women are the family caretakers

HELPFUL SUGGESTIONS

The necessary articles for preparing formula are:
16-ounce graduate or measuring cup
A tablespoon and a saucepan
Funnel of glass or aluminum
Can opener or ice pick

Prepare the formula for the 24-hour feeding period, using clean, sterile containers. Rinse off top of Carnation Milk can with hot water just before opening with sterile ice pick.

For the ordinary type of formula, use water that has been boiled 10 minutes. Cool the water until warm, and to the required amount add and stir in the carbohydrate indicated. Into this water-carbohydrate mixture, pour the required amount of Carnation Milk and stir. The formula is then ready to be poured into sterile nursing bottles. Stopper the bottles with sterile cotton, corks or rubber caps, and place in the refrigerator until needed.

Bottles and nipples should be rinsed in cold water immediately after using as they will be much easier to clean and sterilize. Before boiling, scrub the nipples with a brush in soap and water, turning inside out to make sure that all milk particles are removed.

Hold the baby in a semi-upright position in the curve of your arm when you feed him. Keep the neck of the bottle full of milk. The holes in the nipple should be large enough to permit the milk to drop about as fast as it can without running out in a stream. Use a red hot needle to enlarge the holes if necessary.

Hold the baby over your shoulder for a few minutes in the middle of the feeding period and after he has finished eating, patting him gently on the back so he can get up any air he has swallowed.

Diaper burns are not usually caused by the diet. They may be quickly healed by exposing the bare buttocks to air, sunlight, or the heat of an ordinary reading lamp. Diapers should be thoroughly cleaned, boiled and rinsed, then dipped in a saturated boric solution before drying, to kill the germs that produce ammonia. Diapers should be changed often.

NOTE: You may continue to give your baby Irradiated Carnation Milk after weaning from the bottle. The same good qualities which have helped make your baby a strong healthy child will continue to help him through all his growing years.

ST. JOHN'S HOSPITAL

1923 S. Utica St.   Tulsa, Okla.

Phone 6-2161

Date 7-8-45

For Baby _Fred_

Birth Date 6-29-45 Birth Weight 7 lbs. 12 oz.

Present Weight 7 lbs. 3 1/2 oz. Height _____ in.

FEEDING FORMULA

1. ___9___ ounces boiled water (boil 10 minutes)
2. Cool water till warm, then add:
3. ___1___ level tablespoons _Certose_
   (Soluble Carbohydrate)
4. ___8___ ounces Irradiated Carnation Milk.

Pour this formula into 6 bottles of 1 1/2 ounces each. Cover each bottle with a sterile stopper and keep in a cool place until needed.

Feed baby every 4 hours, or 6 times daily.

Hours for feeding 2-6-10 A. M. 2-6-10 P. M.

Orange or Tomato Juice _____ teaspoons in _____ ounces of water at _____

Cod Liver Oil _____ teaspoons _____ daily.
Give Sterile Water, one to two ounces, at least twice daily between feedings. (To sterilize, boil 10 minutes)

Additional Instructions

_____

_____

_____

_____

_____ M. D.

Irradiated Carnation Milk is used by more people throughout the world than any other brand and may be obtained at any grocery store.
(over)

Figure 7.3. Front and back of Carnation Milk formula feeding card, 1945. Courtesy of the Price family

responsible for the health and well-being of their children; women's most important role in society is motherhood. But mothers are not capable of carrying out their duties alone; mothers need direction from experts, usually medical practitioners, from whom they must learn the "scientific" principles of childrearing. A few child-care educators, like Spock, acknowledged that in certain situations a mother could safely "trust" her own "instincts." But such soothing advice was almost invariably followed with the admonition to "follow the directions that your doctor gives you." Particularly in the area of infant feeding, scientific mothers, modern mothers, whether breast feeding or bottle feeding, would rely on the expertise of physicians.

Even in the early years of the twentieth century, when artificial infant feeding had gained some measure of acceptability, breast milk remained the preferred nutrient, recommended by physicians and child-care educators alike. Over the three decades following World War I, however, the situation changed. More and more articles on infant feeding began with a nod to the advantages and benefits of maternal nursing, and then discussed bottle feeding in great detail. Symbolic of the increasing identification of infant feeding with artificial feeding was a 1938 article in *Hygeia:* simply entitled

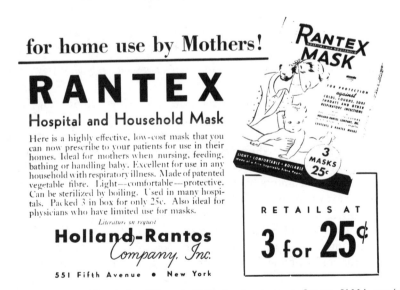

Figure 7.4. Rantex Hospital and Household Mask advertisement. Source: *JAMA, 122* (3) (1943), adv. 8

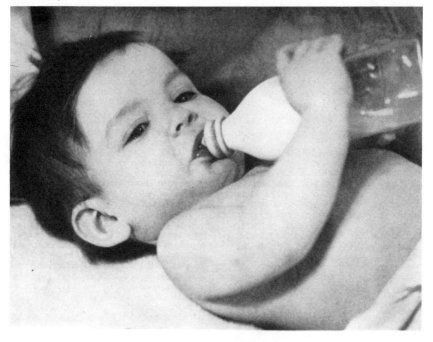

INFANT FEEDING

Figure 7.5. Photograph heading article on infant feeding. Source: *Hygeia, 16* (1938), 406

"Infant feeding," it had at its head a picture of a bottle-feeding baby (figure 7.5).

Despite paeans to breast feeding, physicians and other writers of advice literature and child-care educators warned of the difficulties faced by nursing mothers and assumed that women would, for a variety of reasons, bottle feed. Some commentators blamed the decline of maternal nursing on false modesty and fashion or on "civilized conditions" that compromised women's ability to breast feed. In particular they indicted peer pressure, "gossip" heard in the hospital ward, or suggestions "gratuitously received from a nurse, an intern, or a neighbor."[21] Psychological theory, too, was used to explain the choice of nonnursing mothers. Claimed one 1949 publication:

> Some women fear that in nursing a baby they lose their attractiveness to men in general and to their husbands in particular. On the contrary such

"womanliness" is actually attractive to most men. Many women who do not want to nurse their babies are sexually frigid which further bespeaks their incomplete understanding and acceptance of sex matters and of their role as mothers.[22]

Yet the most frequently cited cause for the abandonment of breast feeding was a practical one: insufficient milk, milk deficient in either quantity or quality. Fortunately, infants who failed to thrive, who did not gain weight rapidly, or who cried after each breast feeding could be safely brought up on bottle feeding when under a doctor's supervision.[23]

Even successful breast feeding demanded a knowledge of scientific and medical discoveries. To ensure production of healthful milk, women had to watch their diets, adjust their lifestyles, and even contain their emotions. Nursing mothers, instructed child-care educators in manuals and classes, must eat a nutritious, well-balanced diet including milk. They must get plenty of fresh air and exercise, but avoid fatigue. Above all, mothers who breast fed must cultivate an easy-going, relaxed attitude because "there is no one thing which more certainly and completely interferes with the secretion of the milk than any overwrought, nervous condition." Another writer warned that a mother worried "about dust under the davenport" could cause colic in her baby. The lesson was clear: unless a nursing mother very carefully monitored her life, she could endanger the well-being of her infant.[24]

Additionally, mothers were advised to institute specific practices to ensure that their infants received a sufficient quantity of breast milk. For example, after each breast feeding a mother could offer her infant some formula; an infant getting sufficient nourishment would simply refuse the bottle. One physician-author explained in minute detail an alternative method:

> The young infant requires at least two ounces of breast milk per pound of body weight in twenty-four hours. Thus, a seven pound infant needs a total of at least fourteen ounces of breast milk; in other words, he needs between two and three ounces, six times in twenty-four hours. . . . By weighing the clothed infant before and after a nursing, the amount of milk obtained from the breast at the feeding can be easily determined; by doing this at each feeding over a twenty-four-hour period and adding up the increase noted in his wieght each time, the total amount of food obtained from the breast in one day is determined.[25]

If the infant was not getting enough milk from the breast, a bottle should be provided for additional nourishment. With either method, the nursing mother should have on hand a prepared bottle filled with a formula prescribed by a physician.[26] As at the turn of the century, even women who were successfully nursing their infants were encouraged to supplement breast feeding with bottle feeding.[27]

By the 1930s discussions of infant feeding in magazines and pamphlets were in general promoting the efficacy and healthfulness of bottle feeding, at times preferring artificial foods to breast milk. One article in *Parents' Magazine* in 1936 described various techniques for treating a colicky baby. If the infant was breast fed, then the condition probably arose from "nervousness in the mother"; solution: a relief bottle to allow the mother time for rest and relaxation and a change in the mother's diet. "In some ways, it is easier to cure" a colicky bottle-fed baby, wrote the physician-author, who proceeded to outline several alternative formulas and feeding schedules. Other writers did not so baldly admire bottle feeding, but they usually considered artificial feeding under a physician's supervision at least equal to breast feeding and frequently noted the inevitability of bottle feeding. "Don't count too heavily on nursing your baby," cautioned one mother writing in 1938. "You hope to nurse him, of course, but there is an alarming number of you mothers today who are unable to breast-feed their babies and you may be one of them. . . . Even if you are breast-feeding you may be ordered by your doctor to give him supplementary feedings by bottle, so it is fairly safe to count on bottles and their attendant equipment."[28]

The emphasis on bottle feeding is also evident in child-care manuals of the period. While praising maternal nursing, the authors of these books often devoted comparatively few pages to breast feeding and many more to the details of artificial feeding. Dr. Louis Sauer, in his *Nursery Guide for Mothers and Nurses,* published in 1923, spent some 23 pages on breast feeding, discussing nursing technique, the mother's routine, and the nutritional problems of breast-fed infants. He then provided the reader with 47 pages on artificial feeding, outlining the preparation of the bottles and formulas, the advantages of mixed feeding, and the nutritional disturbances of the bottle-fed. Significantly, even though in the text Sauer clearly preferred breast feeding, his suggested daily schedule treated breast and bottle feeding as equivalent. Spock's chapter on breast feeding is 23 pages long, compared with 29 pages on bottle feeding. Much of his discussion of maternal nursing, moreover, concerns insufficiency of breast milk and weaning. And despite Spock's support of breast feeding, he is as careful as other child-care advisors to assure his readers that bottle-fed babies are no less healthy, no less happy, than breast-fed infants.[29]

The stress on artificial feeding and a concomitant de-emphasizing of breast feeding is likewise apparent in public school home-economics education. According to extant syllabi, students received much more instruction on bottle feeding than on maternal nursing. In 1924 Wisconsin initiated a series of ten one-hour lessons on infant hygiene for the state's school-age girls. One lesson outlined the various foods suitable for infants, including breast milk and bottle formulas. Three other lessons described the preparation of artificial food, what utensils were needed, and how to give a bottle feeding. If the student successfully completed the course, passed a written or oral examination, and gave demonstrations of infant bathing and "putting up a bottle formula," she received a diploma naming her one of "Wisconsin's Little Mothers."[30]

Hospital routines also taught new mothers to appreciate medically directed bottle feeding and discouraged maternal nursing. For instance, mothers received their babies for feeding on a strict time schedule, usually every four hours, but sometimes every eight. It did not matter if an infant awoke a half-hour early and cried with hunger in the nursery or if the infant was sleepy at the prescribed feeding time. Furthermore, many doctors expressed fear over the initial weight loss often exhibited by newborns, especially in the early days of life before a mother's milk supply came in and was successfully established. Practitioners wrote glowingly about their solution to the problem: they would follow insufficient breast milk feedings with complementary bottles. One 1935 survey analyzing the feeding of 250 infants at three San Diego hospitals reported that only 19 percent of the newborns had been fed exclusively at the breast. Of the remaining infants, 48 percent had been offered bottle feedings on the first day of life; 40 percent on the second; and the remaining 12 percent on the third. The writer commented that the general public and the medical profession "have both accepted the idea that artificial feeding of the new-born can replace breast milk without deleterious effect upon the growth and health of the infant." A study of the feeding of over a thousand infants at the Beth Israel and Jewish Maternity Hospital, New York, went even further in stating that "unless there is prompt establishment of breast milk, the infant should be given complementary feedings." Such reports reflect the hospital practice—routine by the 1930s—of giving newborns supplemental bottles.[31]

At Madison General Hospital in Wisconsin, physicians could specify infant-feeding orders, but most doctors followed the hospital's routines. Infants in the first twenty-four hours of life regularly received a glucose solution supplement. Women could, if they wanted, nurse their infants, but breast-fed infants were weighed before and after each feeding to determine how much bottle formula was needed to supplement the mother's milk supply. If nursing mothers wanted to sleep through the night—and they were encouraged to get the rest—they were not awakened, and their babies received night bottle feedings. At another institution, a large eastern hospital connected with the University of Pennsylvania, at the scheduled feeding time the nurse brought a bottle along with the baby to the mother's room. After the infant had nursed, the mother automatically offered the bottle. These supplemental bottle-feeding procedures were common in hospitals, despite the recognition that such feeding could decrease the stimulation of the mother's breasts needed to promote maternal nursing.[32]

Obviously feeding routines among hospitals were not identical in all parts of the country, or unchanging over time; however, hospital procedures were relatively homogenous. Mothers and infants were separated and saw each other primarily during scheduled feeding times. Bottle feeding was standard fare either before the mother's milk supply came in or as a supplement for infants who did not gain sufficient weight. Therefore, despite the express message that "breast is best," supplementary feeding in the hospitals implied not only that mother's milk was insufficient but also that formulas were healthful. Similarly, hospital classes for postpartum women, which included a demonstration of how to prepare a baby's formula, and the bottle of prepared formula given mothers when they left the hospital advanced the idea that bottle feeding was a suitable alternative to mother's milk, if not the expected mode of infant feeding. As one women reported to me, such activity suggested to her that the "bottle was just as good as [the] breast."[35]

The various scientific motherhood forums not only accepted and applauded artificial feeding but also promoted the importance of the physician in the successful, healthful rearing of children, particularly in the area of infant feeding. Kenyon, in her "Health and Happiness Club" in *Good Housekeeping*, stressed that mothers should visit a doctor regularly; she warned her readers that the magazine's column was not intended to replace the private physician. Child-care columns in other popular magazines and domestic medical manuals, while sometimes providing detailed instructions on bottle feeding, directed readers to medical practitioners. Even some advertisements, such as those of the Mead Johnson Company (figure 7.6) and KLIM, a dried milk product, directed women to physicians for infant-feeding information. And, of course, after the AMA's decision on infant-food advertising in the 1930s, almost all infant-food companies gave women the same advice.[34]

By the 1920s, 1930s, and 1940s, much of the advice literature consciously avoided any detailed directions about artificial feeding. In a 1927 booklet he

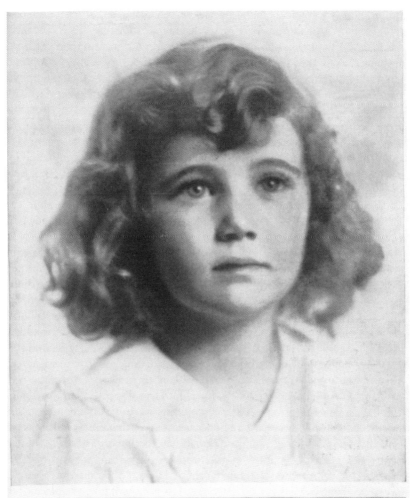

Figure 7.6. Mead Johnson advertisement. Source: *Hygeia, 16* (1938), 1057

published for his patients, one Chicago physician stated flatly that each baby is an individual case and that infant feeding "cannot be put into routine form." Therefore his booklet included no specific information on bottle feeding.[35] A mother-writer, in her chatty book *Common Sense for Mothers,* succinctly described the relationship between scientific mothers and physicians in the area of infant feeding: "We mothers can aid and abet our native intelligence today with all sorts of expert information about child rearing, from doctors and nurses, from books and magazines and radio." But, she went on, "Don't misunderstand me; in important matters [e.g., infant feeding], the doctor should decide—you must rely on his advice completely; he must lay down the laws you are to follow out and you are to ask no one else about them."[36]

With his maxim "mind your doctor," Bundesen summed up the child-care advice of the 1930s.[37] His book provides a good example of the typical, and sometimes contradictory, information women received in the period. Of course, "babies thrive best if they are given breast milk," but breast feeding was not simple; mothers had to be taught the correct nursing techniques. Furthermore, Bundesen explained, "When the baby cannot get breast milk, he can, as a rule, be safely brought up, if the milk mixtures are properly planned by a doctor." Since "not all babies are alike," Bundesen often reminded his readers that "the mother should consult a doctor." However, he added, "for the well baby of average weight for his age, certain general rules can be given for figuring the number of ounces of milk, water, and sugar to be used in the milk mixture." He then told mothers how to estimate these amounts for an appropriate bottle formula. His full-page "Plan for Feeding the Baby from Month to Month" graphically illustrates the contradictions embedded in his advice. Despite Bundesen's claims that breast milk was best and that mothers should consult physicians about bottle feeding, he presented a chart listing suitable bottle formulas for various ages on which he relegated to a footnote the reminder that "the baby should be breast fed, if possible. If the baby is breast fed, the breast milk will take the place of the milk mixtures in the daily feedings."

Over the decades, discussions of the positive value of physician-directed artificial feeding dominated infant-care advice in the United States. L. Emmett Holt, Jr., in *The Good Housekeeping Book of Baby and Child Care,* carried on the tradition established by his father in 1895 with *The Care and Feeding of Children,* neatly expressing mid-twentieth-century views of infant feeding and scientific motherhood. First he admits that bottle feeding may have been dangerous before pasteurization, refrigeration, and sanitation and before doctors had learned to modify milk to make it suitable for infant feeding. Now, however, "if bottle feeding is carried out under good medical guidance by a reasonably intelligent and careful mother—two very important 'ifs'—the risk becomes negligible." An intelligent, knowledgeable mother who bottle feeds according to her doctor's instructions need not feel that she is neglecting an important duty. "A bottle mother," he assured readers, "may still be a perfect mother."[38]

The content and tone of articles and advertisements in women's magazines and of child-care education in general, as well as women's experiences in the hospital, all point to an accelerating shift in the pattern of infant-feeding advice. Obviously by the middle of this century mothers were hearing and learning more about the importance of medical supervision in child care and the acceptability of artificial feeding, and they were exposed to more information about bottle-feeding techniques than breast feeding. Typically women were exhorted to nurse their infants, to provide them with "nature's food." Yet throughout the twentieth century, mothers were hearing and learning more and more about artificial infant feeding and the limitations of breast feeding. Mother's milk may be slow to come in; supplementary feedings should be instituted. Mothers should know how to prepare bottles because even apparently sufficient milk supplies may dry up. In any case, relief bottles should be employed to allow nursing mothers a few free hours.

Despite its praise for maternal nursing, the ideology of scientific motherhood, mirroring the claims of contemporary medical science and medical practitioners, equated "scientific" infant feeding and physician-directed bottle feeding. Women's magazines, child-care manuals by individuals, governmental agencies, and infant-food manufacturers, advertisements, and maternal- and child-health classes increasingly promoted the efficacy of "scientific" infant feeding, which often meant bottle feeding under a doctor's supervision. Hospitals taught this lesson by example, establishing routines that discouraged breast feeding and encouraged artificial feeding, demonstrating the procedures for modifying milk, and providing prepared bottles for mothers leaving the maternity ward.

The growing emphasis on the need for scientific and medical expertise in infant feeding created contradictions within the ideology of scientific motherhood. On the one hand it accorded women status; they were responsible for the health and well-being of children and, by extension, for the nation's future. Modern mothers, responsible mothers, scientific mothers should use the advances of science and medicine to shape their infant-care routines. On the other hand, scientific motherhood denied women control over their own mothering practices; women were incapable of successfully fulfilling their maternal duties without expert advice. Modern mothers, responsible mothers, scientific mothers, whether bottle feeding or breast feeding, should look to medical experts to direct their infants' feeding. That is, the ideology of scientific motherhood gave women even greater responsibility in the area of infant feeding but refused them the power to decide how to feed their infants. The extent to which women were able to resolve these contradictions in their own infant-feeding practices, what choices they made, and how they made them are the subjects of the next section.

PART FOUR

Mothers and Infant-Feeding Practices

VIII

"A Word of Comfort"
1890–1920

"Jamie, the poor little fellow is six months old and has been sick almost since birth," confided Julia Carpenter to her diary in January 1889.[1] Carpenter had had little breast milk, and the "nurse Mrs. Baker advised me to dry." Then Carpenter, who lived on a claim in LaMoure County, Dakota Territory, a few miles north of the Edgeley town site, began her search for a healthful alternative to mother's milk. "For five or six weeks we tried *fresh cow's milk,* different cows and different strengths, but he continually had a diarrhea— green undigested stools and grew thinner. When he was about six weeks old we commenced condensed milk, but with no better effect." The sources from which Carpenter learned about cow's-milk and condensed-milk formulas are never identified, but she soon sought expert help. On 17 September, as "Jamie grew rapidly worse, we finally telegraphed to Grand Rapids for Dr. Anderson who reached us on the NP train the twentieth."

> Doctor put him on Ridges Food which did not agree with him. We then tried one teaspoon of cream, one teaspoon of sugar and one half cup of water. We next tried a tablespoon of oat milk cooked in one pint of water then mixed two thirds of this with one third milk. But none of these agreed with him.

Despairing, Carpenter took the baby and her two other children to Aberdeen, South Dakota, where they spent nearly two months trying various means of feeding Jamie. First they used Lactated Food. Then they "procured a wet nurse for days" but used condensed milk for nights:

> He picked up on the breast for a month then I thought I must find some kind of food that I might get home. I tried Peptinized milk for a week but he did not improve. . . .

I had employed Dr. Coyine but at this point changed to Dr. Backe. He put the baby on oatmeal diet. He improved somewhat so that on the sixth of December we came home, but he ran down very fast. I thought again he could not live, but January first and fourth teeth came through and then he again to pick up a little. A portion of the time he weighed less than when born. The first week he was sick Lydia French, Mrs. F. Campbell, Mr. Ed Campbell, Mrs. Pratt, Mrs. Kesler and Mrs. Salisbury watch with him.

During the next several months, Jamie's diet included, at various times, fresh cow's milk, "Cod Scotts Emulsion of Cod Liver Oil, hypophosphites and soda"; oatmeal; Swiss Milk Food and cod liver oil; and even wine because "at Christmas time he vomited so dreadfully that by Dr. Backe's order we gave him from four to eight drops of wine until the vomiting was somewhat controlled. From that time on I gave him wine eight drops before each feeding sherry afterwards port."

Then one night in March 1889 she fed Jamie and laid him to sleep in his cradle:

when I got into my cot [next to the cradle in the sitting room], looked at Jamie boy, he had his food, his eyes were open and his bottle still in his mouth. He was perfectly quiet. . . . I went right off to sleep supposing of course that my darling was going off to sleep all night, but whether he did or not I never knew. He usually awakened somewhere between two and four o'clock waking me immediately. This night I slept from 12 until 6 AM when I was awakened by him. He seemed to breathe funny yet I warmed his dinner and gave him but he did not take it although I had thought he took the wine. He kept gasping. . . . I took him in my arms calling Jamie, Jamie, he did not look at me, but his eye gradually closed, he gasped a few times and was *dead, my* baby, *my* darling, *my* boy Jamie all without a moments warning.

"Died. James Lucien Carpenter, March 13th, 1889, aged 8 months. Youngest child of James D. and Julia L. Gage Carpenter. Edgeley, Lamoure County, North Dakota."

The dilemmas encountered by Julia Carpenter in her search for an infant food for her Jamie dramatically exemplify the situation faced by many American women in the late nineteenth and early twentieth centuries. For a variety of reasons and under various circumstances, mothers decided that they could not breast feed their infants; they needed a healthful infant food. Whether Carpenter learned of different foods from publications or from neighbors and friends is not clear; some women did specifically acknowledge such nonmedical sources, and even the promotions of infant-food manufacturers informed their infant-feeding practices. Physicians were another source, but their authority was not unquestioned. Carpenter names at least three doctors, each of whom gave her different advice, which she accepted or rejected as conditions changed. The history of James Lucien Carpenter is more complete than many other extant reports describing artificial infant feeding in the period, but Julia Carpenter's course was not unique.

Although most women have left little or no direct evidence of their child-care practices and beliefs, particularly as they relate to infant feeding, some felt impelled to write up their experiences, usually in the hope that their solutions would be instructive to other mothers. In a few instances women recorded significant, traumatic incidents in their diaries. On the whole, such sources directly inform us only about white, middle-class, literate mothers. The histories of these women and mothers outside this select class can, however, be inferred through careful analysis and interpretation of indirect sources, such as public-health workers' reports, statistics, and prescriptive literature.

Growing numbers of women, whether or not they consciously articulated the ideology of scientific motherhood, acted on its basic tenets. Mothers accepted the centrality of motherhood in their lives and appreciated the need for scientific advice for healthful child rearing. They read about scientific child care in magazines and books, they attended classes, and from the late nineteenth century onward, they increasingly looked to the medical profession for direction in their infant-feeding practices.

Women sought out expert advice on infant care. The growing number of books and pamphlets on child care demonstrates that women were eager for guidance. The numerous editions and printings of, for example, Holt's *Care and Feeding of Children* and the federal government's *Infant Care* indicate that a market existed for these manuals. In addition, correspondence published in women's magazines attests to the desire to learn the most up-to-date and scientific information, and the content of the letters tells of women also seeking out the assistance of physicians and nurses. Moreover, hundreds of thousands of parents from all over the country sent letters to the Children's Bureau; they not only requested pamphlets but also solicited advice on specific problems. According to a study done by Nancy Pottisham Weiss, these letters document two important points: "First, they demonstrate that the pamphlet *Infant Care* circulated among the poor. Secondly, they show that working class women felt sufficiently interested in the advice to ask for more information." In 1917 and 1918 alone the Bureau received 73,837 letters.[2] Contemporary studies too document that women read this general child-care literature. Of the approximately 460 women who participated in a Children's Bureau investigation in Montana in 1919, more than 35 percent reported literature as their source for information on child care. The material ranged from Holt and various federal and state publications to what the surveyor termed "quite worthless patent medicine advertising matter." Only 34 of these women received information from physicians, and 20 from trained or practical nurses.[3]

Of course, reading advice literature and even actively seeking out information does not necessarily mean that women followed the instructions they were given.[4] Other evidence, though, demonstrates that women appreciated and in many instances depended upon expert advice. For example, mothers wrote to the Children's Bureau that *Infant Care* "saved my baby's life" and that "without your books I would have been like a ship on a strange sea without a compass."[5] Women related in their diaries and in letters to magazines situations in which they utilized the assistance of medical practitioners.

Moreover, sociologists and historians have demonstrated that changes in values and practices in infant care reflected those advocated in the advice literature. And those segments of society having the closest access to agencies of change tend to alter their childrearing practices most quickly. These agents include the public media, clinics, medical practitioners, and the like. Urie Bronfenbrenner and Nancy Pottisham Weiss found specifically that shifts in infant-care practices corresponded to the advice published in Children's Bureau pamphlets and similar sources of "expert opinion." This does not mean that changes in advice literature caused shifts in parental values and practices. The ideas of "experts" at least in part grow out of and reflect contemporary cultural values, as do the beliefs of parents. Nevertheless, promotion by professionals can accelerate the acceptance of a set of beliefs and values.[6] There is, therefore, sufficient evidence to warrant the supposition that parents were affected by the advice they read and that the prescriptive literature represents, in broad terms, contemporary child-care practices.

One of the most important trends noted in the scientific motherhood literature was the increasing discussion and acceptability of artificial infant feeding. The hypothesis that mothers' practices reflected the basic values of this literature suggests that mothers increasingly bottle fed their infants. What statistical data exist substantiate this conclusion.

There are no studies of the percentages of breast-fed and bottle-fed babies for the nineteenth century, but commentators did discuss the size of the infant-food industry. The *American Analyst* in 1889 estimated that "the quantity of artificial food annually consumed in the United States amounts, in money value, to about $8,000,000 to $10,000,000." Similarly, several years later an article in the *Journal of Medicine and Science* pointed to "the immense plants [for the production of infant foods] and enormous capital devoted to the manufacture of these plants." More direct, though highly selective, statistics further document the relative importance of artificial feeding. A 1914 report from the Vanderbilt Clinic described the 1,500 infants who visited the milk station. Nine hundred were bottle-fed, 300 were breast-fed, and 300 others received mixed feedings.[7].

In addition to these statistical claims, various other measures point to the increased use of artificial feeding in the late nineteenth and early twentieth centuries. Impressionistic evidence documents the widespread acceptance of bottle feeding. Many of the letters and articles written by mothers in women's magazines about their child-care practices discussed infant feeding, including artificial feeding. Similarly, these journals devoted a tremendous amount of space to instructing women in the latest, most scientific modes of infant feeding. The *Ladies' Home Journal,* under the long-time editorship of Edward Bok, exemplified the close relationship between a mass-circulation journal and its reader. Bok, according to his biographer Salme Harju Steinberg, "shrewdly measured the needs and wishes of his female audience" and kept "pace with their developing interests and expanding roles":

> Bok's successful editorship was the result of his carefully attuning himself to his readers, sensing their fears, and giving them what they wanted to read and a little bit more. This combination, more than any other factor, assured the *Journal*'s large circulation and its consequent choice by advertisers for spending their revenue.

This conscious attempt, on the part of the *Journal* and other women's magazines, to present images acceptable to their readers suggests that when the sum total of the editorial content of a variety of magazines points to a general trend, one can and must assume that it is congruent with the beliefs and values of the readership.[8]

There is no doubt that women's magazines of the period moved from acceptance of bottle feeding as an alternative to breast feeding when necessary to a notion that many women had experience with bottle feeding. Numerous articles from the late nineteenth century onward discussed both modes of feeding. (See Chapters 6 and 7.) Furthermore, mothers writing in these journals frequently made statements to the effect that fewer and fewer women were capable of nursing and that for many artificial feeding was, therefore, a necessity. In 1889 one mother offered the opinion that "the majority" of American women could not "afford to get along without that useful article," the bottle. Another mother, in *Modern Priscilla* in 1909, described the situation from her perspective:

> In the olden days every mother nursed her baby as a matter of course, and strong sturdy men and women grew from this gentle, capable motherhood which reared large families in the comparative shelter of rural or semi-populous towns; but times have changed, and in this nervous high strung age it often happens that a mother is not able to nurse her little ones, or even when she is it is not deemed advisable, for her's or the children's health, for her to do so.

Thus, by the turn of the century, many mothers admitted the need for artificial feeding and sought out healthful infant foods.[9]

Articles and advertisements not directly related to infant feeding exhibited similar, more subtle, assumptions about the readers' familiarity with artificial feeding. Elizabeth Robinson Scovil, in an 1899 column, discussed baby's first birthday party. She suggested as appropriate party favors for the guests "doll feeding-bottles" with pink ribbons for the girls and blue ribbons for the boys. In 1904 an advertisement for Ivory Soap pictured a woman carefully washing out nursing bottles (figure 8.1). The copy assured the reader that for this task "there is nothing quite so good as Ivory Soap." Since the product itself was not directly connected with artificial feeding, the fact that the soap company promoted Ivory to clean bottles indicates that the company believed the magazines' readers would recognize the task. Several years later in *Good Housekeeping,* the column "Discovery" printed directions for making a flannel "bottle bag." The baby's bottle would be easier to grasp and would stay warm longer, making the bag a good gift for a "tiny baby." The 1915 Christmas cover of the *Ladies' Home Journal* pictured a chubby, smiling baby holding a bottle; it was titled "His First Christmas Dinner."[10] Additional evidence for the growing popularity of bottle feeding comes from the extensive advertising campaigns for infant foods and equipment for artificial feeding. If the use of these products had been totally alien to mothers, companies would not have been able to create and sustain a demand for their products.[11]

One could argue that an analysis focusing on the editorial and advertising content of women's magazines, especially in the late nineteenth and early twentieth centuries, has a built-in bias toward middle-class, urban values. The promotional materials of mail-order companies are, however, indicative of the values of nonurban women. David L. Cohen, historian of the Sears, Roebuck Company, insists (with perhaps some hyperbole) that this com-

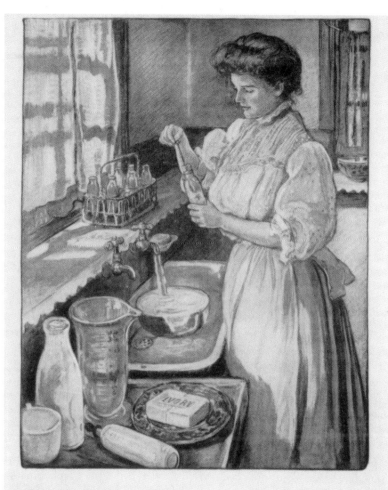

The most exquisite cleanliness is necessary in the care of bottles and other utensils used in the preparation of a baby's food.

For this purpose, there is nothing quite so good as Ivory Soap.

Dissolve a few shavings of Ivory Soap in a quart of hot water. Rinse the bottles with cold water, wash them inside and out in the Ivory Soap suds, and then scald with boiling water. Pitchers, bowls and spoons should be cleansed in the same way. Boil the rubber tops of nursing-bottles once a day besides washing them turned inside out.

"How to Bring Up a Baby" contains 40 pages of valuable information about the care of children. Every phase of the subject is covered—Food, Sleep, Dress, Cleanliness, Ventilation, The Care of the Eyes, Ears, Nose, Teeth, Hair and Nails. Full of helpful suggestions and sound advice. Charmingly illustrated. Sent free on application to THE PROCTER & GAMBLE CO., Cincinnati, Ohio.

Ivory Soap - 99 44/100 Per Cent. Pure.

Figure 8.1. Ivory Soap advertisement. Source: *Ladies' Home Journal, 23* (9) (1905–1906), 4

pany's catalogue provides a reasonable gauge of the buying habits of rural America:

> The catalogue is based not upon hope but upon experience. There is no room in it for guessing, wishing, or, save occasionally and conservatively, experimenting. It does not attempt to cram down the throats of the public its own ideas of taste or merchandise. The catalog never leads, never crusades. It is based purely upon public acceptance of the goods it offers, but not until the public has clearly signified that it wants a thing does that thing appear in its pages. We know, therefore, beyond all doubt, that the catalog's pictures of American life are drawn not from the imagination but from the living model.

The catalogue's original printing in 1879 ran only 318,000 copies, but the company sent out over one million copies of its spring catalogue in 1904 and double that number the following year. In the 1920s the circulation reached over seven million for each of the two annual seasons. Throughout the early decades of this century, the consumer could order through the catalogue all the equipment needed for artificial infant feeding: bottles, nipples, sterilizers, and the like. Various brands of infant foods, like Horlick's Malted Milk, Mellin's Food, Dextri-Maltose, Nestlé's Milk Food, and, later, S.M.A., were available. Sears also offered canned milks; from the 1909 catalogue, for example, the buyer could order "Specially adapted for infants, For cooking and For Ice Cream, Iris Brand, 3 cans @ 27 cents, 6 cans @ 53 cents, 12 cans @ $1.05."[12]

Manufacturing statistics and advertising data provide a barometer of changing infant-feeding practices and the growing utilization of bottle feeding. To understand why individual women chose artificial feeding and how they decided which food to use we must look at more fragmentary evidence. In popular journals, mothers discussed their fears and problems and rationalized their solutions. Women wrote detailed letters and articles in which they described their successes and failures and asked questions about difficulties they faced. The content of women's magazines demonstrates the difficulty in separating out the "informers of consciousness" and the "reflections of consciousness" (see Chapter 1). In much of this material, the two are inextricably entwined. Mothers used their experiences to instruct other women who might face similar situations; they described their lives to present others with cautionary tales or prescriptions. Consequently, these sources acted simultaneously as "reflections" and "informers." In addition to this published material, accounts gleaned from diaries and from interviews with mothers give insights into mothers' concerns and choices.

In particular women worried that their breast milk was insufficient, claiming, as did T. G. of Cedar Rapids, Iowa, in *Babyhood* in 1898, "I nurse my baby for four months, but fear that my supply of milk is failing, as she does not gain in flesh as she ought, and is rather puny." In 1907 A. W. reported to *American Motherhood* that she was expecting her second child:

> When my first baby came, I had plenty of good milk for four weeks, then the quality became poor and the quantity diminished until at six weeks I had to wean him entirely. . . . I was under great strain at the time of the first baby's coming, and had a severe fright with chill, severe cold, flooding and fainting spells at the time the milk first became poor.

She worried that she would not be able to nurse the second child. In other cases the onset of menstruation or the infant's failure to gain weight suggested to women that bottle feeding was needed.[13] Mothers also commented that physicians recommended that they wean their infants and use bottle formulas instead.[14]

In this period, however, there was no one generally accepted authority to which women would turn for advice on how to feed the baby. Mothers used magazines as extensions of the traditional female network of relatives, neighbors, and friends. In writing books for young mothers, women employed a supportive, sisterly tone. But there were other sources for information on infant feeding. Mothers even looked to manufacturers for their infant feeding instructions, as well as physicians. In 1887 a correspondent asked the editor of *Babyhood* to recommend the best books on the "raising of children by artificial means." F.W.P. of New York City wrote that because it was difficult to obtain "pure, fresh milk" in the city, she had been using Borden's condensed milk. Now she was worried because "after reading a book sent to me by Mellin's Food Company [I] am afraid there is something wrong about using condensed milk for children." Another woman from Penn Yan, New York, asked how to judge the correct temperature for pasteurization. Obviously aware of the discussions concerning the relative merits of milk from different breeds of cow, H.C. of Normandy, Missouri, asked, "Will you kindly tell me how cow's milk should be fed to a baby eight months old? . . . The cow it comes from is a Jersey and the milk is very rich. My baby boy has been nursed by the mother but must be weaned now." These and other women recognized the difficulties involved in artificial infant feeding and wanted answers from a source they felt they could trust.[15]

At the *Ladies' Home Journal,* Emelyn Lincoln Coolidge frequently answered questions on the subject. S.H.L. wrote, "I am about to make a change in my baby's food and want to try modified milk, but do not know the correct proportions. Will you please help me? My baby is just three months old." Another mother was concerned; she had always fed her six-month-old infant condensed milk, but he did not thrive and was constipated. "It is necessary to stop nursing my two-weeks-old baby," Mrs. H.S.K. told Coolidge. "Will you kindly tell me whether a patent food or cow's milk will be best to give him and how to prepare it?" In all these instances, Coolidge recommended that the mothers use a mixture of cream, milk, water, and cereal gruel with sugar and bicarbonate of soda added. Mrs. J.S. worried because her one-year-old daughter "seems to be tender all over and screams when I lift her." She explained to Coolidge that the child had always been fed satisfactorily with an unnamed patent food. Though Coolidge was leery of making a diagnosis without seeing the child, she replied that this must be a case of scurvy. She advised switching to cow's milk mixtures and supplementing the child's diet with beef juice and orange juice.[16]

Mothers used the articles in women's and child-care magazines almost as textbooks for information on infant feeding. "I used sterilized milk for my first baby. Now that the pasteurized milk is thought superior I will try it, using my 'Arnold Sterilizer' in the manner described by Dr. Yale (July 1892)," wrote E.V.D. of Brooklyn, New York, in 1893. This mother had bottle fed her first child, but she requested information from *Babyhood* because "I do not know the quantity of milk, etc., for an average child, for my first, having scarlet fever and measles before she was two, was fed as a sick child directed by my physician." In other words, in ill health she turned to a doctor; otherwise she expected to feed her child without medical oversight. Mothers typically combined various sources of information, balancing and questioning the recommendations from one with what they learned from others. They saved and then "searched carefully through" back issues of journals to find information they needed. For example, P.H.C. of Woburn, Massachusetts, read with interest "the queries of 'Anxious Mother' in the August number of your magazine concerning 'nursing beyond a year'" because "questions of an almost similar nature had arisen in my own mind in regard to the weaning of my ten-months-old baby." Women also expected the editors of journals like *Babyhood* to interpret advice found in other sources, such as advertisements and child-care manuals. Since P.H.C could not obtain the barley flour that had been recommended in the magazine, she inquired, "Would you use Robinson's preparation, such as I have seen advertised?" From Atlanta, Georgia, F.B.S. wrote, "I notice that Dr. Holt gives five as the proper number of meals a day for one year, but does not approve night feedings after 9 months. . . . What do you advise?" Because "your valuable magazine has done much toward teaching me the necessity of watching the minutest detail in the care of children," F.B.S. was confident that the editorial staff of *Babyhood* would "gladly answer my numerous questions."[17]

Mothers used magazines not only to receive advice but also to give it. When they found a satisfactory alternative to breast milk, they wanted other mothers to learn from their experiences. H.E.H. wrote to the editor of *Babyhood* in 1886 that she had been "obliged to wean" her son when he was four months old. For six weeks she fed him Mellin's Food, and the baby grew thin, sickly, and fretful:

> I tried one cow's milk, and also milk mixed from different cows. There was no improvement, and I became convinced that he could not digest new milk. Then I tried Mellin's food in connection with Anglo-Swiss condensed milk. It worked to a charm, and in a week from the time I began its use he was a happy, well-satisfied baby, gaining steadily in flesh, and so he has continued ever since.

In the "Mothers' Council" of the *Ladies' Home Journal* in 1890, Rosamond E. generously offered "many scraps gathered up over an experience of twenty years of caring for my babies, all of whom were bottle fed." Her letter gave detailed instructions on the preparation of artificial food and the care of bottles and nipples. Two years later "Bell" wrote the "Mothers' Council" that it had taken her five months to discover the food that agreed with her infant son. She now used a mixture of cream and water and advised other mothers to try this food before going "through the whole catalogue of 'Baby Food.'" Another mother explained in 1891 in the *Herald of Health* that because city milk could not be trusted, she had found that condensed milk provided satisfactory nutrition. This sisterly advice continued into the early years of the twentieth century. Mrs. J.J. wrote in *American Motherhood* in 1914, "I would like to tell mothers of constipated babies that a bottle of Horlick's Malted Milk the first thing in the morning is just fine."[18]

Around the turn of the century, the content of letters to women's magazines began to shift. Mothers continued to report experimenting with various patent foods and bottle formulas recommended in articles published in the magazines and in child-care manuals. But they also mentioned more frequently that their babies were "under physician care" and that "the physician recommended" a certain food. When the children had been fed successfully according to physicians' advice, women praised the profession. Evidently some women were beginning to accept the medical supervision of infant feeding, but mothers did not necessarily believe that physicians personally had to direct the feeding of all infants. In 1891 one correspondent wrote to the "Mothers' Council" so that other mothers might "benefit" from her experience:

> I have tried nearly all kinds of prepared foods, and all ways of preparing milk, and the only one which agreed perfectly with [the baby] was a prepared milk powder [no name given]. . . . She is a thoroughly well, good baby. All that I have done for her has been in accordance with a doctor's orders.

This mother's letter implied that other readers of the *Journal* could profit from the experiments conducted by her doctor and would not have to call in their own physicians.[19]

Other letterwriters seemed dissatisfied with their doctors' suggestions and inquired whether the foods prescribed by the physicians were adequate or correct.[20] For example, E.B.W. related in *Home Science* in 1903 the problems she was having with her five-month-old daughter. Originally breast-fed, the baby stopped gaining weight at six weeks. Her doctor advised various bottle formulas, but nothing seemed to be satisfactory. The columnist, a physician, suggested consulting the doctor again. Similarly, a year later, Mrs. P.J.L. wrote to Coolidge at the *Ladies' Home Journal* complaining that she had fed her six-month-old infant seven different infant foods but he did not gain weight. The doctor had told her that there was nothing organically wrong with her son; they simply had not found the correct food. Coolidge advised using a series of plain milk formulas.[21]

Mothers, especially those who had successfully bottle fed, were stimulated to write of their experiences, in part at least, by a desire to assuage the fears of other mothers who might also find it necessary to feed their infants artificially. These writers often considered mother's milk was, according to S.M.L. of Northampton, Massachusetts, writing in *Babyhood* in 1886, the "natural and proper food" for an infant.[22] They accepted, though, that for various reasons many women were incapable of nursing their children healthfully. An 1888 article by Ada E. Hazell, a mother, in the *Ladies' Home Journal* poignantly described the possible difficulties late nineteenth-century mothers faced:

> The alarming mortality among infants strikes a chill to the heart of the inexperienced mother, who, as she gazes fondly at the tiny being so recently entrusted to her care, feels her own eyes grow dim as she realizes her great responsibility, not only as regards his future moral and mental development, but also his present physical welfare. . . . This will prove no light burden,

but if it save the life of the beloved one what true mother will not feel amply repaid for long, weary hours of self-denying vigil?

If the mother is so fortunate as to be able to nurse her child—a blessing all too uncommon now-a-days—let her govern her diet with extreme care. . . .

Aside from diet, many other causes affect breast milk, and that mother who values the health of her child will persistently endeavor to preserve a cheerful, even temperament, and to avoid becoming overheated from violent or too prolonged exercise, manual labor, etc. Anything that unfavorably affects her milk will manifest itself in the fretting and indisposition of the babe.[23]

Similarly, S.M.L. warned that with modern lifestyles

the tranquil and placid existence which is absolutely necessary to a nursing mother is impossible. Nerves are rampant; neuralgia, that worst of enemies, acts like a thunderstorm in the dog day's [sic] of the mother's milk. The mother eats some apparently innocent article of food and poor Baby is rewarded with colic.

For these reasons, both Hazell and S.M.L. had deemed it necessary to resort to bottle feeding and had found that their infants thrived with artificial food. S.M.L. proclaimed:

I have never yet seen the baby who could not be well and strong and happy with good, sweet cow's milk, with, perhaps, a little "Mellin's Food" mixed with it, and always, and above all things, a sweet and *clean* bottle.

She went on, however, to assure readers of the primacy of breast feeding:

Let no one imagine that I am trying to give the bottle the place of honor which a healthy nursing-mother holds by right, but only a word of comfort to the many mothers who sadly and trembling feel that the death warrant is signed when the bottle is prescribed.

Other mothers echoed these sentiments. They acknowledged the superiority of mother's milk but cautioned that in many instances mothers could not supply it in the proper quantity or quality. In an 1889 article aptly titled "In Defense of the Bottle-fed Baby and His Mother," one mother comfortingly asserted:

I confidently believe that it is far better to feed a child carefully and intelligently, on artificial food, than to give it mother's milk which is poor in quality or deficient in quantity, or which, good in itself, is given at the expense of the mother's vitality. . . . to those who stand, as I myself stood, dreading the obnoxious bottle for the dear baby, I will say one earnest word, I wish it might be of comfort. Regard the bottle as your baby's friend, not his foe. You can make it so, unless the odds are fearfully against you. If one kind of food will not suit the child, some other will. Only give the matter your intelligent thought.[24]

These late nineteenth-century mothers had read, seen, and believed that bottle feeding was dangerous to infants. They gave preference to breast feeding but were grateful to learn from their own experience that artificial feeding could be healthful. In circumstances where they had had to use "the much abused patent nursing bottle," in the words of one writer in the *Ladies' Home Journal* in 1891, they discovered that

a careful intelligent mother may bring up her children in perfect health by so-called artificial feeding, sanitary and other conditions being good. I have cared for two children, and I am familiar with the catalogue of evils attendant upon the use of the nursing bottle only through the columns of various periodicals.

Women who had successfully bottle fed their infants encouraged other mothers not to despair if artificial feeding was necessary.[25]

By the twentieth century, "if artificial feeding is necessary" apparently had become "when artificial feeding is necessary." Many women seemingly expected that at some point they would be obliged to bottle feed. In a 1912 article, "How I Raised My First Baby," one mother dramatically described her experience for the edification of others.

From the Day of My Baby's Birth I had feared that she might have to be a bottle baby. So fearful was I that, before my nurse left, I had her tell me explicitly how to care for the bottle, and these directions I wrote in my notebook. . . .

When Baby was four months old the worst had happened: bottles had become a necessity! That first preparation of modified milk—shall I ever forget it? I had bought eight nursing bottles with nipples, a graduated pitcher that held two quarts, a box of sugar of milk, and some limewater, and with this outfit and the formula my physician had given me, I prepared the milk. . . .

After This First Preparation I drew a long breath; with my doctor to give me a new formula every month I felt that I could overcome the dangers of bottles. . . .

No mother can tell how soon it may happen that her baby will have to become a bottle baby; and this hint ought never to be forgotten.[26]

In the few decades before and after the turn of this century, mothers' views of infant feeding and their practices had undergone a transformation. More and more women were reporting the "necessity" of artificial feeding. Julia Carpenter was not alone; others believed that they could not nurse their infants healthfully. Some mothers began to bottle feed shortly after birth; others were "obliged to wean" after a few months of nursing. Recognition of this need impelled women to search for the best substitute for mother's milk, and they learned of alternatives to maternal nursing through new and rapidly multiplying sources. The content and tone of the advice given mothers, and the forms of women's inquiries, reflect the state of medical and scientific knowledge of the period and the basic tenets of the ideology of scientific motherhood. Mothers accepted responsibility for the health and welfare of their children. But they also acknowledged that they required expert scientific and medical advice in order to be successful. However, opinions differed on who were the experts. A plethora of sources promoted different answers to the question, How shall I feed my baby? Child-care manuals and manufacturers of infant foods provided information for the successful feeding of "bottle babies." Mothers found help in the growing number of women's magazines; women wrote letters of inquiry and described their experiences in articles that document the use of a wide variety of resources and formulations. At times mothers called upon physicians for assistance, typically for sick babies. By the second decade of the twentieth century, as greater numbers of women bottle fed their infants, physician-supervised infant feeding became increasingly common but was not yet the norm for American mothers. This situation would change significantly in the next several decades.

IX

"Count on Bottles"
1920–1950

More and more women in the twentieth century answered the question of how to feed the baby in the same way: they bottle fed their infants under medical supervision. This solution was a logical extension of the ideology of scientific motherhood, of the education women received, and of the circumstances under which increasing numbers of women gave bith. Child-care literature continued to stress the need for expert advice; women read these publications and also attended classes that promulgated a similar philosophy of motherhood. In addition, the growing popularity of hospitalized childbirth introduced a new form of mothercraft instruction, one in which many more mothers directly encountered the influence of medical authority in infant care.

As earlier twentieth-century studies had documented, women actively sought out child-care information from a variety of sources. The Lynds' study of Middletown in the 1920s described many "working class" and "business class" mothers who felt the need to study childrearing techniques. Women read booklets and pamphlets; a few obtained informal assistance from the head of the home economics department of the local school and from occasional state health department demonstrations on child care. One business-class mother took a course in Montessori methods in a nearby city before the birth of her daughter; some working-class mothers received advice on the physical care of children from the Visiting Nurses' Association. In Middletown, Holt's *Care and Feeding of Infants* was used, although women's magazines were the "most important" sources. "And yet a prevalent mood among Middletown parents," reported the Lynds, "is of bewilderment, a feeling that their difficulties outrun their best efforts to cope with them." The authors quoted one woman who clearly felt the strain imposed by the ideology of scientific motherhood on twentieth-century women:

"Life was simpler for mother," said a thoughtful mother. "In those days one did not realize that there was so much to be known about the care of children. I realize that I ought to be half a dozen experts, but I am afraid of making mistakes and usually do not know where to go for advice."[1]

Middletown women could and did obtain advice from a multitude of sources. But in the 1920s at least, women had not yet identified a single, generally accepted expert to whom they would turn automatically for assistance. In a 1936 study incorporated into the White House Conference on Child Health and Protection, John E. Anderson published a survey of 3,000 families. Its sample represented a broad cross-section of socioeconomic levels of American society. Anderson found that over 50 percent of the families surveyed had read at least one book on child care during the year, and over 70 percent had read at least one pamphlet. Though only a small proportion of these families subscribed to child-care magazines, almost three-quarters of the mothers in the survey reported reading magazine and newspaper articles on the subject.[2]

Women not only read about child-care techniques and attended classes; they also acted on the advice they received. In a 1925 issue of *Farmer's Wife*, a Virginian described her six-month-old baby, whom she was "raising by the book." She recommended to other mothers that they utilize the information available in books and magazines "to help you and you in turn to give the baby the best chance possible for a good start in life."[3] Mothers did more than urge women to read child-care literature. Mrs. P.O., Iowa, was so appreciative of *Infant Care* that she wrote to the Children's Bureau in 1928, "The government books which I obtained from your department have been of such wonderful help to me in raising my three lovely children that two friends of mine would like a copy of them also."[4] Relating her child-care experiences, another woman wrote in *Cosmopolitan* in 1940,

> My constant companion was that Bible of the 1940 young mother, the "Infant Care" pamphlet printed by the United States Government. The title was just too prosaic for the singing hearts of the mothers, so someone rechristened it "The Good Book," and by that name it is generally known.[5]

Visiting health professionals in Wisconsin in the 1930s reported the ease with which women in poor rural areas of the state discussed *Infant Care*. After a visit to a tar-paper shack in Spooner, one nurse recorded:

> During my discussion with the mother in regard to health habits, I was surprised at the freedom with which she discussed tomato juice and cod-

liver oil. It was evident that she had read her "Infant Care" which had been sent her following the twins' birth registration.

One doctor was pleased to note that in DeForest, Wisconsin, "we found quite a few mothers following their Infant Care books and giving babies cod liver oil and orange juice."[6]

In print and in interviews, mothers reported "religiously" following the instructions they had been taught in prenatal and postnatal classes, the advice they had read in books and pamphlets, or the information they had received from physicians.[7] One interviewee fondly remembered the course she had taken at the University of Wisconsin, popularly called "The Bride's Course." Taught by a physician, it had included instruction in prenatal and postnatal care. Ten years later, after the birth of her second child, she still continued to refer to her class notes.[8] Another mother recalled that the doctor told her what to do "every step of the way . . . and I did it."[9] Women not only visited medical practitioners and baby clinics, but they also "tried to follow the latest advice" from pamphlets and books.[10] Interviewed when their children were thirty or more years old, many of these women still remembered vividly the books they had read, the classes they had attended, the doctors and clinics who had counseled them, and how important this advice had been.

Several common themes permeated the child-care literature and education of the period. Most significantly, they all expressed to a greater or lesser degree the growing acceptance and even assumption of artificial infant feeding. The hypothesis that women's experiences reflected the content of the published advice they read and the instruction they received suggests that mothers turned more frequently to bottle feeding in the twentieth century. Statistical studies from the period substantiate this supposition. Unfortunately, the extant data are usually not directly comparable. Surveys typically focused on small populations, limited either geographically or by the class of the patient. (The earliest national statistics, limited to hospital births, appeared in 1948.) Some did not differentiate between infants fed exclusively at the breast and those who received some supplemental bottle feedings. Despite the problem of incommensurable data, however, these studies do provide some indication of contemporary infant-feeding practices.

Table 9.1 lists the results of the more detailed surveys published between 1917 and 1948.[11] These data represent the percentages of women who exclusively breast fed or exclusively bottle fed their infants. From the Children's Bureau data (1917–1919), one point is readily apparent: at any given time infant-feeding practices differed significantly across the country. In rural

Table 9.1. Modes of infant feeding in the United States, 1917–1948: Percentage of infants exclusively breast- or bottle-fed

Year/Source of Data	1 week or hospital discharge		1 month or less		3 months		6 months	
	breast	bottle	breast	bottle	breast	bottle	breast	bottle
1917–1919/Children's Bureau Studies								
Rural Kans.			92	2	83	6	61	13
Rural southern Wis.			92	6	82	11	51	16
Rural northern Wis.			89	6	76	9	49	16
Saginaw, Mich.			88	9	75	16	54	24
Akron, Ohio			88	8	73	19	55	27
Johnstown, Pa.					67	20	41	26
New Bedford, Mass.			83	12	66	25	45	37
Manchester, N.H.			82	15	61	33	36	47
1930/Boston, Mass.								
Private patients		11	26		51		85	
Clinic patients		9	25		42		53	
Composite		10	25		46		69	
1934/Rural New York State		12			31			
1948/U.S. Hospital Births								
Northeast	23	61						
East and Central	36	34						
Southeast	55	18						
Southwest	47	18						
Mountain and Plains	44	28						
Pacific	31	40						
National	38	35						

Note: Because breast-feeding mothers who gave their infants supplementary bottles are not included, figures do not add up to 100 percent.

Sources: Data for rural Kansas, Johnstown, Manchester, and Akron, from Elizabeth Moore, *Maternity and infant care in a rural county of Kansas,* Children's Bureau Publication no. 2 (Washington, D.C.: Government Printing Office, 1917), reprinted in *Child care in rural America* (New York: Arno Press and the New York Times, 1972), p. 42. Wisconsin, Saginaw, and New Bedford, data from Florence Brown Sherbon and Elizabeth Moore, *Maternity and infant care in two rural counties in Wisconsin,* Children's Bureau Publication no. 46 (Washington, D.C.: Government Printing Office, 1919), reprinted in *Child care in rural America,* p. 92. Boston data from Joseph Garland and Mabel B. Rich, "Duration of breast feeding: A comparative study," *New England Journal of Medicine, 203* (1930), 1279–1282. Rural New York State data from Rachael Sanders Bizal, "Our babies: What they are fed," *Medical Woman's Journal, 41* (1934), 158–162. Hospital births data from Katherine Bain, "Incidence of breast feedings in hospitals in the United States," *Pediatrics, 2* (1948), 313–320; Herman F. Meyer, "Breast feeding in the United States: Extent and possible trend," *Pediatrics, 22* (1958), 116–121.

Kansas mothers overwhelmingly nursed their babies. Though increasing numbers of that state's mothers artifically fed after the third month, over 60 percent continued to breast feed their infants at six months. This contrasts with mothers in Manchester, New Hampshire, 15 percent of whom were already bottle feeding their infants in the first month. By three months 61 percent, and by six months only 36 percent, of these more urban women nursed their children. Data from other areas demonstrate less difference between urban and rural practices but do suggest that maternal nursing was more common in the Midwest than in the Northeast during the late 1910s. Statistics from the 1940s reflect a similar differentiation between regions. In a study of infant feeding at the time of discharge from the hospital nursery, infants in the Northeast (including Massachusetts, Connecticut, Maine, New York, New Hampshire, Vermont, and Rhode Island) were overwhelmingly bottle fed.

When one analyzes the use of bottle feeding, a slightly different picture emerges. Though the proportion of women who exclusively breast fed older infants declined in all studies, increased artificial feeding did not necessarily signal weaning. On the one hand, in rural Wisconsin only 16 percent of the mothers relied on bottle formulas alone to feed their six-month-old babies. On the other hand, 37 percent of the mothers of New Bedford, Massachusetts, had totally weaned their six-month-olds. Evidently mothers in rural areas of the Midwest tended to supplement their breast milk with artificial food; those in the urban Northeast frequently stopped nursing entirely and only bottle fed. In 1930 Joseph Garland, M.D., and Mabel B. Rich, R.N., studied 200 mothers from private practices in Boston and 200 from the Out Patient Department Clinic of the Massachusetts General Hospital. They discovered that in the early months of life both groups bottle fed in approximately the same proportions, but that in the later period, specifically after three months, private patients were less likely to breast feed than clinic patients.

Taken as a whole, the table illustrates two broad trends. First, women in the United States increasingly declined to breast feed and instead depended on artificial food to nourish their babies. The 1930 figures sharply contrast with those from 1917 to 1919. In the earlier period, at most one-third of the mothers bottle fed at three months, and by six months less than one-half did so. By 1930 the percentage of babies fed no breast milk was dramatically higher at both ages. Second, over time American mothers tended to replace maternal nursing with bottle feeding at an earlier age. For example, before 1930 weaning typically occured sometime after age one month, yet a 1934 study in rural New York State documented that 12 percent of the mothers never even attempted to breast feed. Similarly, more than one-quarter of the Boston patients studied in 1930 had stopped nursing by one month; in the 1910s this figure was much lower.

The popularity of artificial feeding continued to grow in the next decades. Since milk was rationed and difficult to obtain during the war, at least one doctor expected to see a resurgence of breast feeding.[12] However, the statistics show otherwise. The 1948 hospital survey (table 9.1), which included more than two-thirds of all hospitals in the United States with twenty-five beds or more admitting women for delivery, disclosed that over one-third of the infants were weaned at the time of discharge, slightly more were exclusively breast fed, and the remainder received both breast and bottle feedings. Though varying widely between regions, the overall trend clearly points to the decrease in breast feeding and the rise in bottle feeding throughout the country. The tendency accelerated; a similar study published in 1958 found that only 21 percent of infants leaving the hospital were exclusively breast fed, while 63 percent received bottle formulas only.[13]

Many factors undoubtedly influenced mothers' decisions to bottle feed rather than breast feed. For one thing, they continued to read and hear much more about artificial feeding than about maternal nursing. And much of what they found in women's magazines seemed to assume that they would be bottle feeding (see Chapter 7). Even if they were breast feeding, or planning to, women were warned to expect to use a bottle at some time in their infants' lives. As one mother counseled prospective mothers in *Parents' Magazine* in 1938:

> You hope to nurse him, of course, but there is an alarming number of young mothers today who are unable to breast-feed their babies and you may be one of them . . . Even if you are breast-feeding you may be ordered by your doctor to give him supplementary feedings by bottle, so it is fairly safe to count on bottles and their attendant equipment in your scheme of things.[14]

Coupled with this advice were the advertisements. Advertising, especially from the 1920s on, consciously manipulated both the "intrinsic and extrinsic properties of goods in use."[15] According to the philosophy of one of the leading "ad-men" of the twentieth century, "The product itself should be its own best salesman. Not the product alone, but the product plus a mental impression, an atmosphere, which you place around it."[16] The evaporated milk companies, for example, promoted their products as safe, scientific, and up-to-date modes of infant feeding. The Dionne Quintuplets, the most carefully supervised babies of the 1930s, were fed Carnation Milk (figure 9.1). The on-the-go, modern mother could trust Pet Milk, which was "scien-

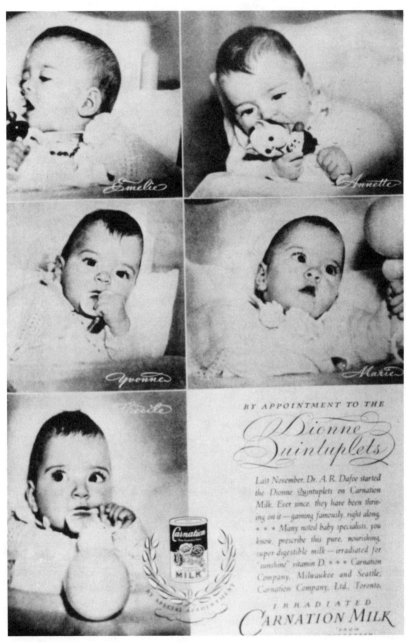

Figure 9.1. Carnation Milk advertisement. Source: *Parents' Magazine, 10* (5) (1935), 47

tifically clean" (figure 9.2). These typical advertisements did not bother to compare artificial feeding and nursing; breast milk apparently was no longer the standard in infant feeding. As with other infant-care literature and education, the examples of infant feeding in the text and advertisements of women's magazines presumed that American mothers bottle fed their babies.

Though more women were bottle feeding by the third, fourth, and fifth decades of this century, magazines published fewer letters of inquiry from mothers about infant feeding. The infant-feeding experiences of women who gave birth in these decades suggest some possible explanations for this decline. The advice literature and domestic-science courses insisted that all babies, especially those artificially fed, should be under the care of a medical practitioner. Mothers increasingly did employ private physicians or attend well-baby clinics. When they had problems or questions, they could call or see a medical person and did not have to correspond with a distant magazine. Instead of asking for advice from journals, they "did what the doctor said," and did it "when the doctor said."[17] Only about 12 percent of the mothers included in Anderson's 1936 survey reported never consulting some medical person.[18]

Magazine editors continued to answer some queries, but they rarely gave specific advice. "I have been feeding my 6 months old baby Dryco [a dried milk] with boiled water only, and would like to know if you advise the use of Dextri-Maltose; or is the Dryco a whole food in itself, all that a baby of this age needs?" asked one concerned reader in *Hygeia* in 1926. The editor explained that Dextri-Maltose was a carbohydrate, plain Dryco was equivalent to "plain milk," and "the only safe way in preparing a formula for infant feeding is to have a physician thoroughly familiar with the case prescribe the formula and alter it from time to time as the child grows older or to meet special indications."[19] Since the AMA published *Hygeia,* it is not surprising to find the editor directing readers to physicians. In responding to similar queries, however, other journals also advised their readership to seek the advice of medical practitioners.

In contrast to the dearth of inquiry letters, magazines included many articles written by mothers in which women described their infant-care experiences and offered suggestions to new mothers. Jane Gilbreth Heppes comfortingly reassured readers: "I am a new mother with a five-months old baby. If someone had been able to convince me as I want to convince you, that having a baby and coming home from the hospital with him to rear is not a staggering problem, I would have been very grateful."[20] The writers did not intend their advice to replace that of medical practitioners. While not always wholeheartedly accepting the instructions of their physicians, nonetheless

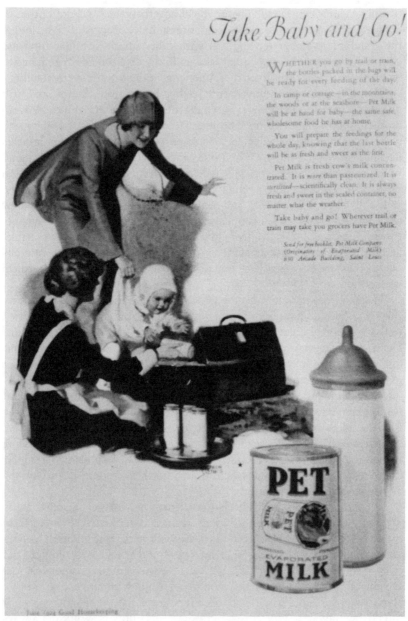

Figure 9.2. Pet Milk advertisement, 1924. Source: Frank Presbrey, *The history and development of advertising* (Garden City, N.Y.: Doubleday, Doran, 1929)

these women respected medical expertise and expected readers to be under the supervision of a medical practitioner. Still, they also sought to assuage the fears of prospective mothers by relating their personal histories and advising new mothers how they could better carry out their physicians' instructions and follow the advice given to increasing numbers of women in hospital nurseries.

In 1920 barely 20 percent of American women gave birth in hospitals. Within just a few decades, by 1950, over 80 percent of U.S. births occurred there. This institutionalization not only led to greater medicalization of birthing procedures, but affected postpartum conditions for mother and child as well. Many of the points taught in hospitals were also stressed in the prescriptive literature and child-care education of the day; therefore, it is difficult to separate out the influence of the hospital from that of literature, schooling, and even social networks. Nevertheless, in both printed sources and in interviews, mothers reported that their infant-care experiences, especially in the first few weeks after returning home from the hospital, were totally unexpected and were influenced by what they had, or had not, encountered in the hospital. One woman was from a large family, and before the birth of her first child in 1943 she had felt fairly confident about her ability to handle infants. But, she stressed, "I will never forget the first week out of the hospital." During her stay she had "felt that the baby didn't belong to me, that the hospital owned him." She complained that the nurses "don't tell you that the baby cried half the night." Despite her prior confidence, she recalled, those first few weeks she was tense, and "that's how I started out motherhood, exhausted."[21]

Through its routines and procedures, its implicit and explicit teachings, the hospital fostered the ideology of scientific motherhood, the need for scientific and medical expertise in the successful rearing of infants. Hospitals were medical institutions which represented the best, most scientific forms of infant care. As one mother commented about hospitalized childbirth and its aftermath, "We were scientific." Fathers, too, recognized the importance of scientific care, even though it meant that they were separated from their infants until the homecoming. Writing for his unborn child, a prospective father drew this picture of modern, scientific childrearing:

> For two weeks you will remain in the hospital in a big room with all the other babies who will have been born about the same time. You will be fed by scientific formulae. Your mother will have her hands and face sterilized before you are brought to her. When I come to see you I will stare through a glass door and a nurse will point you out.

> [At home] you will eat, sleep, play, and be bathed in the sterilized
> atmosphere of an operating room.

Sarah M. Privette of Brooklyn, New York, claimed that her husband had been content to see his daughter through glass during her hospital stay because "he could see the wisdom of this strict rule, so he accepted it, as most people do, without much protest." Parents believed that the hospital knew what was best medically, scientifically, for the baby.[22]

Hospital conditions and practices discouraged breast feeding and encouraged the belief that bottle feeding was as good as, if not better than, mother's milk. As we have seen (Chapter 7), hospital routines could inhibit lactation. Mothers and babies were separated for most of the day. Often women saw their children only at fixed feeding intervals, and even then the fear of cross-infection dictated stringent controls over the interaction between mother and child. Women were instructed to use face masks. Nurses would wash the mothers' nipples before bringing the infants from the nursery. At one Madison, Wisconsin, hospital, the mothers were not even allowed to hold their children after feeding. The nurses would pick up the babies, burp them, and return them to the nursery.[23] Acting on the medical professions' concern about the initial weight loss exhibited by many newborns, hospitals often instituted automatic supplemental feeding programs. Nursing mothers were encouraged to sleep through the night; babies received night bottle feedings (see Chapter 7). It is easy to imagine that such routines did "not provide an atmosphere which encourages breast feeding."[24]

A 1950 investigation undertaken at a University of Pennsylvania hospital demonstrates the effect of such supplemental feedings, particularly with mothers not fully committed to maternal nursing. Some of the 91 women in this study had a positive attitude toward breast feeding, another group was ambivalent, and a third group was negative but agreed to attempt maternal nursing. (Excluded from the study were mothers who flatly refused to consider breast feeding.) At this hospital nurses brought the babies to their mothers six times a day. For the first four days, a bottle accompanied each infant, and following the breast feeding the mother automatically offered her child this supplemental glucose solution or formula feeding. On the fourth day, the bottle ceased to accompany the baby routinely, but the infant was weighed before and after each breast feeding to determine the need for any additional nourishment. The study's results are not surprising: in circumstances where bottle feeding was easily available, the mother's attitude toward maternal nursing had a significant affect on her ability to breast feed. Of those with a positive attitude, 74 percent were breast feeding with no supplemental bottles after four days; of the negative mothers, 26 percent were successful; and of those ambivalent about the need for or desirability of maternal nursing, only 35 percent were successfully breast feeding without supplemental bottles at the time of hospital discharge. Women committed to maternal nursing probably found comfort in the ready availability of an alternative to mother's milk; they did not worry about "starving" their babies and thus were more relaxed and successful. For women undecided or uneasy about maternal nursing, however, the hospital's provisions discouraged serious breast-feeding attempts.[25]

Other, more common hospital practices undoubtedly affected women's ability to nurse their infants. Mothers received their infants on a fixed schedule, usually every four hours, and were instructed to offer alternate breasts at each feeding. Furthermore, to allow the mothers to rest, the nurses bottle fed the infants in the nursery for the 2 A.M. feeding. Thus a mother saw her infant five times a day, and each breast would be stimulated only two or three times in a twenty-four-hour period. Moreover, her newborn would rarely empty the breast completely. These physical conditions are not conducive to successful maternal nursing, especially in the early days when a mother is attempting to establish the flow of her milk.[26]

Mary McCarthy's account of postpartum care in her novel *The Group* captures the problems of breast feeding under hospital conditions. Priss Hartshorn Crockett is married to a doctor who insists that she nurse their son, Stephen, the only infant in the nursery not bottle-fed. The baby is, of course, brought to his mother for feedings only, and on a strict schedule. Visitors often hear Stephen's loud cries from the nursery, and Priss and the nurses hear him through most of the day and night.

> At eight o'clock that night, right on the dot, down in the nursery Stephen started to cry. She knew his voice—the whole floor knew it. Sometimes he would whimper and then go back to sleep for a while, but when he began noisily, as he was doing now, he might cry for two solid hours—a scandal . . . But if he woke up shortly after a feeding, it was horrible: after an hour's cry, he would get his water, sleep, wake up and cry again without stopping—his record, so far, was two hours and three-quarters.

Eventually the hospital staff and her husband decide that Stephen needs some supplemental bottles. A short time later, Priss receives a phone call from an old college friend, now in publishing, who asks her to write a magazine article about her breast-feeding experience. Priss declines, claiming that such an article would be "in poor taste." "Is it in poor taste to talk about it?" responds her friend. "Why, it's the most natural thing in the world." To which

Crockett retorts, "If it's so natural, why are you so excited about putting it in a magazine?" After hanging up the phone, Priss reflects:

> She was doing "the most natural thing in the world," suckling her young, and for some peculiar reason it was completely unnatural, strained, and false, like a posed photograph. . . . In reality, what she had been doing was horrid, and right now, in the nursery, a baby's voice was rising to tell her so—the voice, in fact, that she had been refusing to listen to, though she had heard it for at least a week. It was making a natural request, in this day and age; it was asking for a bottle.[27]

Women unable to provide "full rations" for their babies felt that their milk supply was inadequate and that they could not, or should not, continue nursing. Mothers often recalled that though they had wanted to nurse, they "never had enough." Women who feared that they were starving their babies were content to bottle feed under their doctor's supervision.[28] Supplementary feeding in the hospital implied not only that mother's milk was insufficient but also that formulas were healthful: the "bottle was just as good as [the] breast." Similarly, hospital classes for postpartum women, including a demonstration on how to prepare a baby's formula, and the bottle of prepared formula given mothers when they left the hospital promoted the idea that bottle feeding was expected.[29]

Hospital routines continued to affect a woman's ability to nurse her child even after she returned home. The separation of mother and child during the lying-in period allowed the woman little opportunity to "get to know her baby." An article in the *Atlantic Monthly* in 1934 poignantly portrays the anxieties that many a mother felt leaving the hospital:

> And then we took the baby home.
> If only mothers were reading this—mothers who have taken home from a hospital their first-born without a nurse—it would be unnecessary to say another word. To be sure, I had read three books on baby care, I had everything in the bathroom cabinet that could possibly be used on a baby, and I had been allowed to *watch* the nurse bathe mine on the last morning. She had bathed a dozen in an hour! I knew all the theory—but theory had no relation to this squirming, crying bundle of humanity we took across town that hot Saturday afternoon.[30]

Everything seemed rosy in the hospital: the baby was healthy, the nurses attended to the needs of mother and child. But, warned a mother of two in a 1938 article, then you go home. . . . Your legs feel as though they would slide out from under you and the mere thought of diapers, formulas and two o'clock feedings sickens you. Oh, to be back again in the comforting, quiet hospital.[31]

In writing these articles women did not seek to replace the medical expertise of the physician nor to suggest methods particularly different from those taught in the hospital or in prescriptive literature. Instead, they were recreating in modern form the female advice network that had supported their foremothers in earlier years. They wanted to prepare the new mother for the burdens she faced upon returning home and to provide routines and hints that would simplify and ease her first few weeks at home as she tried to replicate "the expert care [the baby] has had in that efficient nursery."[32]

Women did try to duplicate in their own homes the lessons they had learned in the hospital. One woman described the problems she faced upon homecoming. Despite her education (she had a doctorate and a professional career), she was unprepared for the reality of the "six-pound bundle of wailing baby in my arms."

To be sure, before the period of hospitalization was over, . . . the nurse had demonstrated how to pin a diaper, how to hold and turn a baby, how to bathe and oil and clothe him, how to prepare a formula, and how to hold a bottle. But copied answers to questions and observation of a single demonstration cannot take the place of background, long acquaintance, or experience. Luckily, Robert [her baby] cannot remember those hours after he was taken to his home. He cannot recall the struggles with that first diaper; or the way which his first bottles of formula had of always getting too hot, in spite of clock-watching obedience to instructions.[33]

Another mother who gave birth in Minneapolis in the late 1940s felt a little "nervous" when she went home. In the hospital she had washed her nipples with boric acid before nursing, a routine she continued at home. She was "very rigid" about feeding her child on a four-hour schedule because she felt more confidence in the doctor and the hospital than in herself.[34]

But in incorporating hospital routines into their daily lives, mothers made pragmatic changes in the procedures to suit their personal situations. One mother of two daughters born in the 1940s remembers feeling that she had a "natural aptitude to handle this kind of thing," explaining that "you either have it or you don't." Consequently, she had read little before entering a large Brooklyn hospital. She did not nurse but after each birth received her infants several times a day for feedings. The nurses wore masks, and the mothers were told to wear masks, so this mother continued to don a face mask even when she returned home until it became "too much of a bother." However, she sterilized all the feeding utensils for five or six months and "fed by the clock," even if the baby cried out earlier. Despite her sense that she had a "natural aptitude," she "assumed if the hospital gave you information that it was the best thing for the baby."[35] Noted another mother in *Better Homes & Gardens* in 1948, "the hospital probably had him on a 6 am, 10 am, 2 pm, and 6 pm schedule." She had instituted this schedule at home with her first two children. However, she counseled, she had discovered with her third child that in a busy household a 7, 11, 3, and 7 schedule was better.[36] The theory remained; only the conditions demanded a slight revision of its application.

Mothers developed various methods for dealing with the pressures, because the pressures did exist. Especially in the first few days after returning home, nervousness and tension caused mothers to "dry up." Even women who had successfully nursed in the hospital had to resort to supplemental bottle feedings. J.B.'s baby had been born three weeks early. The girl was small and weak and could not nurse; in five days she had lost one of her five pounds. "My breasts were bound; I was told I would nurse her no more," reported the mother. Knowing the mortality rate of premature babies and considering mother's milk like "life insurance," J.B. argued and finally persuaded the doctor to allow her to use a breast pump and to nurse her daughter with an eye dropper. The baby regained her health. Yet committed as J.B. was to maternal nursing, once she was out of the hospital her milk supply diminished and her baby was bottle fed.[37] Sometimes mothers successfully nursed for a few months and then discovered that they needed supplemental bottles. Mrs. C.A. wrote to the Children's Bureau in 1926 about her problem:

> I have a fine baby boy, age 12 weeks, weight 12 pounds 6 oz. At first I had more than enough milk for him but the last 2 weeks I have not had enough, and had my doctor give me a formula for to feed him part time—about 2 or 3 feedings a day. I do not understand why I cannot nurse him as at first. . . .
> . . . When I asked my doctor again about it, he said, "Why don't you wean him altogether?"

Clearly the physician believed that it was easier to bottle feed than to worry about breast feeding, though Mrs. C.A. thought differently.[38] For other mothers, supplemental bottles signaled the end of breast feeding. Given the time and energy involved in preparing a few bottles a day, mothers who employed supplemental bottle feeding often quickly weaned their babies. One mother of eight discovered that when her "milk seemed to dry up" and she had to supplement with Carnation milk and Karo Syrup, "it was easier" to stop nursing entirely.[39]

Obviously not all women bottle fed their infants. However, the available statistics and mothers' reports of infant-feeding practices in written sources and interviews document that mothers turned more frequently and more easily to artificial feeding after about 1920. And they did so under medical supervision. By the middle of this century, mothers generally expected to conduct their infant feeding, even breast feeding, with the assistance of medical practitioners.[40] But most mothers bottle fed their babies. The case of one mother of four from Madison, Wisconsin, is fairly typical.[41] All her children were born in a hospital, and all received regular medical supervision. She started to nurse her first child, born in 1934. When the baby was less than six weeks old, she feared that her milk supply was insufficient. This mother went to a well-baby clinic run by a local physician and there received a formula. She tried to nurse her second child, born in 1935, but she quickly decided that she could not; the hospital put the baby on a formula. With her subsequent children she did not even attempt nursing.

Most mothers who bottle fed their infants in the twentieth century did not consciously decide against nursing. Rather, they discovered that their breast milk was somehow deficient; bottle feeding, they felt, was necessary.[42] In the 1930 study of Boston mothers by Garland and Rich, the most cited reason for weaning was "insufficient milk." Of those who bottle fed, more than 50 percent claimed that they did not have enough breast milk to satisfy their infants. Several mothers attempted to stimulate the flow of milk by following procedures similar to those advocated by Sedgwick in the 1910s: they employed breast pumps or manually stripped their breasts. Although these techniques were often effective in the short term, according to Garland and Rich, they "were rarely tolerated for any period of time," and these mothers usually artificially fed their infants.[43]

In interviews women remembered that they bottle fed because they did not have sufficient breast milk. They claimed, however, that some of their friends bottle fed because they "didn't want to be bothered with breast feeding" or feared that with nursing they "couldn't go out much."[44] One mother, who had breast fed all her children "because I had so much milk it would have been a crime if I didn't," recalled that after about six months she "got tired." She instituted bottles at that time to decrease her milk flow and to wean the baby.[45] Acknowledging that breast feeding was the most "natural thing to do," these women accepted the efficacy of medically directed bottle feeding.[46]

In many respects women's experiences in infant feeding mirrored the assumptions and scenarios presented to them in the literature, in child-care courses, and by medical practitioners. Women read books, pamphlets, and magazines and attended infant-care classes, and they increasingly sought out and accepted direction from private physicians and well-baby clinics. Even women who wanted to breast feed often discovered in the hospital that their milk supply was inadequate or found that it dwindled shortly after coming home or several months later. And though these mothers were sorry that they could not nurse their children, they considered bottle feeding "all right" if they had a "good formula" prescribed by a doctor.[47] Most women reported that doctors and hospitals did not particularly encourage breast feeding and sometimes specifically discouraged women from attempting or continuing to nurse. By mid-century, mothers no longer regarded breast feeding as the norm; they approved of bottle feeding, found it satisfactory and generally accepted it as standard infant-feeding practice.[48] As one interviewee recalled: some of her friends nursed, and some did not. She herself did not nurse. With both her children, supplemental bottle feeding began in the hospital; by the time she left, they were bottle-fed babies. But the fact that her infants were not breast fed did not worry her in the least because she believed that physician-supervised "bottle feeding was O.K."[49]

During the first half of the twentieth century, increasing numbers of American women appreciated and practiced artificial infant feeding. Mothers typically expressed the belief that maternal nursing represented the best nourishment for the baby. Nevertheless, experience tempered their faith as women recognized possible limitations in breast feeding. Worried that they had insufficient or deficient milk, exhausted and faced with a crying baby, mothers more and more frequently, and more and more easily, turned to bottle feeding. After all, artificial feeding had apparently aided other mothers who encountered difficulties in nursing, who could not provide "full rations" for their babies. Experts recommended alternatives to mother's milk, and hospitals demonstrated formula preparation; both tacitly and overtly promoted the use of bottles in infant feeding. Although mothers affirmed that breast feeding was "natural," they did not deny the need for artificial infant feeding and the benefits of bottle feeding. By mid-century, artificial infant feeding had become the norm, and rather than fearing the loss of mother's milk, women found it reassuring to know that they could "count on bottles."

Infant Feeding in the Twentieth Century

X

"According to Your Own Preferences"

The general acceptance of medically directed bottle feeding by the mid-twentieth century signaled a striking transformation in child-care values and practices in the United States and a significant shift in the relationship between medical practitioners and mothers. As I have shown, the impulse to develop efficacious bottle feeding often originated in a concern for high rates of infant mortality and morbidity, yet the search for healthful alternatives to mother's milk affected the nutrition of all infants, not just ill ones. The creation of nutritious infant foods consequently enlarged the scope of medical practice, created a new industry, and altered women's views and mothering practices.

Though no one single cause satisfactorily explains the growing employment of artificial infant feeding, the factors associated with the increased use of bottle formulas are clear. Physicians wanted to alleviate the problems of infant mortality and morbidity and to expand the arena of medical practice. Manufacturers, though sometimes developing their products for humanitarian reasons, needed to build consumer demand for infant foods. And mothers, concerned for the health and well-being of children and uncertain of their own abilities, came to believe that doctor-supervised artificial feeding was best for their infants. In the United States from the late nineteenth century to the twentieth century, changing ideology, developments in medical practice, and ongoing scientific research all played a part in the medicalization and commercialization of infant feeding and the redefinition of women's maternal role.

Nineteenth-century physicians correlated high rates of infant mortality, specifically from gastrointestinal diseases, with poor nutrition, often the result of bad artificial feeding. The limited statistics available give credence to physicians' concerns about this relationship and to their assertion that improved artificial feeding in some instances reduced the infant death rate. In the 1890s the mortality rate from diarrheal diseases usually declined after the establishment of Straus-type milk depots in cities (see Chapter 4). Similarly, twentieth-century pediatric textbooks often pointed to the precipitous drop in the mortality rate of children under one year of age from the late nineteenth century onward. Figure 10.1 shows that in New York City the mortality rate fell dramatically from the late 1890s, with a particularly steep decline in deaths from gastrointestinal diseases. Physicians proudly claimed that this reduction resulted from improved milk supplies, better maternal education in infant feeding and hygiene, and increased medical supervision of infants.[1]

Still, the relationship between the increasing employment of bottle feeding and the decrease in infant mortality remains an open question. Did the mortality rate decline because of or in spite of the rise in artificial feeding? No definitive answer is possible. On the one hand, we know that bottle feeding apparently benefited some infants. Ill babies and premature infants, according to studies from the 1920s and 1930s, did better with evaporated milk formulas than breast milk (Chapter 3). Undoubtedly artificial feeding saved

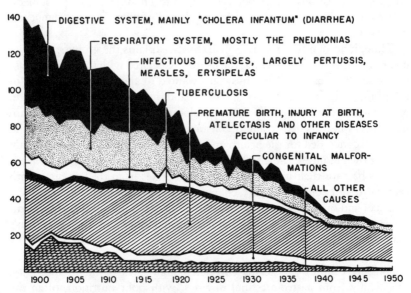

Figure 10.1. Infant mortality rate in New York City, 1898–1950: Deaths under one year of age per 1,000 live births. Source: L. Emmett Holt, Jr., and Rustin McIntosh, *Pediatrics,* 12th ed. (New York: Appleton-Century-Crofts, 1953), p. 61

some lives. Moreover, the availability of clean milk made bottle feeding safer than previously; that is, a smaller proportion of bottle-fed infants died.

On the other hand, the sharp decline in infant mortality, specifically from gastrointestinal diseases, may well have resulted from changes other than the growing popularity of bottle feeding. For example, the diets of infants in the first year of life include more than breast milk or bottle formulas. In the 1890s physicians discovered that infants from "poor" families less frequently exhibited signs of scurvy than babies in the households of the "well-to-do." To explain this difference, doctors pointed out that the former were fed table scraps, fresh fruit, and similar items more often than the latter. In the twentieth century, diet lists for both the breast-fed and the bottle-fed recommended various fruits, vegetables, and other foods in the first year of life. The effects of varied diets, both in introducing infection and in changing the flora of the digestive tract, are unclear. Moreover, throughout the period, mothers were advised, especially in the summer months, to give their infants water periodically. The improvement in supplies of water and foodstuffs certainly contributed to a decline in gastrointestinal diseases.[2]

Yet it is true that in the 1910s and 1920s, various studies revealed that the overwhelming majority of infants who died from diarrheal diseases were bottle-fed. But while documenting higher mortality rates for bottle-fed babies, investigators usually recognized the importance of other conditions. Analyses like those of Glazier and Garland and Rich demonstrated that, all else being equal, bottle-fed infants were as healthy as breast-fed babies. These researchers claimed that an infant's well-being depended more on the socioeconomic and educational status of the household than the mode of feeding. Pointing to the effects of "bad care and neglect," they frequently concluded that neither the improvement of artificial feeding nor the promotion of breast feeding was sufficient to solve the problem of infant mortality, especially from diarrheal diseases. They called for better living conditions and maternal education.[3]

Evaluating the positive and negative aspects of increased bottle feeding remains difficult. In 1984 the American Academy of Pediatrics' Task Force on the Assessment of the Scientific Evidence Relating to Infant-feeding Practices and Infant Health reported on the epidemiological evidence gathered primarily since 1970. Its analysis echoes the conclusions of earlier researchers:

> If there are health benefits associated with breast-feeding in populations
> with good sanitation, nutrition, and medical care, the benefits are
> apparently modest. In middle and upper class populations in developed
> countries where rates of serious illness are already low, it would be difficult

to unequivocally demonstrate effects of breast-feeding on health by the observational methods most frequently used.

In certain U.S. subpopulations in which good sanitation and nutrition are not universal and mothers and infants may not receive optimal medical care, infants have higher morbidity and mortality rates than those seen among the general population. Any health benefits associated with breast-feeding would more likely appear in these populations than in groups of higher socioeconomic status. Such is the case with the few studies on native North American populations, which suggest that substantial health benefits accrue to breast-fed infants, especially in terms of protection from gastroenteritis.

Thus, despite decades of investigations and even with today's more sophisticated and large-scale studies, researchers continue to have difficulty controlling the myriad of socioeconomic, environmental, and dietary factors associated with infant morbidity and mortality. For example, several recent studies suggest that the reduction in rates of respiratory illness among breast-fed infants may be attributable to socioeconomic and other differences, such as parental smoking, rather than the feeding method. Time and again the Task Force comments:

> It is unlikely that a large proportion of postnatal deaths in the United States could be averted by universal breast-feeding. However, the lack of good epidemiologic studies in this area suggests that studies of specific causes of death and infant-feeding methods are warranted.[4]

Given these conclusions, it is likely that the rising standard of living, greater access to medical care, and improved food and water supplies in the United States in the first half of this century at least in part masked the negative effects of the growing utilization of artificial infant feeding.

Accordingly, one cannot claim that the increased use of artificial feeding was an unqualified blessing for the American infant. The complexity of the issue and the limitations of historical data make a definitive evaluation of the impact of the growing popularity of bottle feeding on infant mortality rates impossible. Though we know that more infants received breast milk than bottle formulas before the 1930s, we do not have any conclusive statistics on the relative proportions. Without such figures we can only hypothesize that improved bottle formulas did alleviate health problems for some infants; but we do not know for how many. Furthermore, later infant foods were more healthful and safer than earlier mixtures. Mortality rates for the bottle-fed evidently did decline; however, this enhancement of infant health reflected not only improved artificial foods but also the general improvement in living conditions. Despite the early twentieth-century conviction that breast feeding was more healthful than bottle feeling, contemporary studies emphasizing the importance of other factors such as living conditions contributed to a perception that bottle feeding was a reasonable substitute for maternal nursing.

Women were aware of the higher mortality rates for bottle-fed infants, yet not every mother could or would nurse her child. Allegedly, increasing numbers of women refused to breast feed because nursing "tied them down," as changes in American society not only altered women's domestic role but also expanded their activities outside the home. Though few women voiced this sentiment themselves, no doubt some mothers felt constrained when they had to stay home to nurse an infant. Other women worried that their milk supplies were inadequate, believing that physical conditions and the effects of modern life could prevent successful lactation (see Chapter 8). Such women wanted a convenient, safe, and healthful alternative to mother's milk. They looked to science for the solution.

Women were not alone in turning to science for answers. Indeed, during this period faith in science affected diverse facets of American culture, including the medical profession and the idealized view of motherhood. These in turn altered the relationship between physicians and mothers in areas such as infant feeding and also childbirth, which provides an instructive comparison.[5]

Before the eighteenth century, physicians only infrequently attended childbirth. Birth then was a women's affair; midwives and female relatives, friends, and neighbors supported and advised the parturient, an experience which historians have labeled "social childbirth." From then until the early twentieth century, however, childbirth became transformed: medical doctors, usually male, gradually replaced female midwives. By the 1920s medical control of birth management—so-called scientific childbirth—was the norm; parturition was seen as a disease. The medicalization of childbirth, with the loss of women's traditional knowledge and expertise, and the demise of the midwife were not simply the result of physicians' eagerness to build their case loads and force women to conform to the ideals of the medical profession; women's perceptions of childbirth contributed too. Childbirth, like lactation, is a natural function, although delivery is not always easy or safe for mother and child. Women turned to doctors because they believed that medicine promised safer and less painful deliveries through the use of forceps, drugs, and anesthesia.

Subsequently, in "scientific childbirth" women lost some control over the birthing process. But this outcome should not obscure the fact that women participated in the decision to involve physicians in that process. In the transition period of the nineteenth and early twentieth centuries, many women wanted the safest, most comfortable form of childbirth that science could provide. They believed that doctors would provide them with the benefits of scientific labor management. Women's goals and physicians' humanitarian concerns and self-interest all worked together to promote the acceptance of physician-directed childbirth.

Advances in bacteriology, chemotherapy, medical technology, and the like enabled physicians to present themselves as scientific birth attendants and provided the basis for the development of the specialty of obstetrics. Similar factors promoted the establishment of other medical specialties. At the same time, medical educators were succeeding in standardizing the medical curriculum, replacing didactic lectures with clinical instruction and more "scientific" laboratory classes. In the process schools that could not afford to institute these changes were forced to close, limiting the number of new graduates. Physicians participated in the push for more stringent licensing laws with examinations based on the new "scientific" curriculum, which also constricted the number of physicians in practice.[6] Though typically more a vaguely defined rhetorical symbol than a clearly articulated body of knowledge, the ideal of science held an esteemed place in American society, and medicine's growing association with science enhanced the prestige of the medical profession. The elevation of science also helps to explain the development of the ideology of scientific motherhood. Scientific principles, not innate instincts or traditions, were to guide women in the performance of their maternal role.

In the case of infant feeding, scientific discoveries in nutrition, physiology, and bacteriology made it appear that medical science could produce an infant food as good as, if not better than, mother's milk. Physicians encouraged the equation between science and medicine and presented themselves as scientific experts on infant feeding. Women who did not nurse their children wanted an efficacious substitute for breast milk. Science seemingly provided the answer, and doctors appeared to have the knowledge to handle the problem of artificial infant feeding. Consequently, women logically and increasingly replaced the traditional knowledge they had learned through female networks with physicians' advice.

Physicians promoted this intrusion of medical management into a previously nonmedical area. They, like mothers, were influenced by the needs of some women for a substitute for mother's milk and often reiterated this humanitarian argument for "scientific" infant feeding. Coupled with their undoubted sincerity on this point, physicians had other professional and economic reasons for engaging in this new aspect of medical practice. Research in infant nutrition and feeding added a new dimension to general medical practice and helped to define and promote the new medical specialty of pediatrics. Though the early members of the American Pediatric Society typically did not limit themselves to pediatrics, the group did provide physicians with a prestigious forum for discussion and debate. The topic of infant feeding dominated the meetings of the society for many years after its founding in 1889.[7]

Humanitarianism, prestige, and economics similarly affected physicians' views of patent foods. Some foods, they believed, were harmful; it was the doctor's duty to warn consumers. Even foods that were satisfactory could be dangerous if used incorrectly; physicians emphasized that only a knowledgeable practitioner could safely direct their employment. In addition to these medical reasons, physicians feared that widespread distribution of patent foods without medical consultation reflected poorly on the profession. If a mother could decide for herself which product to buy, what did this say for the vaunted scientific expertise of the physician? Moreover, such a mother had little or no need to see a doctor about her infant's food. This could eliminate a potentially lucrative aspect of medical practice.

Infant-food companies also contributed to the rise of bottle feeding in the United States. Their products were widely advertised and purchased throughout the country. Many users, both medical practitioners and mothers, praised them. How persuasive advertising campaigns were in a woman's initial decision to bottle feed, or in her choice of which food to use, we can not ascertain. Undoubtedly, though, infant-food companies influenced the increasing popularity of physician-directed bottle feeding. Manufacturers' marketing efforts helped to persuade doctors to use their infant foods. Their advertisements and booklets, as well as articles written about their products, helped to make mothers and doctors more aware of the possibilities and advantages of artificial feeding. Their promotions strengthened the idea that bottle feeding could be scientific. By the twentieth century, manufacturers' advertisements directing mothers to doctors and their agreement to distribute bottle-feeding directions only to medical practitioners explicitly affirmed that infant feeding was a medical function.

The responses of physicians, mothers, and infant-food companies to the perceived need for and availability of bottle formulas in the late nineteenth and early twentieth centuries established the legitimacy of artificial infant feeding as a substitute for maternal nursing and as an integral part of medical practice. Subsequently, the domination of physicians in the area of bottle feeding resulted from a series of new medical, cultural, and institutional factors.

The scientific orientation of medical education in the first half of this century meant that physicians increasingly learned more about "scientific" infant feeding—that is, bottle feeding—than breast feeding. Lack of knowledge about lactation made physicians at best indifferent to, if not uncomfortable with, mothers who breast fed. When nursing mothers had problems, their doctors apparently found it easier to suggest weaning than to attempt to correct the problem. Furthermore, though doctors acclaimed breast milk as the best nutrient for the infant, they considered it highly variable and often incomplete. The composition of artificial food, on the other hand, was known and uniform. Additionally, when infants had digestive problems, bottle formulas were easier to manipulate. By the 1920s and 1930s, physicians insisted that the uncertain vitamin content of mother's milk necessitated giving even breast-fed infants supplements of cod-liver oil and orange juice. Since artificial food was safe and healthful and the composition of breast milk was uncertain and incomplete, most doctors did not encourage their patients to breast feed and often preferred bottle feeding.

The assumption that artificial food was a healthful alternative to breast milk at least inadvertently discouraged mothers from a commitment to breast feeding. Especially through publications, but also in classrooms and doctors' offices, women learned about the acceptability and availability of artificial infant feeding. And the specifics of this feeding advice often weakened the dictum that breast milk was the food for infants. For example, all infants, even the breast-fed, needed supplemental food, especially cod-liver oil and orange juice. Also, the widespread promotion of mixed feeding in the early months of life to eliminate the "tied down" feeling suggested that nursing was a chore. Once a mother added a bottle or two a day to her infant's diet, it was less work to wean the child and only feed artificially. Most babies experience some digestive upset or colic; since healthful, safe artificial foods were available and more easily modified than breast milk, some mothers opted to wean their babies who showed signs of gastrointestinal problems. Hospital births too placed mothers in situations in which they observed the ready use of bottle formulas at the slightest hint of insufficient breast milk. Hospital routines and schedules, moreover, created conditions that made lactation failure more likely. Finally, one cannot overlook the symbolism of giving the mother a ready-made bottle of formula as she left the hospital. The message was clear: a bottle was as good as the breast.

Statistics and studies from the third quarter of the twentieth century document that bottle feeding in the United States continued to increase.

Whether citing national or regional studies, whether focusing on urban or rural populations, investigators point to the overwhelming number of bottle-fed babies. One 1972 study reported that in the first week of life less than 30 percent of American infants were fed exclusively at the breast and that by two months more than 80 percent were exclusively on the bottle. Significantly, the authors declared that these statistics were consistent across income levels.[8]

The explanations given for the continued decline of breast feeding were similar to those discussed earlier in the century.[9] In addition, according to a "founding mother" of the La Leche League, mothers in this period who wanted to nurse had little or no information about lactation. Observing that few women had seen babies breast fed, she asserted that even if mothers did know someone who had nursed, usually that woman employed bottle feeding sooner or later. Therefore, the La Leche organizer hypothesized, other women concluded that they might as well start out with a bottle "and save all the switching."[10]

Though artificial infant feeding continued to rise after 1950, the founding of the La Leche League in 1956 suggests a growing reaction against the widespread employment of physician-directed bottle feeding. The organiz-ers recognized that mothers interested in maternal nursing had only limited access to information and could benefit greatly from the experiences of women who had successfully breast fed their infants. In essence, the informal networks of female relatives, neighbors, and friends who had earlier helped women through nursing problems no longer existed. Marian Tompson had tried unsuccessfully to nurse three children. With the encouragement of Gregory White, a family physician, Tompson succeeded in nursing her fourth child. Years later she recalled, "It just didn't seem fair that mothers who bottle feed . . . were given all sorts of help . . . but . . . when a mother was breastfeeding, the only advice she was given was to give the baby cow's milk."[11]

In the summer of 1956, in order to help other women in the community, Tompson and her friend Mary White, wife of Gregory White, decided to offer encouragement and advice to their friends and neighbors through informal classes and an instruction pamphlet. From this small beginning La Leche League groups spread throughout the country. The fact that the leaders of the league were not medical people has been taken as a sign of "demedicalization of breast feeding,"[12] yet the organization did not reject the assistance or imprimatur of the medical profession. From the beginning, the organization included medical consultants and popularized medical research that showed the superiority of breast feeding. However, though the league accepted medical involvement, its primary goal was to reach out, woman to woman, to provide a network of female sharing to counteract the sense of isolation faced by many mothers and to teach new mothers by example in an informal atmosphere. In much the same way that turn-of-the-century mothers described their experiences for the edification of other women, the league sought to give new mothers "the benefit of what we had learned and experienced." Unlike their earlier sisters, though, league members go beyond personal experience and include medical and scientific conclusions to support their work.[13]

For the La Leche League, the decline in breast feeding resulted from women's unfamiliarity with the practice. Others at mid-century connected women's failure to nurse to the hospital experience. Segregated from their infants in the hospital, new mothers had little opportunity to become acquainted with them and to establish lactation during the lying-in period. To ease the transition from hospital to home and to create an environment more conducive to breast feeding, some hospitals in the late 1940s instituted "rooming-in."

Hospitals constructed small nurseries of four to six cribs adjacent to the mothers' rooms. (Still concerned with the possibility of contagion, hospitals hoped that such arrangements would reduce the chance of cross-infection). With the exception of visiting hours, when the nurse would remove the babies to the nursery behind glass walls, the infant and mother, and even the father, could spend the entire day together. One mother interviewed in 1948 remarked, "My baby girl, Diane Margaret, and I will be going home tomorrow, and I know that if I had not been given the privilege of being in Rooming-in, I would be a nervous wreck tonight." No matter how many classes she had attended or how many manuals she had read, she believed that there was no substitute for the experience she had gained through rooming-in. This experience she found especially helpful in the establishment of maternal nursing: "There are many girls today who sincerely want to breast feed their babies, but they are never given the right start in the hospital, and they find themselves going home with a bottle fed baby."[14]

The American Academy of Pediatrics *Standards of Hospital Care* for 1949 declared that with rooming-in hospital attendants could better instruct the mother in "the correct care of her baby before she goes home."[15] And mothers who initially tried rooming-in agreed. One commented, "It's wonderful from a practical point of view to learn how to take care of the baby while you're still in the hospital. Then you have the baby but not the anxiety. You know if there's something you don't understand, the nurse is there to help you." Rooming-in eased the tensions of new motherhood and allowed the mother to become familiar with her infant before leaving the hospital; yet at the same time it enhanced the medicalization of infant feeding by promoting physicians and hospital personnel as the experts on child care.[16]

Organizational and institutional efforts such as the La Leche League and rooming-in apparently did little to slow the increasing employment of bottle feeding in the 1950s and 1960s. However, in the 1970s there appeared a resurgence of breast feeding in the United States. The many infant-feeding surveys of the past decade suffer various methodological shortcomings and are not directly comparable, but all document a similar trend: since the 1970s the proportion of mothers breast feeding has steadily increased, and women are breast feeding their infants longer.

Researchers connected with Ross Laboratories, manufacturers of a popular infant formula, Similac, have published the most complete, comparable set of statistics.[17] They show that in 1970 less than 25 percent of the infants in hospitals were breast fed; by 1978 this figure had climbed to over 46 percent; and by 1981 to 58 percent. Furthermore, mothers continued to breast feed. In 1971 less than 14 percent of infants aged two months received breast milk; within a decade this had more than trebled to over 42 percent. The increased incidence of breast feeding is even more pronounced in the later months. In 1971 at the age of five and six months little more than 5 percent of infants were breast-fed; by 1980 this had more than quadrupled to nearly 25 percent.

The reasons for this upward trend in breast feeding in the United States are not clear, though recent surveys have demonstrated the relationship between infant-feeding practices and various demographic variables. Education and family income are positively associated with the incidence and duration of breast feeding. Social networks play a role in the choice: a woman whose friends are breast feeding is more likely to breast feed. Other investigations have attempted to analyze relationships between ethnicity and employment patterns and infant-feeding practices. All these studies observe many factors associated with the choice of bottle or breast feeding, but causality cannot be inferred from such observations. True, a college-educated woman is more likely to breast feed, yet she does not decide to breast feed because she attended college.[18] Without a clear understanding of the causal factors involved in infant-feeding decisions, it is difficult to design plans to revive interest in maternal nursing. The need for such efforts is more evident outside the United States, in countries where the choice of artificial infant feeding can have a profound effect on infant mortality and morbidity.

"The Baby Killer," a pamphlet produced by War on Want and first published in Britain in March, 1974, focused international attention on the rise of bottle feeding in Third World countries. It particularly condemned the promotion of commercial infant foods. The report and follow-up studies published in the popular press correlated high rates of infant mortality and morbidity with the decline and early termination of breast feeding in communities with poor sanitation, inadequate medical care, and low income levels.[19] In contrast to the United States, for which the task force found it difficult to assess the potential benefits of universal breast feeding,

> the weight of the evidence from less-developed countries strongly supports an inverse association between breast-feeding and overall mortality, between breast-feeding and diarrheal-related mortality and morbidity, and between breast-feeding and mortality and morbidity in the high-risk newborn.

Environmental factors (that is, water supply, food contamination, crowding, personal hygiene, and the like), susceptibility, access to health care, immune status, and nutritional status all contribute to the spread of infection and illness. Obviously, breast feeding alone cannot solve the high rates of infant mortality and morbidity. Nonetheless, the research does suggest that reversing the trend toward bottle feeding and encouraging maternal nursing "can contribute to reducing overall infant and child mortality, morbidity and mortality associated with diarrheal illness, and illness or death in high-risk (low-birth-weight) newborns."[20]

On the surface, the situation evolving in the Third World appears to be recapitulating that which occurred in the United States in the first half of this century, but in a much shorter time span. Though comprehensive longitudinal studies do not exist for most of these countries, the available evidence does document that over the past several decades increasing numbers of Third World women have turned to bottle feeding. The reasons cited for this increase reflect those discussed in this country throughout the twentieth century. Mothers decide to bottle feed because they fear that their milk supplies are deficient or inadequate. The bottle is a status symbol, "the modern thing to do." Urbanization has accelerated the breakup of the extended family and social networks; thus women have less opportunity to learn from the experience of other women. Practices such as separating the mother and child in maternity wards tend to discourage the establishment of breast feeding. Infant-food companies widely advertise their products in promotions that have increasingly come under attack.[21] More research could determine the similarities and differences between the rising popularity of bottle feeding across cultures.[22] And, perhaps, women in Third World countries will in the future also express a renewed interest in breast feeding.

It is not at all certain, however, that the shift to breast feeding among American women represents the beginning of a long-term trend. Moreover, nursing mothers in the 1970s and 1980s are not merely reverting to nine-teenth-century values of infant feeding. True, the call for breast feeding echoes those in the previous century: lactation is "nature's way"; and breast-fed infants are considered healthier than bottle-fed infants. But now proponents also point to scientific evidence, emphasizing the psychological as well as the physiological benefits of breast feeding for both the mother and the child. One physician writes, in a booklet distributed to women through doctors' offices:

> The "new" modern women turns to breast feeding almost as if it were a
> "new" modern method of feeding baby. She regards it as a way to free
> herself from dependence upon mechanical things in what should be a close,
> personal relationship with her baby. This is but one of the many signs about
> us that man [!] is rebelling against the machine and our computerized age.

The author goes on to explain that not only does "Nature" attest to the superiority of breast milk, but so too does "Modern Medical Science." The importance of "science" remains, though the conclusions drawn from contemporary research differ markedly from those expounded just a few decades earlier. Accompanying the scientific rationale for breast feeding is a definitive affirmation of the physician's role in infant feeding. The reader is told that a woman should discuss her infant's nutrition with her physician or clinic and take her instruction in infant feeding, whether breast or bottle, from the medical profession.[23]

Sources as diverse as the Children's Bureau *Infant Care* pamphlet and booklets from infant-food manufacturers present women with similar advice. Mothers have the "privilege to choose" how they will feed their children. Either method, advisors claim, "is highly effective and satisfacory."[24] With both breast feeding and bottle feeding, these publications caution, there may be problems, but doctors can help solve them. A woman should not feel compelled to feed her infant in a manner with which she is uncomfortable:

> Should you breast feed? Yes, if you think it will be comfortable and
> convenient. No, if you have any strong objections to the idea. Modern
> infant formulas and bottle feeding are convenient and safe as a substitute for
> breast feeding. Human milk is probably a little better, especially if members
> of the family have been allergic to cow's milk. Otherwise there is really no
> strong medical, psychological, or economic reason for choosing either breast
> feeding or bottle feeding, so the choice can be made according to your own
> preferences.[25]

Infant-feeding practices have undergone dramatic changes since the last century, when nursing was a mother's duty and artificial feeding an inferior alternative to be used only where breast milk was insufficient. By the early years of the twentieth century, physician-directed bottle feeding had become a satisfactory substitute for mothers unable or unwilling to nurse their infants. The very success of bottle formulas made the use of artificial food increasingly acceptable and popular. In the middle decades of this century, medically controlled infant foods were considered as good as, if not better than, mother's milk; most babies were bottle-fed.

The shift from breast feeding to doctor-supervised bottle feeding resulted, in large part, from the self-conscious promotion of applied science in American life. Yet, as we have seen, this elevation of science had contradictory and unanticipated effects. On the positive side, doctors were better equipped to handle a variety of infant-feeding problems, and the nutrition of some infants improved. Manufacturers produced safer and more healthful artificial foods than had been available. Mothers unable or unwilling to breast feed had better artificial foods for their infants. But, on the negative side, with the widespread use of "scientific" infant foods, not all babies received the food best for them. Not that manufacturers or physicians forced women to bottle feed. Rather, a combination of the ideology of scientific motherhood, confidence in the medical profession, and shrewd media presentation altered the relationship between mothers and physicians and encouraged mothers to seek out commercial and medical solutions to the problems of infant feeding.

The convergence of many forces helped to reshape women's lives in American society and to redefine the parameters of infant feeding by mid-century. The mass media disseminated "scientific" solutions for all sorts of domestic problems and thus sanctioned the importance of science in daily life. The growing household-technology and food industries commercialized women's domestic labor; at the same time, manufacturers provided mothers with simple-to-use artificial infant foods. The medical profession, claiming particular scientific expertise, expanded the role of the private physician and the clinic into preventive, as well as curative, medicine. Widening educational, organizational, and occupational opportunities, which resulted from women's social and political action, drew women outside the home. Still, various forums reinforced the belief that motherhood, especially scientific motherhood, was woman's principal role.

Despite renewed interest in maternal nursing, in the late twentieth century we are living with the legacy of this conjunction of commercial and medical interests with the emerging ideology of scientific motherhood. The majority of American infants are still bottle-fed, the overwhelming proportion of them with commercial foods. And whether women decide to breast feed or to bottle feed, they do so under medical supervision. The history of infant feeding from the late nineteenth century to the mid-twentieth century documents the growing commercialization and medicalization of infant care, raising questions about the interaction of science, medicine, and commerce and illustrating the complexity of cultural change. Above all, it reveals that in their search for healthful infant care, women participated in a redefinition of the maternal role. The ideological, economic, and medical factors that transformed motherhood earlier in the century continue to influence the lives of American women and our sisters throughout the world.

Journal Abbreviations

Alabama Med. & Surg. Age: *Alabama Medical and Surgical Age*

Am. Analyst: *American Analyst*

Am. Assoc. Study & Prev. Inf. Mort.: *American Association for the Study and Prevention of Infant Mortality*

Am. Child Hyg. Assoc.: *American Child Hygiene Association*

Am. Hist. Rev.: *American Historical Review*

Am. J. Dis. Child.: *American Journal of Diseases of Children*

Am. J. Hygiene: *American Journal of Hygiene*

Am. J. Med. Sci.: *American Journal of the Medical Sciences*

Am. J. Obst. & Dis. Women & Children: *American Journal of Obstetrics and Diseases of Women and Children*

Am. J. Obst. & Gynec.: *American Journal of Obstetrics and Gynecology*

Am. J. Pub. Health: *American Journal of Public Health*

Am. Kitchen: *American Kitchen*

Am. Med.: *American Medicine*

Am. Med. Compend: *American Medical Compend*

Am. Med. Month.: *American Medical Monthly*

Am. Med. Quart.: *American Medical Quarterly*

Am. Motherhood: *American Motherhood*

Am. Pub. Health Assoc., Papers & Rep.: *American Public Health Association, Papers and Reports*

Am. Quart.: *American Quarterly*

Am. Studies: *American Studies*

Am. Therapist: *American Therapist*

Ann. Gyn. & Ped.: *Annals of Gynecology and Pediatrics*

Ann. Hyg.: *Annals of Hygiene*

Arch. Dis. Child.: *Archives of Disease in Childhood*

Arch. Ped.: *Archives of Pediatrics*

Atlanta Med. & Surg. J.: *Atlanta Medical and Surgical Journal*

Atlanta Med. Reg.: *Atlanta Medical Register*

Atlantic Med. J.: *Atlantic Medical Journal*

Boston Med. & Surg. J.: *Boston Medical and Surgical Journal*

Brit. Med. J.: *British Medical Journal*

Brooklyn Med. J.: *Brooklyn Medical Journal*

Bull. Hist. Med.: *Bulletin of the History of Medicine*

Chicago Med. Rec.: *Chicago Medical Recorder*

Child Health Bull.: *Child Health Bulletin*

Cleveland Med. Gaz.: *Cleveland Medical Gazette*

Colorado Med.: *Colorado Medicine*

Columbus Med. J.: *Columbus Medical Journal*

Denver Med. Times: *Denver Medical Times*

Diet. Gaz.: *Dietetic Gazette*

Gaillard's Med. J.: *Gaillard's Medical Journal*

Hahneman. Month.: *Hahnemannian Monthly*

Harvard Ed. Rev.: *Harvard Educational Review*

Home Sci.: *Home Science*

Homeo. J. Obst. & Dis. Women & Children: *Homeopathic Journal of Obstetrics and the Diseases of Women and Children*

Hosp. Soc. Serv.: *Hospital Social Service*

Household Mag.: *Household Magazine*

Housewives Mag.: *Housewives Magazine*

Internat. Clinics: *International Clinics*

Internat. J. Health Services: *International Journal of Health Services*

Iowa Med. J.: *Iowa Medical Journal*

J. Am. Culture: *Journal of American Culture*

J. Am. Dietet. Assoc.: *Journal of the American Dietetic Association*

J. Am. Hist.: *Journal of American History*

J. Florida Med. Assoc.: *Journal of the Florida Medical Association*

J. Hist. Med.: *Journal of the History of Medicine and Allied Sciences*

J. Indiana St. Med. Assoc.: *Journal of the Indiana State Medical Association*

Journal Interdisciplinary Hist.: *Journal of Interdisciplinary History*

J. Maine Med. Assoc.: *Journal of the Maine Medical Association*

J. Med. & Sci.: *Journal of Medicine and Science*

J. Med. Ed.: *Journal of Medical Education*

J. Michigan State Med. Soc.: *Journal of the Michigan State Medical Society*

J. Missouri State Med. Assoc.: *Journal of the Missouri State Medical Association*

J. Ped.: *Journal of Pediatrics*

J. Soc. Hist.: *Journal of Social History*

J. South. Hist.: *Journal of Southern History*

JAMA: *Journal of the American Medical Association*

Kentucky Med. J.: *Kentucky Medical Journal*

Ladies' Home J.: *Ladies' Home Journal*

Maryland Med. J.: *Maryland Medical Journal*

Med. Era: *Medical Era*

Med. J. & Rec.: *Medical Journal and Record*

Med. News: *Medical News*

Med. Rec.: *Medical Record*

Med. Times: *Medical Times*

Med. Woman's J.: *Medical Woman's Journal*

Mod. Hosp.: *Modern Hospital*

N.Y. Analyst: *New York Analyst*

N.Y. Med. J.: *New York Medical Journal*

N.Y. St. J. Med.: *New York State Journal of Medicine*

New Eng. J. Med.: *New England Journal of Medicine*

New Eng. Kitchen Mag.: *New England Kitchen Magazine*

New Orleans Med. & Surg. J.: *New Orleans Medical and Surgical Journal*

Pac. Med. J.: *Pacific Medical Journal*

Parents' Mag.: *Parents' Magazine*

Ped.: *Pediatrics*

Pennsylvania Med. J.: *Pennsylvania Medical Journal*

Phila. Med. J.: *Philadelphia Medical Journal*

Pub. Health Reports: *Public Health Reports*

Soc. Rev.: *Socialist Revolution*

South. Med. Rec.: *Southern Medical Record*

Southwestern Med.: *Southwestern Medicine*

Tr. Am. Child Hyg. Assoc.: *Transactions of the American Child Hygiene Association*

Tr. Am. Ped. Soc.: *Transactions of the American Pediatric Society*

Tr. Coll. Physicians Phila.: *Transactions of the College of Physicians of Philadelphia*

Tr. Med. Soc. Wisc.: *Transactions of the Medical Society of Wisconsin*

Tr. Sec. Dis. Child., AMA: *Transactions of the Section on Diseases of Children, American Medical Association*

Virginia Med. Month.: *Virginia Medical Monthly:*

Notes

Chapter I. "The Grand Prerogative of Woman"

1 T. L. Nichols, *Esoteric anthropology: A comprehensive and confidential treatise . . . anatomical, physiological, pathological, therapeutical and obstetrical, hygienic and hydropathic* (New York: T. L. Nichols, 1855), p. 455.

2 L. Emmett Holt, Jr., *The Good Housekeeping book of baby and child care* (New York: Popular Library, 1957, 1959), p. 65.

3 William Buchan, *Advice to mothers, on the subject of their own health; and of the means of promoting the health, strength, and beauty of their offspring* (Boston: Joseph Bumstead, 1809), p. 3.

4 William H. Cook, *Woman's handbook of health: A guide for the wife, mother and nurse*, 5th ed. (Cincinnati: W. H. Cook, 1866), p. 229. See also William P. Dewees, *A treatise on the physical and medical treatment of children* (Philadelphia: Carey, Lea & Carey, 1829); Barbara Welter, "The cult of true womanhood: 1820–1860," *Am. Quart., 18* (2) (1966), 151–174; Carl N. Degler, *At odds: Women and the family in America from the Revolution to the present* (New York: Oxford University Press, 1980), pp. 66–83; Nancy F. Cott, *The bonds of womanhood: "Woman's sphere" in New England, 1780–1835* (New Haven: Yale University Press, 1977); Shelia M. Rothman, *Woman's proper place: A history of changing ideals and practices, 1870 to the present* (New York: Basic Books, 1978); Maxine L. Margolis, *Mothers and such: Views of American women and why they changed* (Berkeley: University of California Press, 1984).

5 Marion Harland [Mrs. Mary Virginia (Hawes) Terhune], *Our baby's first and second years* (New York: Reed & Carnrick, [1887?]), p. 17.

6 Ellen H. Goodell, "Responsibilities of mothers," *Herald of Health, 39* (1865), 42–43.

7 Harmon Knox Root, *The people's medical lighthouse; A series of popular and*

192

scientific essays . . . , 8th ed. (New York: n.p., 1854), p. 171. For more on the importance of the mother's role in the health of her family, see Martha H. Verbrugge, "The social meaning of personal health: The Ladies' Physiological Institute of Boston and vicinity in the 1850s," in Susan Reverby and David Rosner, eds., *Health care in America: Essays in social history* (Philadelphia: Temple University Press, 1979), pp. 45–66; Regina Markell Morantz, "Nineteenth-century health reform and women: A program of self help," in Guenter B. Risse et al., eds., *Medicine without doctors: Home health care in American history* (New York: Science History/USA, 1977), pp. 73–94; Robert Sunley, "Early nineteenth-century American literature on child rearing," in Margaret Mead and Martha Wolfenstein, eds., *Childhood in contemporary cultures* (Chicago: University of Chicago Press, 1955), pp. 150–167; Mary P. Ryan, *Womanhood in America: From colonial times to the present* (New York: New Viewpoints, 1975), pp. 164–168; Regina Markell Morantz, "The 'connecting link': The case for the woman doctor in nineteenth-century America," in Judith Walzer Leavitt and Ronald L. Numbers, eds., 2nd ed., *Sickness and health in America: Readings in the history of medicine and public health* (Madison: University of Wisconsin Press, 1985), pp. 161–172.

8 Lawrence D. Longo, "Obstetrics and gynecology," in Ronald L. Numbers, ed., *The education of American physicians: Historical essays* (Berkeley: University of California Press, 1980), pp. 215–225; Rosemary Stevens, *American medicine and the public interest* (New Haven: Yale University Press, 1971), p. 219; Thomas E. Cone, Jr., *History of American pediatrics* (Boston: Little, Brown, 1979). A small number of physicians already interested in pediatrics in the late nineteenth century founded organizations and publications to disseminate their early research and to promote their emerging specialty. In 1880 such a group announced the formation of the American Pediatric Society. As early as 1868 the *American Journal of Obstetrics and Diseases of Women and Children* included a special section for papers on children's diseases, and separate journals appeared in the 1880s and 1890s: the *Archives of Pediatrics* (1884), the *Transactions of the American Pediatric Society* (1889), and *Pediatrics* (1896).

9 Joel Shew, *Children: Their hydropathic management in health and disease: A descriptive and practical work, designed as a guide for families and physicians* (New York: Fowler and Wells, 1852), p. vii. See also Dorothy Jefferies, "Child feeding in the United States in the nineteenth century," *J. Am. Dietet. Assoc.*, 30 (1954), 335–344; Root, *The people's medical lighthouse* (n. 7), p. 229; H. C. Haven, "A study of infant feeding," *Arch. Ped.*, 3 (1886), 541–542; Charles Warrington Earle, "Society proceedings, 18 August 1884 meeting of the Chicago Medical Society," *JAMA*, 3 (1884), 303; William Henry Cumming, "Artificial human milk," *Atlanta Med. Reg.*, n.s. 2 (1883), 434.

10 J. B. Dunham, *The baby: How to keep it well* (Chicago: Gross & Delbridge, 1885), pp. 34–35. See also H. F. Routh, *Infant feeding and its influence on life; Or, the causes and prevention of infant mortality* (New York: William Wood, 1879), pp. 8–12; Haven, "A study" (n. 9), pp. 541–542; Abraham Jacobi, *Infant diet: A paper read before the Public Health Association of New York* (New York: G. P. Putnam's Sons, 1873), pp. 23–24.

11 H. L. Waldo, "Conditions requiring artificial feeding," *Homeo. J. Obst. & Dis. Women & Children*, *1* (1879–1880), 148–159; Dunham, *The baby* (n. 10), p. 34.

12 Root, *The people's medical lighthouse* (n. 7), p. 337.

13 Thomas Morgan Rotch, "The management of human breast-milk in cases of difficult infantile digestion," *Tr. Am. Ped. Soc.*, *2* (1890), 92–99. See also Robert P. Harris, "Milk as a diet during lactation" *Am. J. Obst. & Dis. Women & Children*, *2* (1869–1870), 675–678.

14 C. Cleveland, "The wet-nurse vs. the bottle," *Arch. Ped.*, *1* (1884), 346. See also "Editorial: Against the wet-nurse," *Boston Med. & Surg. J.*, *113* (1885), 308–309; Shew, *Children* (n. 9), 129, 132–135; George Henry Napheys, *The physical life of woman: Advice to the maiden, wife, and mother* (Philadelphia: George Maclean, 1866), 228–230.

15 J. Lewis Smith, "Recent improvements in infant feeding," *Arch. Ped.*, *6* (1889), 848. Some physicians also sought to bring wet-nursing under medical supervision, claiming that their expert knowledge, particularly through the "scientific" analysis of human milk, made physicians necessary advisors in the selection of wet-nurses as well as infant foods. For more on this point, see Janet Golden, "Medical science and domestic problems: Criticism of wet nurses in the late nineteenth century," paper presented at the Berkshire Conference on the History of Women, June 1984.

16 William H. Cumming, "On a substitute for human milk," *Am. Med. Month.*, *9* (1858), 193–199; William H. Cumming and J. M. Johnson, "The nourishment of children," *Atlanta Med. & Surg. J.*, *7* (1867), 532–540; Cumming, "Artificial human milk" (n. 9), 385–434.

17 Jacobi, *Infant diet* (n. 10), pp. 5–8, 14–23; Albert R. Leeds, "Infant foods," *Tr. Coll. Physicians Phila.*, 3rd ser. 6 (1883), 385–386; J. Lewis Smith, "The hygienic management of the summer diarrhea of infants, I," *Arch. Ped.*, *1* (1884), 425; Cook, *Woman's Handbook* (n. 3), pp. 367–377; Napheys, *The physical life* (n. 14), pp. 230–233; J. F. Gould, "Infant diet," *Arch. Ped.*, *1* (1884), 137–138.

18 The basic formula consisted of two parts cream, one part milk, two parts lime-water, and three parts plain water, with the milk sugar dissolved in the plain water in a ration of 17.75 drachms milk sugar to each pint of plain water. Arthur V. Meigs, "Proof that human milk contains only about one percent casein, with remarks on infant feeding," *Arch. Ped.*, *1* (1884), 219–227, 241: idem, *Milk analysis and infant feeding: A practical treatise on the examination of human and cow's milk, cream,*

194

condensed milk, etc., and directions as to the diet of young infants (Philadelphia: P. Blakiston, 1885), pp. 26, 38–48, 61–86: Cone, *History* (n. 8), pp. 135–136. Pediatric writers of the period often used the terms "casein," "proteid," and "albumenoids" interchangeably. As much as possible I have retained the vocabulary of the original source.

19 "Important facts for the people, published by the officers of the Milk Dealers' Association," Chicago, 1879; Bennett F. Davenport, "Physical and chemical qualities of ordinary cows' milk," presented at the Massachusetts Medical Society, Suffolk District, Section for Clinical Medicine, Pathology and Hygiene, *Boston Med. & Surg. J., 115* (1886), 180–181; Norman Shaftel, "A history of the purification of milk in New York: Or, 'How now, brown cow,'" *N. Y. St. J. Med., 58* (1958), 911–928; Judith Walzer Leavitt, *The healthiest city: Milwaukee and the politics of health reform* (Princeton: Princeton University Press, 1982), pp. 156–189.

20 W. S. Christopher, "Infant feeding," *JAMA, 18* (1892), 644; "Boiled and unboiled milk," *JAMA, 7* (1886), 266; John M. Keating, "The artificial feeding of infants," *Ann. Hyg., 1* (1884–1885), 157; Charles Warrington Earle, "The sterilization of food for infants," *Chicago Med. Rec., 3* (1892), 472–480; J. Amory Jeffries, "On the sterilization of milk and foods for infants," *Am. J. Med. Sci., 95* (1888), 486–496; "Medical progress: Infant feeding," *JAMA, 8* (1887), 320; "New York Academy of Medicine, Section of Pediatrics," *Boston Med. & Surg. J., 119* (1888), 16–17. On the problem of scurvy, see Jack Cecil Drummond and Anne Wilbraham, *The Englishman's food: A history of five centuries of English diet* (London: Jonathan Cape, 1939), pp. 378–379; Ian G. Wickes, "A history of infant feeding: Part V—Nineteenth century concluded and twentieth century," *Arch. Dis. Child., 28* (1953), 495–496; Thomas E. Cone, Jr., *Two hundred years of feeding infants in America* (Columbus, Ohio: Ross Laboratories, 1976), 44–48.

21 Reay Tannahill, *Food in history* (New York: Stein and Day, 1973), pp. 345–346; Drummond and Wilbraham, *The Englishman's food* (n. 20), pp. 375–376; Alice Wood, "The history of artificial feeding of infants," *J. Am. Dietet. Assoc., 31* (1955), 477; W. A. Greene, "The value of malt and Loefland's concentrated Liebig's Food for infants, and an account of their introduction to the medical profession," *South. Med. Rec., 8* (1878), 225–227; Cone, *History* (n. 8), pp. 144–145. On the importance of Liebig's research in the American context, see Margaret W. Rossiter, *The emergence of agricultural science: Justus Liebig and the Americans, 1840–1880* (New Haven: Yale University Press, 1975).

Actually Liebig's formula was not the first commercial infant food. In 1862 an Englishman named Ridge had patented an infant food made from cooked flour, sugar, and bicarbonate of potash. However, Liebig condemned this product because it lacked any cow's milk, an ingredient he considered essential for infant nutrition. He created his own food, in part, as a reaction against this infant food, which he believed to be unsuitable. Though manufactured in England, Ridge's Food was also available in the United States. See Drummond and Wilbraham, *The Englishman's food* (n. 20), p. 376; Cone, *History* (n. 8), p. 145.

22 Henri Nestlé, *Memorial on the nutrition of infants* (Vevey: n.p., 1875), pp. 1–3; Hermann Lebert, *A treatise on milk and Henri Nestlé's Milk Food* (New York: n.p., 1887); Nestlé and Anglo-Swiss Holding Company Limited, *This is your company* (1946), pp. 3–6, 71; Jean Heer, *World events, 1866–1966: The first hundred years of Nestlé*, trans. A. Bradley, et al., (Lausanne, Switzerland: Nestlé, 1966), pp. 29–35, 39–43, 58–64, 78–79.

23 Frank Presbrey, *The history and development of advertising* (Garden City, N.Y.: Doubleday, Doran, 1929), pp. 390–391; *Am. Analyst*, 4 (1888), 257; *The care and feeding of infants* (Boston: Mellin's Food Company, 1904), pp. 11–13.

24 J. S. Hawley, "Liebig's Food for Infants: Remarks made before the Medical Society of the County of Kings" (Brooklyn, c. 1875), p. 12; William C. Wagner, "A few remarks upon Wagner's Infant Food" (Brooklyn: n.p., [1890]), pp. 11–13; Harland, *Our baby's first and second years* (n. 5), pp. 18–20, 35–36; Joe B. Frantz, *Gail Borden: Dairyman to a nation* (Norman: University of Oklahoma Press, 1951), pp. 224–255; George J. Kienzle, *The birth of an industry: The story of Gail Borden* (New York: n.p., 1947); Tannahill, *Food in history* (n. 21), pp. 373–374; "How condensed milk is made," *N. Y. Analyst*, n.s. *1* (7) (1885), 11; "Condensed milk," *Am. Analyst*, n.s. *1* (20) (1885), 9; Francis Marion, *The fine old house* (Philadelphia: Smith Kline, 1980), pp. 7–75.

25 Patrick Campbell, typescript history of the Horlick's Corporation, undated, no pagination, in the Horlick's Corporation Papers, 1873–1974, State Historical Society of Wisconsin, Division of Archives and Manuscripts, Madison, Wisconsin (hereafter referred to as HCP), box 1, folder 1; letter from Frank E. Hartman, executive vice-president, to Harry Hanson, editor of the *New York World-Telegram Almanac,* dated 31 January 1949, in HCP, box 1, folder 1; and patent application, in HCP, box 1, folder 10.

26 *Mellin's Food for Infants and Invalids* (Boston: Doliber-Goodale & Co., 1884).

27 Heer, *World events* (n. 22), pp. 40–42.

28 Hawley, "Liebig's Food" (n. 24).

29 Letter from Hartman to Hanson (n. 25).

30 Compare, for example, Nestlé's advertisement in *Am. Analyst*, 4 (1888), 130, with the one in *Babyhood*, 4 (40) (1888), iv; and that in *JAMA, 12* (1888), 14, with the one in *Babyhood, 5* (52) (1889), viii.

31 Reed & Carnrick advertisement, *JAMA, 13* (1889), 25.

32 Charles Warrington Earle, "Infant feeding," *JAMA, 11* (1888), 154; Simon Baruch, "Artificial infant foods," *Diet. Gaz., 3* (1888), 1–3.

33 "An extensive food laboratory," *Am. Analyst, 2* (1886), 393–398.

34 See, for example, Nestlé's advertisements in *JAMA, 7* (1886).

35 C. P. Putnam, "Nestlé's Food for babies," *Boston Med. & Surg. J., 95* (1876), 551–552.

36 Patent application in HCP, box 1, folder 10; advertisements in journals such as the *Am. Analyst* and *JAMA*.

37 Leeds, "Infant foods" (n. 17); Mellin's advertisement, *JAMA, 4* (1885), iv.

38 Jacobi, *Infant diet* (n. 10), 28–30.

39 George B. Fowler, "Farineous infant foods," *Am. J. Obst. & Dis. Women & Children, 15* (1882), 458–464.

40 Horatio R. Bigelow, "Infant digestion," *Arch. Ped., 1* (1884), 434–436; I. N. Love, *Practical points in the management of some of the diseases of children* (Detroit: George S. Davis, 1891), pp. 22–23; idem, "The problem of infant feeding: Intestinal diseases of children and cholera infantum," *Arch. Ped., 6* (1889), 585–586.

41 "Report of Sub-Committee on Infant Feeding of the American Medical Association, May 1888," *JAMA, 11* (1888), 208.

42 Sylvia D. Hoffert, "Private matters: Attitudes toward childbearing and infant nurture in early-nineteenth-century America," Ph.D. dissertation, Indiana University, 1984; Sally McMillen, "Mothers' sacred duty: Breast-feeding patterns among middle- and upper-class women in the antebellum South," *J. South. Hist., 51* (1985), 333–356.

43 By a mother, "How to prepare cow's milk for babes," *Herald of Health, 51* (1871), 172–173.

44 Fanny B. Workman, "The wet-nurse in the household," *Babyhood, 2* (1886), 142–144; Louise J., "Nursery problems," *Babyhood, 2* (1886), 245–246; A.B.C., "The mother's parliament," *Babyhood, 3* (1887), 352.

45 Helen Maxwell, "Baby's early days," *Ladies' Home J., 5* (7) (1888), 7; Ada E. Hazell, "Timely hints about baby," *Ladies' Home J., 5* (4) (1888), 5.

46 Charles E. Rosenberg, *No other gods: On science and American social thought* (Baltimore: Johns Hopkins University Press, 1976), pp. 2, 4. For more on the relationship between science and medicine in American culture, see Matthew D. Whalen and Mary F. Tobin, "Periodicals and the popularization of science in America, 1860–1910," *J. Am. Culture, 3* (1980), 195–203; Andrew McClary, "Germs are everywhere: The germ threat as seen in magazine articles, 1890–1920," *J. Am. Culture, 3* (1980), 33–46; John Harley Warner, "Science in medicine," in Sally Kohlstedt and Margaret Rossiter, *Osiris: Historical writings on American science,* 2nd ser. *1* (1985): 37–58; Barbara Gutmann Rosenkrantz, "The search for professional order in nineteenth-century American medicine," in Leavitt and Numbers, *Sickness and health* (n. 7), pp. 219–232; Richard Harrison Shryock, *The development of modern medicine: An interpretation of the social and scientific factors involved* (New York: Alfred Knopf, 1947), pp. 273–303; Bar-

bara Ehrenreich and Deirdre English, *For her own good: One hundred fifty years of experts' advice to women* (Garden City, N.Y.: Anchor Press/Doubleday, 1979), 28–82; Paul Starr, *The social transformation of American medicine: The rise of a sovereign profession and the making of a vast industry* (New York: Basic Books, 1982), 4–19, 135–140.

47 Nancy F. Cott, "Introduction," in Nancy F. Cott, ed., *Root of bitterness: Documents of the social history of American women* (New York: E. P. Dutton, 1972), p. 5.

Chapter II. "Establishing the Rules for Substitute Feeding"

1 E. A. Wood, "Address on dietetics," *JAMA, 11* (1888), 38–39. For more on the high rates of infant mortality, see, for example, J. A. Work, "Some of the causes of the great mortality in infancy and childhood," *JAMA, 25* (1895), 618; T. B. Greenley, "The management of infants under a year old, hygienic, dietetic and medicinal," *JAMA, 13* (1889), 507–512; Victor C. Vaughan, "Infantile mortality: Its causation and restriction," *JAMA, 14* (1890), 181–183; Thomas E. Cone, Jr., *History of American pediatrics* (Boston: Little, Brown, 1979), pp. 99–128; Judith Walzer Leavitt, *The healthiest city: Milwaukee and the politics of health reform* (Princeton: Princeton University Press, 1982), 28–30, 174–175, 188–189.

2 Thomas Morgan Rotch, "The general principles underlying all good methods of infant feeding," *Boston Med. & Surg. J., 129* (1893), 505.

3 This was a typical argument for pediatric research in the late nineteenth and early twentieth centuries. See, for example, L. Emmett Holt, "Where does the medical profession stand to-day upon the question of infant feeding?" *Arch. Ped., 14* (1897), 816; Thomas Morgan Rotch, "The artificial feeding of infants," *Arch. Ped., 4* (1887), 458; Wood, "Address on dietetics" (n. 1), pp. 38–39; Arthur V. Meigs, "The artificial feeding of infants," *Tr. Am. Ped. Soc., 1* (1889), 7; A. C. Cotton, "Has the milk laboratory come to stay?" *JAMA, 28* (1897), 1065–1067; Isaac A. Abt, ed., *Abt-Garrison history of pediatrics* (Philadelphia: W. B. Saunders, 1965), p. 130; Harold Kniest Faber and Rustin McIntosh, *History of the American Pediatric Society, 1887–1965* (New York: McGraw-Hill, 1966), pp. 19–20; Cone, *History* (n. 1), pp. 99–101, 131–132.

4 For a few examples, see Albert R. Leeds, "Infant foods," *Tr. Coll. Physicians Phila.,* 3rd ser. 6 (1883), 385–386; George B. Fowler, "Farineous infant foods," *Am. J. Obst. & Dis. Women & Children, 15* (1882), 449–465; Henry Trimble, "An analysis of seven of the most prominent foods for infants and invalids," *Ann. Hyg., 2* (1887), 243–246.

5 Fritz Talbot, "Thomas Morgan Rotch (1849–1914)," in Borden S. Veeder, ed., *Pediatric profiles* (St. Louis, Mo.: C. V. Mosby, 1957), pp. 29–32; "Obituary: Thomas

198

Morgan Rotch, M.D.," *Boston Med. & Surg. J., 170* (1914), 596–597; Charles Hunter Dunn, "Thomas Morgan Rotch, M.D.," *Boston Med. & Surg. J., 172* (1915), 82–84; Abt, *Abt-Garrison history of pediatrics* (n. 3), p. 141; Cone, *History* (n. 1), pp. 104, 126.

6 Rotch, "The general principles" (n. 2), p. 506.

7 Thomas Morgan Rotch, "The value of milk laboratories for the advancement of our knowledge of artificial feeding," *Arch. Ped., 10* (1893), 97–98. Similar sentiments from other physicians may be found in A. C. Cotton, "How shall we feed the baby?" *JAMA, 29* (1897), 1195; E. F. Brush, "The relationship of food to scorbutus in children," *JAMA, 19* (1892), 736; Thomas D. Parke, "The modification of milk," *Alabama Med. & Surg. Age, 10* (1897–1898), 359.

8 Rotch, "The general principles" (n. 2), 505; idem, "Infant-feeding—Weaning," in John M. Keating, ed., *Cyclopaedia of the diseases of children* (Philadelphia: J. B. Lippincott, 1889), vol. 1, pp. 274, 280–281. See also idem, "The management of human breast-milk in cases of difficult infantile digestion," *Tr. Am. Ped. Soc., 2* (1890), 92–99; idem, *Pediatrics: The hygienic and medical treatment of children,* 1st ed. (Philadelphia: J. B. Lippincott, 1895), pp. 159, 181–182, and subsequent editions (1901, 1906). This was not a new claim, but Rotch gave it new urgency. For earlier physicians' calls, see, for example, H. L. Waldo, "Conditions requiring artificial feeding," *Homeo. J. Obst. & Dis. Women & Children, 1* (1879–1880), 148–150; [John] Binnie, "A plea for the artificial feeding of infants with cow's milk," *Arch. Ped., 1* (1884), 648–649; Robert P. Harris, "Milk as a diet during lactation," *Am. J. Obst. & Dis. Women & Children, 2* (1869–1870), 675–678.

9 Rotch, *Pediatrics,* 1895 (n. 8), pp. 153–154.

10 Rotch, "The artificial feeding of infants" (n. 3), 479; Rotch, "Infant-feeding—Weaning" (n. 8), p. 323.

11 Thomas Morgan Rotch, "Proceedings of the Obstetrical Society of Boston: The artificial feeding of infants," *Boston Med. & Surg. J., 117* (1887), 307; Rotch, "Infant-feeding—Weaning," (n. 8), p. 323; Rotch, "Artificial feeding of infants" (n. 3), pp. 479–480. See also Rotch, *Pediatrics,* 1901 (n. 8), p. 156; Rotch, *Pediatrics,* 1906 (n. 8), p. 150.

12 Thomas Morgan Rotch, "Improved methods of modifying milk for infant feeding," *Boston Med. & Surg. J., 127* (1892), 56–59; idem, "The value of milk laboratories for the advancement of our knowledge of artificial feeding," *JAMA, 19* (1892), 56–57. See also idem, "An historical sketch of the development of percentage feeding," *N. Y. Med. J., 85* (1907), 532–537. For more on the development of milk laboratories, see Chapter 4 below.

13 Rotch, *Pediatrics,* 1895 (n. 8), pp. 267–270; and subsequent editions.

14 Rotch, *Pediatrics,* 1895 (n. 8), pp. 231, 270; and subsequent editions.

15 "Review of Thomas Morgan Rotch, *Pediatrics* (1896)," *Boston Med. & Surg. J.,*

133 (1895), 572–573; Henry Dwight Chapin, *The theory and practice of infant feeding, with notes in development* (New York: William Wood, 1902), pp. 205–213; Frank Spooner Churchill, "Observations on infant feeding, with report of cases," *JAMA, 44* (1905), 1653.

16 Cotton, "How shall we feed" (n. 7), p. 1196; Parke, "The modification of milk" (n. 7), 361; Thompson S. Westcott, "The scientific modification of milk," *Internat. Clinics, 3* (1900), 235. For similar praise, see George M. Kober, "Impure milk in relation to infant mortality," *JAMA, 25* (1895), 986–987; C. G. Jennings, "Some recent advances in pediatrics," *JAMA, 21* (1893), 832; Samuel S. Adams, "The evolution of pediatric literature in the United States," *Tr. Am. Ped. Soc., 9* (1897), 30; L. Emmett Holt, *The diseases of infancy and childhood: For the use of students and practitioners of medicine* (New York: D. Appleton, 1897), pp. 172–173; R. O. Beard, "Physiologic principles underlying infant dietary," *JAMA,31* (1898), 1448; William A. Dickey, "The care and feeding of infants," *Am. Med. Compend, 15* (1899), 448–449.

17 Rotch, *Pediatrics,* 1895 (n. 8), pp. 276–281.

18 Holt, *Diseases of infancy,* 1897 (n. 16), pp. 174–177; idem, *Diseases of infancy,* 1902 (n. 16), pp. 148–149, 186–192; idem, "A new method of calculating milk percentages," *Am. J. Obst. & Dis. Women & Children, 64* (1911), 555–558. For other examples, see John Lovett Morse, "The home modification of milk," *Boston Med. & Surg. J., 134* (1896), 557–559; idem, "The principle and limitations of the home modification of milk," *Boston Med. & Surg. J., 139* (1898), 291–293; J. C. Gittings, "The importance of the first steps in artificial feeding of infants," *JAMA, 45* (1905), 1724; Godfrey R. Pisek, "A presentation of the subject of artificial infant feeding for the general practitioner," *Am. J. Obst. & Dis. Women & Children, 58* (1908), 694–704.

19 William L. Baner, "The home modification of milk," *N. Y. Med. J., 67* (1898), 345; Charles W. Townsend, "Remarks on infant feeding, with special reference to the home modification of milk," *Boston Med. & Surg. J., 140* (1899), 275–276.

20 Townsend, "Remarks on infant feeding" (n. 19), 277.

21 Baner, "Home modification" (n. 19), pp. 346–348; Robert S. McCombs, *Diseases of children for nurses,* 4th ed. (Philadelphia: W. B. Saunders, 1923), pp. 399–402.

22 Thomas Morgan Rotch, "The essential principles of infant feeding and the modern methods of applying them," *JAMA, 41* (1903), 418–421; Rotch, *Pediatrics,* 1901 (n. 8), pp. 229–230; Rotch, *Pediatrics,* 1906 (n. 8), p. 189. This chart first appeared in Maynard Ladd, "Percentage modification of milk in infant feeding," *Boston Med. & Surg. J., 148* (1903), 8. In the 1906 edition of *Pediatrics,* Rotch informed his readers that the card "may be obtained of F. H. Thomas Co., 703 Boylston Street, Boston."

23 O. N. Torian, "The evolution and present-day status of infant feeding," *J. Indiana*

St. Med. Assoc., 25 (1932), 78; Lewis Webb Hill and Jesse Robert Gerstley, *Clinical lectures on infant feeding* (Philadelphia: W. B. Saunders, 1917).

24 Some examples of this literature include: Charles W. Townsend, "The use of fat-free milk in infant feeding," *Boston Med. & Surg. J., 158* (1908), 379–381; "Clinical section of the Suffolk District Medical Society," *Boston Med. & Surg. J., 158* (1908), 383–384; Abraham Jacobi, "The gospel of top milk," *JAMA, 51* (1908), 1216–1219; Charles W. Townsend, "Case of fat-free milk in infant feeding," *Am. J. Obst. & Dis. Women & Children,* 57 (1908), 933–934; Thomas S. Southworth, "High fat percentages in infant feeding," *JAMA, 51* (1908), 1219–1222.

25 Frank X. Walls, "Question of the proteids of cow's milk in infancy," *JAMA, 48* (1907), 1391; Joseph Brennemann, "Nutritional disturbances in infancy due to overfeeding," *JAMA, 48* (1907), 1344.

26 Henry Dwight Chapin, "Limitations of caloric method of infant feeding," *Am. J. Obst. & Dis. Women & Children,* 62 (1910), 594–595.

27 Churchill, "Observations on infant feeding," (n. 15), p. 1653.

28 J. S. Fowler, *Infant feeding: A practical guide to the artificial feeding of infants* (London: Oxford University Press, 1909), pp. 113–115. For similar American rationales, see Thomas S. Southworth, "Some important but often neglected factors in infant feeding," *Am. J. Obst. & Dis. Women & Children,* 60 (1909), 1062; Ladd, "Percentage modification" (n. 22), p. 6; Rotch, "The essential principles" (n. 22), p. 353; Thomas S. Southworth, "The trend of pediatric opinion concerning the artificial feeding of infants," *JAMA, 47* (1906), 1085.

29 Rotch, *Pediatrics,* 1906 (n. 8), p. 201.

30 Rotch, "Infant-feeding—Weaning" (n. 8), pp. 324–325; Rotch, *Pediatrics,* 1895 (n. 8), pp. 237–238; Rotch, *Pediatrics,* 1901 (n. 8), p. 177; Rotch, *Pediatrics,* 1906 (n. 8), p. 171.

31 Abraham Jacobi, "Discussion at the New York Academy of Medicine, Section in Pediatrics, 12 May 1892," *Boston Med. & Surg. J., 127* (1892), 460; Rotch, *Pediatrics,* 1895 (n. 8), p. 238. See also Abraham Jacobi, "Milk-sugar in infant feeding," *Tr. Am. Ped. Soc., 13* (1901), 150.

32 Holt, *Diseases of infancy,* 1897 (n. 16), pp. 171–172; E. H. Bartley, "Some points in the chemistry of cow's milk, with reference to infant feeding; with a description of a method for home modification of cow's milk," *Brooklyn Med. J., 14* (1900), 341; B. F. Davenport, "The chemical difference in composition between cow and human milk," *Boston Med. & Surg. J., 129* (1893), 93–96.

33 Brennemann, "Nutritional disturbances" (n. 25), p. 1343. See also Henry Helmholz, "Studies on milk sugar," *Am. Assoc. Study & Prev. Inf. Mort., 1* (1910), 107–114.

34 Thomas Morgan Rotch and John Lovett Morse, "Recent advances made in the scientific study of food stuffs," *Boston Med. & Surg. J., 160* (1909), 244.

35 *The Mellin's Food method of percentage feeding* (Boston: Mellin's Food Company, 1908).

36 Eskay's advertisement, *JAMA, 54* (1910), 52. See also Eskay's advertisement, *JAMA, 56* (1911), 52.

37 Jerome S. Leopold, "The Finkelstein-Meyer method of infant feeding by 'casein milk,'" *Arch. Ped., 27* (1910), 604. For similar discussions, see also Frank C. Neff, "Recent experiences in the artificial feeding of one hundred infants," *JAMA, 57* (1911), 2068-2071; Jules M. Brady, "Experience with albumin milk," *JAMA, 57* (1911), 1970-1972; Thomas S. Southworth, "The dextrins and maltose in infant feeding," *Arch. Ped., 29* (1912), 646-653.

38 Several years earlier, Jacobi had prescribed a gruel made by boiling wheat flour, cooling it, and stirring in a malt extract. Remembering how successful this food had been, Johnson agreed to manufacture a malt sugar.

39 "A glimpse of Mead Johnson" (Evansville, Ind.: Mead Johnson & Company, [1961?]), pp. 8-9; L[ambert] S. Johnson, "Your company—Past, present and future," undated typescript located in "History-Documents" folder, box 2C of Mead Johnson & Company Business Records, 1895-1971, Indiana State University–Evansville, Special Collections, Evansville, Indiana (hereafter referred to as the MJ Collection), pp. 1-2; and "Pablum: A brief history," typescript history in "Pablum" folder, box 25a of MJ Collection.

40 Talbot, "Thomas Morgan Rotch" (n. 5), p. 31.

41 Joseph Brennemann, "Periods in the life of the American Pediatric Society: Adolescence, 1900-1915," *Tr. Am. Ped. Soc., 50* (1938), 65. See also Cone, *History* (n. 1), pp. 137-138; Ladd, "Percentage modification" (n. 22), p. 6; Frederick Fraley, "A rapid and simple method for calculating the caloric value of percentage mixtures," *Arch. Ped., 29* (1912), 123-125.

42 Harry Lowenburg, "Best artificial food mixtures for hospital babies," *Am. J. Obst. & Dis. Women & Children, 71* (1915), 847: John Lovett Morse, commenting on Fritz B. Talbot, "Extremes in infant feeding, the present tendencies," *Boston Med. & Surg. J., 179* (1918), 38; Ralph R. Scobey, "A practical method in infant feeding," *Arch. Ped., 47* (1930), 355-356.

43 Charles Hunter Dunn, *Pediatrics: The hygienic and medical treatment of children (founded upon the teachings of Thomas Morgan Rotch)* (Troy, N.Y.: Southworth, 1917), pp. iii–iv, 277-283; Hill, *Clinical lectures* (n. 23), pp. 17-19; John Lovett Morse and Fritz B. Talbot, *Diseases of nutrition and infant feeding,* 2nd ed. (New York: Macmillan, 1920), pp. 192-193, 214-215; Lewis Webb Hill, "A critical discussion of certain phases in the development of modern infant feeding: Their influence upon present tendencies," *Boston Med. & Surg. J., 182* (1920), 311-320.

202

Chapter III. "A Rational Means of Feeding the Baby"

1 Lewis Webb Hill and Jesse Robert Gerstley, *Clinical lectures on infant feeding* (Philadelphia: W. B. Saunders, 1917), pp. 1, 151.

2 See, for a few examples, Joseph Garland, "Pediatrics in general practice," *Boston Med. & Surg. J.*, *195* (1926), 108; Robert S. McCombs, *Diseases of children for nurses*, 3rd ed. (Philadelphia: W. B. Saunders, 1917), p. 356; Julius Hess, *Principles and practice of infant feeding*, 3rd ed. (Philadelphia: F. A. Davis, 1922), p. xv; and Philip S. Potter, "Basic feeding principles," *Arch. Ped.*, *45* (1928), 718.

3 Simon M. Skole, "Lactose in the treatment of diarrhea and vomiting in infants, with illustrative case reports," *Arch. Ped.*, *50* (1933), 395; see also C. Anderson Aldrich, "Looking forward in pediatrics," *JAMA*, *97* (1931), 363; John Lovett Morse, "Progress in pediatrics," *New Eng. J. Med.*, *206* (1932), 685; Borden S. Veeder, "Third annual meeting of the American Academy of Pediatrics: Round-table discussion on attitudes of and toward children," *J. Ped.*, *5* (1934), 128–129.

4 See, for example, H. M. McClanahan, "The relative morbidity of breast and bottle fed infants," *Tr. Am. Ped. Soc.*, *30* (1918), 185–195; Harold K. Faber and T. Leonard Sutton, "A statistical comparison of weight, growth and morbidity during the first year in breast-fed and bottle-fed babies," *Tr. Am. Ped. Soc.*, *42* (1930), 44–46; Roger H. Dennett and John Dorsey Craig, "A comparative study of infant feeds," *Med. J. & Rec.*, *136* (1932), 133–135; Carl C. Fischer, "The artificial feeding of the healthy normal infant," *Hahneman. Month.*, *69* (1934), 529; Edward T. Wilkes, "Whole milk plus carbohydrates in early infant feeding," *Arch. Ped.*, *56* (1939), 106–113; Arthur M. Yudkin, "Vitamin A research and its clinical application in pediatrics," *J. Ped.*, *12* (1938), 714–715; Philip C. Jeans, "The feeding of healthy infants and children," *JAMA*, *120* (1942), 913–921.

5 Hill, *Clinical lectures* (n. 1), pp. 21–23; J. B. Stone, "Care and feeding of the newborn and the premature from the pediatric viewpoint," *Virginia Med. Month.*, *66* (1939), 159; H. J. Gerstenberger, "Preventive infant feeding—Its simplification," *Am. J. Pub. Health*, *13* (1923), 186–188; Roger H. Dennett, *Simplified infant feeding with seventy-five illustrative cases*, 1st ed. (Philadelphia: J. B. Lippincott, 1915), pp. 250–251; Cornelia Kennedy et al., "The vitamin content of breast milk," *Tr. Am. Ped. Soc.*, *35* (1923), 26–33; Lafred F. Hess et al., "Antirachitic properties developed in human milk by irradiating the mother," *JAMA*, *88* (1927), 24–26; Esther B. Hardisty, "Sunshine and irradiated milk therapy to reduce high incidence of rickets," *Arch. Ped.*, *50* (1933), 549–550; Ralph M. Tyson, "Immediate care of the newborn in relation to neonatal mortality," *JAMA*, *124* (1944), esp. 353–354.

6 Edwards A. Park, "New viewpoints in infant feeding," *Boston Med. & Surg. J.*, *192* (1925), 120–121; "Editorial: Some current views on infant feeding," *JAMA*, *84*

(1925), 752; Edwin A. Riesenfeld, with the assistance of H. L. Lichtenberg, "A comparative study of complementary feedings in 1,182 newborn infants," *Arch. Ped.*, *55* (1938), 553–559; Stone, "Care and feeding" (n. 5), p. 159.

7 Abraham Tow, "Simplified infant feeding: A four hour feeding schedule," *Arch. Ped.*, *51* (1934), 49–50.

8 Manuel M. Glazier, "Comparing the breast-fed and the bottle-fed infant," *New Eng. J. Med.*, *203* (1930), 626–631; Joseph Garland and Mabel B. Rich, "Duration of breast feeding: A comparative study," *New Eng. J. Med.*, *203* (1930), 1279–1282. For similar analyses in which more emphasis is given to environment and education and less to the mode of feeding, see also Rowland Godfrey Freeman, "Infant milk depots," *Arch. Ped.*, *29* (1912), 724–736; George T. Palmer and G. Arthur Blakeslee, "Infant mortality in Detroit," *Am. J. Pub. Health*, *11* (1921), 502–507; Robert Morse Woodbury, *Infant mortality and its causes* (Baltimore: William Wilkins, 1926), p. 149; Samuel Friedman, "Progress in pediatrics: Infant feeding and nutrition," *Am. J. Dis. Child.*, *49* (1935), 153–155. Similar results were reported for Australia and England. See Milton Lewis, "The problem of infant feeding: The Australian experience from the mid-nineteenth century to the 1920s," *J. Hist. Med.*, *35* (1980), 174–187; Carol Dyhouse, "Working class mothers and infant mortality in England, 1895–1914," *J. Soc. Hist.*, *12* (1978), 248–267.

9 Joseph Brennemann, "A contribution to our knowledge of the etiology and nature of hard curds in infants' stools," *Am. J. Dis. Child.*, *1* (1911), 341–359; idem, "Boiled versus raw milk: A experimental study of milk coagulation in the stomach, together with clinical observations on the use of raw and boiled milk," *JAMA*, 60 (1913), 575–582.

10 Brennemann, "Boiled versus raw milk" (n. 9).

11 Brennemann, "Boiled versus raw milk" (n. 9); idem, "The coagulation of cow's milk in the human stomach," *Arch. Ped.*, *34* (1917), 81–117; idem, "Artificial feeding of infants," in Isaac A. Abt, ed., *Pediatrics* (Philadelphia: W. B. Saunders, 1923), vol. 2, pp. 635–636, 651–656; Dr. H. Kent Tenney, interview, 24 September 1979, Madison, Wisconsin.

12 Brennemann, "Artificial feeding" (n. 11), p. 654; idem, *Notes on infant feeding: Maternal and artificial* (Chicago: Harry R. Franham, [1919]), pp. 31–32.

13 Gerstenberger, "Preventive infant feeding" (n. 5), pp. 195, 186.

14 H. J. Gerstenberger et al., "Studies in the adaptation of an artificial food to human milk," *Am. J. Dis. Child.*, *10* (1915), 249–265; H.J. Gerstenberger et al., "A further step in the adaptation of an artificial food to human milk," *Am. J. Obst. & Dis. Women & Children*, *72* (1915), 374–375; H. J. Gerstenberger and H. O. Ruh, "Studies in the adaptation of an artifical food to human milk: II. A report of three years' clinical experience with the feeding of S.M.A. (Synthetic Milk Adapted)," *Am. J. Dis. Child.*, *17* (1919), 1–37; S.M.A. advertisement, *JAMA*, 95

204

(1930), 16; "Unravelling the mysteries of breast milk," *Pulse of pharmacy,* [1962?], p. 11; Harold Kniest Faber and Rustin McIntosh, *History of the American Pediatric Society, 1887–1965* (New York: McGraw-Hill, 1966), p. 98; Thomas E. Cone, Jr., *Two hundred years of feeding infants in America* (Columbus, Ohio: Ross Laboratories, 1976), p. 85.

15 G. F. Fowler et al., "The prevention of the development of rickets in rats by sunlight," *Am. Child. Hyg. Assoc., 12* (1921), 74–91; Ruth A. Guy, "The history of cod liver oil as a remedy," *Am. J. Dis. Child., 26* (1923), 112–116; Henry C. Sherman, "Vitamin D," in *Chemistry of food and nutrition,* 5th ed. (New York: Macmillan, 1937), pp. 446–467; Genevieve Stearns et al., "The effect of vitamin D on linear growth in infancy," *J. Ped., 9* (1939), 1–10; Richard Gubner, "Metabolic background of rickets: An interpretative review," *New Eng. J. Med., 216* (1937), 879–887; Elmer Verner McCollum, *A history of nutrition: The sequence of ideas in nutrition investigations* (Boston: Houghton Mifflin, 1957), pp. 266–290; Cone, *Two hundred years* (n. 14), pp. 6–70.

16 For an interesting example of the controversy, see the correspondence pages of *Boston Med. & Surg. J., 194* (1926), 1196–1197; *195* (1926), 246; and *195* (1926), 292–293.

17 See, for example, Benjamin Kramer and Isaac C. Gittleman, "Vitamin D milk in the treatment of infantile rickets: A clinical assay," *New Eng. J. Med., 209* (1933), 906–916; J. M. Lewis, "Clinical experience with crystalline vitamin D: The influence of the menstruum on the effectiveness of the antirachitic factor," *J. Ped., 6* (1935), 362–373; "Miscellany: Academy of Pediatrics, Symposium on vitamin D milk," *New Eng. J. Med., 212* (1935), 125–126; Milton Rapoport, "The antirachitic value of irradiated evaporated milk and irradiated whole fluid milk in infants," *J. Ped., 8* (1936), 154–160; Martha M. Eliot et al., "A study of the comparative value of cod liver oil, viosterol, and vitamin D milks in the prevention of rickets and of certain basic factors influencing their efficacy," *J. Ped., 9* (1936), 355–376; Cone, *Two hundred years* (n. 14), pp. 70–72.

18 Maurice Ostheimer, "The prevention of summer diarrhea," *JAMA, 45* (1905), 594–597.

19 Clifford Groselle Grulee, *Infant feeding,* 1st ed. (Philadelphia: W. B. Saunders, 1912), p. 115. See also subsequent editions of Grulee's text (1914, 1917, 1922); Rowland G. Freeman, "Pasteurization of milk," *JAMA, 54* (1910), 372–373; Eugene A. Darling, "The use of whole milk and fat diminished milk in infant feeding," *Boston Med. & Surg. J., 165* (1911), 747–753.

20 Grulee, *Infant feeding,* 1917 (n. 19), pp. 133–135; "Therapeutics: The care of infants," *JAMA, 59* (1912), 720–721; Brennemann, "Artificial feeding" (n. 11), pp. 667–679.

21 See, for example, Joseph Garland, "Milk and the public health" *Boston Med. &*

Surg. J., 189 (1923), 460–464; "Editorial department: Raw vs. heated milk, *New Eng. J. Med., 207* (1932), 849.

22 "Editorial: Milk—Safe or unsafe?" *Boston Med. & Surg. J., 188* (1923), 177; M. J. Rosenau, "Vitamins in milk," *Boston Med. & Surg. J., 184* (1921), 455–458; Brennemann, "Artificial feeding" (n. 11), 667–679; S. V. Layson, "Facts and fallacies about milk," *Hygeia, 13* (1935), 350–352.

23 Henry J. Gerstenberger et al., "Observations on the effect of aging on the potency of spray-dried antiscorbutic material," *J. Ped., 3* (1933), 93–111.

24 Williams McKim Marriott, *Infant nutrition: A textbook of infant feeding for students and practitioners of medicine* (St. Louis, Mo.: C. V. Mosby, 1930), pp. 129–130; Borden S. Veeder, "Williams McKim Marriott (1885-1936)," in Borden S. Veeder, ed., *Pediatric profiles* (St. Louis, Mo.: C. V. Mosby, 1957), p. 222.

25 Lewis Webb Hill, "A critical discussion of sugar in its relation to infant feeding," *Boston Med. & Surg. J., 179* (1918), 14; John Lovett Morse and Fritz B. Talbot, *Diseases of nutrition and infant feeding,* 2nd ed. (New York: Macmillan, 1920), pp. 205–210; Brennemann, "Artificial feeding" (n. 11), p. 644; Cone, *Two hundred years* (n. 14), p. 79.

26 Veeder, "Marriott" (n. 24), p. 223; Marriott, *Infant nutrition* (n. 24), pp. 41–47; F. W. Schlutz and Elizabeth M. Knott, "The use of honey as carbohydrate in infant feeding," *J. Ped., 12* (1938), 465–473; F. W. Schlutz et al., "The comparative values of various carbohydrates used in infant feeding," *J. Ped., 12* (1938), 716–724.

27 Martin L. Bell, *A portrait of progress: A business history of Pet Milk Company from 1885 to 1960* (St. Louis, Mo.: Pet Milk Company, 1962), pp. 101–102.

28 Bell, *Portrait* (n. 27), pp. 26–35, 41–42, 160; John D. Weaver, *Carnation: The first seventy-five years, 1899-1974* (Los Angeles: Carnation Company, 1974), pp. 23–28, 221–227; James Marshall, *Elbridge A. Stuart: Founder of Carnation Company* (Los Angeles: Carnation Company, 1970), pp. 52–57, 66–84; O. L. Stringfield and James Tobey, "The advantages and limitations of condensed milk in infant feeding," *Arch. Ped., 47* (1930), 769–778.

29 Williams McKim Marriott and Ludwig Schoenthal, "An experimental study of the use of unsweetened evaporated milk for the preparation of infant feeding," *Arch. Ped., 46* (1929), 135–148; Williams McKim Marriott, "Preparation of lactic acid milk mixtures for infant feeding," *JAMA, 89* (1927), 862–863; idem, "Practical points in the feeding and care of infants," *J. Missouri State Med. Assoc., 25* (1928), 411–415; Cone, *Two hundred years* (n. 14), pp. 83–84.

30 Frank E. Rice, "The use of unsweetened evaporated milk in infant feeding," *Arch. Ped., 44* (1927), 758–765; Lillian Kositza, "A comparative study on the use of unsweetened evaporated milk and bottled cow's milk in infant feeding," *J. Ped., 1* (1932), 426–434: W. Quillian, "Evaporated milk in infant feeding: A clinical study

of 340 cases," *J. Florida Med. Assoc.*, 20 (1934), 291–295; C. T. Williams and A. O. Kastler, "A comparison of the nutritional and growth values of certain infant foods," *J. Ped.*, 4 (1934), 454–464; Charles Gilmore Kerley, "Evaporated milk in infant feeding," *Arch. Ped.*, 49 (1932), 22–26.

31 Marriott and Schoenthal, "An experimental study" (n. 29), pp. 146–147; Marriott, *Infant nutrition* (n. 24), pp. 141–144; Julian Deigh Boyd, *Nutrition of the infant and child* (New York: National Medical Book Co., 1937), pp. 92–95.

32 Robert A. Strong et al., "The antirachitic properties of irradiated evaporated milk fed to normal babies under home conditions," *J. Ped.*, 7 (1935), 21–36; Clifford G. Grulee et al., "Irradiated evaporated milk as a food for infants: A study of growth, elimination, protection from rickets and morbidity in upper respiratory infections in comparative groups fed on irradiated and nonirradiated evaporated milk," *J. Ped.*, 14 (1939), 725–729; Marshall, *Elbridge A. Stuart* (n. 28), pp. 185–186, 253–254; Weaver, *Carnation* (n. 28), pp. 84–86; Bell, *Portrait* (n. 27), pp. 146–147.

33 Alice D. Weber, "Dried milks for infant feeding—A resume," *Arch. Ped.*, 42 (1925), 735–742; James A. Tobey, "Recent clinical experiences with 3,800 infants on evaporated, powdered and condensed milks: A review," *Arch. Ped.*, 50 (1933), 183–191.

34 M.C.P., "Obituaries: Roger H. Dennett, M.D., 1876–1935," *Am. J. Dis. Child.*, 49 (1935), 742–743; Dennett, *Simplified infant feeding* (n. 5), p. 37. By the 1930s other professors of pediatrics had published articles on the simplified methods they taught their students. See, for example, Ralph R. Scobey, "The importance of infant feeding to the general practitioner," *Arch Ped.*, 50 (1933), 110–122; Louis Sauer, "A simple, inexpensive stock formula for young infants," *J. Ped.*, 1 (1932), 194–202.

35 Roger H. Dennett, "The teaching of infant feeding: Past and present," *Arch. Ped.*, 48 (1931), 226.

36 Dennett, *Simplified infant feeding* (n. 5), pp. 4–9.

37 See, for example, Morse and Talbot, *Diseases of nutrition* (n. 25), pp. 229–235; Maynard Ladd, "The feeding of the normal infant at birth," *Boston Med. & Surg. J.*, 196 (1927), 50–53.

38 Ralph R. Scobey, "A practical method in infant feeding," *Arch. Ped.*, 47 (1930), 355–368; Tyson, "Immediate care" (n. 5), p. 354.

39 For example, Dennett, *Simplified infant feeding* (n. 5), pp. 327–338; Hill, *Clinical lectures* (n. 1), p. 53.

40 Marriott, *Infant nutrition* (n. 24), pp. 155–159; Grulee, *Infant feeding*, 1922 (n. 19), pp. 182–184, 186: Louis Webb Hill, "A critical discussion of certain phases in the development of modern infant feeding: Their influence upon present tendencies," *Boston Med. & Surg. J.*, 182 (1920), 11–12.

41 Ralph N. Shapiro, "A critical study of 97 infants fed on Lactogen," *Arch. Ped.*, 50 (1933), 437–440; Adolph G. DeSanctis et al., "A critical clinical study of concen-

trated and dried infant foods: II. Modified dried milk," J. Ped., 1 (1932), 704–718. (Though this article does not mention Lactogen by name, internal evidence and the Lactogen advertisement in *JAMA, 100* (1933), 8, indicate that the product studied was Lactogen.) Another clinical test of Lactogen is reported in H. R. Litchfield, "Value of properly modified powdered milk in infant feeding," *Arch. Ped., 49* (1932), 327–329. For instances of research funded by commercial concerns, see P. C. Jeans et al., "Factors possibly influencing the retention of calcium, phosphorus, and nitrogen by infants given whole milk feedings," *J. Ped., 8* (1936), 403–414 (funded by Mead Johnson); Harold E. Harrison, "The retentions of nitrogen, calcium, and phosphorus of infants fed sweetened condensed milk," *J. Ped., 8* (1936), 415–419 (funded by Borden's); C. Dixon Fowler, "Observations on feeding infants with low fat and otherwise modified evaporated milk," *Arch. Ped., 56* (1939), 535–538 (funded by Borden's); William H. Clark, "The value of irradiated milk in infant feeding," *Arch. Ped., 55* (1938), 178–184 (funded by the Wisconsin Alumni Research Foundation).

42 Lewis Webb Hill, *Practical infant feeding* (Philadelphia: W. B. Saunders, 1920), pp. 225–226; Morse and Talbot, *Diseases of nutrition* (n. 25); and Charles Hunter Dunn, *Pediatrics: The hygienic and medical treatment of children (Founded upon the teachings of Thomas Morgan Rotch)* (Troy, N.Y.: Southworth, 1917), pp. 291–292, 299.

43 Tow, "Simplified infant feeding" (n. 7), pp. 49–50.

44 R. Cannon Eley, "Medical progress: Artificial feeding of infants," *New Eng. J. Med., 225* (1941), 232.

Chapter IV. "For Humanity's Sake"

1 J. B. Casebeer, "Who shall treat the children?" *Arch. Ped., 1* (1884), 735–743.

2 Augustus Caillé, "The need for post-graduate instruction in pediatrics," *Tr. Am. Ped. Soc., 20* (1908), 171–173.

3 E. W. Saunders, "Infant feeding," *Med. Rec., 33* (1888), 421. See also, for example, W. Thornton Parker, "The mother's parliament," *Babyhood, 3* (1887), 313–314; William Z. Holliday, "Bottle-fed babies," *Ped., 13* (1902), 43–54.

4 Nineteenth- and twentieth-century practitioners expressed their views on infant feeding and described their personal experiences with bottle feeding in letters and articles in medical and nonmedical journals, as well as papers and comments at national and local medical meetings. For the opinions of twentieth-century doctors, these published data can be supplemented with interviews with physicians in practice from the third decade of this century to the present.

5 J. Noer, "Substitute infant feeding in general practice," *Tr. Med. Soc. Wisc., 34* (1900), 384. See also Frederic M. Warner, "The sterilization of milk," *Med. Rec.,*

34 (1888), 244; Cyrus Edson, "Artificial feeding of infants," *Gaillard's Med. J., 56* (1893), 557; George Byrd Harrison, "A lecture on artificial feeding," *Arch. Ped., 3* (1886), 346; H. M. McClanahan, "Artificial feeding of infants," *Am. J. Obst. & Dis. Women & Children, 33* (1896), 660; L. Boorse, "Substitute feeding of infants, with special reference to the percentage method, and home modification of cow's milk, *Tr. Med. Soc. Wisc., 34* (1900), 372; Isaac A. Abt, *Baby doctor* (New York: Whittlesey House, McGraw-Hill, 1944), pp. 109–110.

6 W. Nicholas Lackey, "Pediatric practice in the small towns and country," *Ped., 25* (1913), 367, 374. For a similar sentiment in an urban setting, see John Zahorsky, *From the hills: An autobiography of a pediatrician* (St. Louis, Mo.: C. V. Mosby, 1949), pp. 134–135.

7 J. M. Keating, "A few practical notes," *Arch. Ped., 10* (1893), 842–843. See also W. A. Edmonds, *A treatise on diseases peculiar to infants and children* (New York: Boericke & Tafel, 1881), p. vii; Louis Fischer, *Infant-feeding in its relation to health and disease* (Philadelphia: F. A. Davis, 1901), p. v.

8 A. W. Kratzsch, "Infant feeding," *Tr. Med. Soc. Wisc., 32* (1898), 411–417. For more on practitioners' views of the relationship between poor nutrition and infant mortality and morbidity, see H. C. Haven, "A study of infant feeding," *Arch. Ped., 3* (1886), 530–532; Frederic M. Warner, "The proper feeding of infants," *Med. Rec., 49* (1893), 78–79; Charles H. S. Davis, "Hints upon the rearing of hand-fed children," *Virginia Med. Month., 6* (1879–1880), 49–55; O. H. Phelps, "Feeding the young," *JAMA, 15* (1890), 744–745; J. A. Work, "Some of the causes of the great mortality in infancy and childhood," *JAMA, 25* (1895), 618–619.

9 R. B. Gilbert commenting at the 1903 AMA meeting, *JAMA, 40* (1903), 1708; James Burns, "The first principles of homo-culture," *Herald of Health, 46* (1868), 163–166; H. L. Waldo, "Conditions requiring artificial feeding," *Homeo. J. Obst. & Dis. Women & Children, 1* (1879–1880), 148–159; Jerome Walker, "Is nursing by the mother to be encouraged?" *Arch. Ped., 2* (1885), 1–10; J. B. Dunham, *The baby: How to keep it well* (Chicago: Gross & Delbridge, 1885), p. 34; I. N. Love, "The problem of infant feeding—Intestinal diseases of children and cholera infantum," *Arch. Ped., 6* (1889), 584; Nathan Allen, "'The decline of suckling power among American women," *Babyhood, 5* (1889), 111–115; W. C. Borden, "The vital statistics of an Apache indian community," *Boston Med. & Surg. J., 129* (1893), 8; Robert Meade Smith, "The modification of cow's milk for infant food," *Denver Med. Times, 16* (1896–1897), 426; A. K. Bond, "The era of the child," *Babyhood, 14* (1898), 107; "Society proceedings: Illinois State Medical Society, 1898," *JAMA, 30* (1898), 1351; David E. Bowman, "The practical application of physiologic principles in infant dietary," *Am. Med. Compend, 15* (1899), 71; William A. Dickey, "The care and feeding of infants," *Am. Med. Compend, 15* (1899), 447; Alexander McAlister, "Infant-feeding," *JAMA, 35* (1900), 209–210; Edward F. Brush, "How to produce milk for infant feeding," *JAMA, 43* (1904), 1385; Loren Johnson, "The

necessity for the artificial feeding of infants," *Am. J. Obst. & Dis. Women & Children, 57* (1908), 671–675; "Washington Obstetrics and Gynecology Society," *Am. J. Obst. & Dis. Women & Children, 57* (1908), 738–739.

10 See, for example, Willard Parker, "A physiological view of the woman question," *Hearth & Home, 1* (1869), 760; Charles G. Kerley, "The management of infants during the summer," *Babyhood, 10* (1894), 225; R. Tunstall Taylor, "Recent improved methods of infant feeding, with especial reference to modified milk," *Med. News, 66* (1895), 572; S. H. Dessau, "Mother's milk as an infant food," *Ped., 5* (1898), 497–498; Edward Hamilton, "Percentage modification of cow's milk for infant feeding," *Am. J. Obst. & Dis. Women and Children, 44* (1901), 487–492; Thomas S. Southworth, "The modification of breast-milk by maternal diet and hygiene," *Med. Rec., 61* (1902), 656–658.

11 Contemporary discussions of wet-nursing and its problems will be found in I. N. Love, *Practical points in the management of some of the diseases of children* (Detroit: George S. Davis, 1891), pp. 17–18; C. Cleveland, "The wet-nurse vs. the bottle," *Arch. Ped., 1* (1884), 346; Charles Warrington Earle, "Summer diseases of children, and infant diet," *Arch. Ped., 1* (1884), 559; R. O. Beard, "The causes of infant mortality," *Am. Pub. Health Assoc., Papers & Rep., 15* (1890), 90–91; Frank Spooner Churchill, "Infant feeding," *Chicago Med. Recorder, 10* (1896), 109; Kratzsch, "Infant feeding" (n. 8), 412–413; J. M. G. Carter, "The artificial feeding of infants in gastro-intestinal disturbances," *JAMA, 31* (1898), 1348; B. F. Gibbs, "Some observations on the artificial feeding of infants," *Am. Med. Month., 16* (1898–1899), 407; Nathan Oppenheim, *The care of the child in health* (New York: Macmillan, 1900), pp. 75–76. See also Chapter 1. For a historical treatment of the topic of wet-nursing, see Janet Golden, "From breast to bottle: The decline of wet nursing in Boston, 1867–1927," Ph.D. dissertation, Boston University, 1884.

12 Benjamin Edson, "Condensed milk for bottle-fed babies," *Arch. Ped., 1* (1884), 745–746. Similar views are expressed in Charles G. Kerley, "Dentition," *Babyhood, 10* (1894), 73; J. P. Crozer Griffith commenting at the 1897 AMA meeting, *JAMA, 29* (1897), 1200; William H. Wells, "Some personal experiences in infant feeding," *JAMA, 31* (1898), 1012–1013; J. P. Crozer Griffith commenting at the 1898 AMA meeting, *JAMA, 31* (1898), 1106; W. F. Boggess commenting at the Falls City Medical Society, *Ped., 8* (1899), 167–169; Edward Reynolds commenting at the Obstetrical Society of Boston, *Boston Med. & Surg. J., 143* (1900), 371; Southworth, "Modification of breast-milk" (n. 10); Effa V. Davis, "Observations on breast feeding from an obstetrician's point of view," *JAMA, 40* (1903), 1697–1700; Carlyle Pope, "Substitute infant feeding," *Am. J. Obst. & Dis. Women & Children 47* (1903), 431–432; "Proceedings of the section on Diseases of children, 1908," *JAMA, 50* (1908), 2089; Nicholas Wade, "Bottle-feeding: Adverse effects of a Western technology," *Science, 184* (1974), 45–48.

13 Brush, "How to produce milk" (n. 9), 1385; Boggess at Falls City Medical Society

(n. 12); John Binnie, "A plea for the artificial feeding of infants with cow's milk," *Med. Rec., 26* (1884), 287; "Maine Medical Association," *Boston Med. & Surg. J., 112* (1885), 626; E. W. Bogardus, "Infant feeding," *Med. Rec., 38* (1890), 139; Beard, "Causes of infant mortality" (n.11); Philip F. Barbour, "The feeding of infants," *Am. Therapist, 4* (1895–1896), 70; Carter, "The artificial feeding" (n. 11), 1349.

14 Waldo, "Conditions requiring artificial feeding" (n. 9), 141–142, 147; "American Pediatric Society," *Boston Med. & Surg. J., 141* (1899), 368; McAlister, "Infant-feeding" (n. 9), 210; John Zahorsky, "Mixed feeding of infants," *Ped., 11* (1901), 208–215; Henry Dwight Chapin, *The theory and practice of infant feeding, with notes on development* (New York: William Wood, 1902), p. 194; Southworth, "Modification of breast-milk" (n. 10); Henry Enos Tuley, "Every-day problems in infant feeding," *JAMA, 40* (1903), 1640; H. M. McClanahan, "What should be taught about mixed feeding?" *JAMA, 53* (1909), 587; Maurice Ostheimer, "Help the mother nurse her child," *JAMA, 53* (1909), 521; Whitridge J. Williams, "What the obstetrician can do to prevent infantile mortality," *Am. Assoc. Study & Prev. Inf. Mort., 1* (1910), 198–199.

15 Edson, "Condensed milk" (n. 12).

16 J. Milton Mabbott, "The theory and practice of infant feeding," *N. Y. Med. J., 53* (1891), 446–452. See also "Report of sub-committee on infant feeding [1888 AMA meeting]," *Boston Med. & Surg. J., 118* (1888), 504–505; "Report on meeting of Oct 20-23, 1891 of American Public Health Association," *JAMA, 17* (1891), 846–847; "Correspondence: Shall we continue to sterilize milk for infants," *JAMA, 25* (1895), 1145–1146; "Societies: Maryland Public Health Association," *JAMA, 34* (1900), 1669; John T. Winter, "How shall we feed the baby?" *Am. J. Obst. & Dis. Women & Children, 33* (1896), 49, 126–127.

17 Joseph Brennemann, "Periods in the life of the American Pediatric Society: Adolescence, 1900–1915," *Tr. Am. Ped. Soc., 50* (1938), 65–66; "Medical progress: Sterilized milk," *JAMA, 11* (1888), 234; "Report of Massachusetts Medical Society, Suffolk County Section for Clinical Medicine, Pathology and Hygiene," *Boston Med. & Surg. J., 119* (1888), 286; Charles Warrington Earle, "The sterilization of food for infants," *Chicago Med. Recorder, 3* (1892), 475; Abraham Jacobi, "Infant feeding—A review," *Ped., 1* (1896), 6–7; Louis Waldstein, "A new apparatus for the sterilization of milk for the feeding of infants and invalids," *Med. Rec., 44* (1893), 140–141; John Lovett Morse, "The home modification of milk," *Boston Med. & Surg. J., 136* (1897), 230; Luther S. Harvey, "Infant feeding," *Ann. Gyn. & Ped., 11* (1897–1898), 854.

18 See, for example, W. C. Bennett, "The hygiene of milk and its relation to infant feeding," *Tr. Med. Soc. Wisc., 32* (1898), 422–423.

19 Leroy M. Yale, "Private interests and public duty in guarding the milk supply,"

Babyhood, 9 (1893), 72–74; "Ohio Medical Society, May 1894," *JAMA,* 22 (1894), 885–886; "Society proceedings: New Jersey State Medical Society, 1897," *JAMA,* 29 (1897), 129–132; Leroy M. Yale, "The meaning of clean milk," *Babyhood, 14* (1898), 183–185; "American Public Health Association, 1899," *Boston Med. & Surg. J., 141* (1899), 577–578; Noer, "Substitute infant feeding" (n. 5), 388–393; J. Ross Snyder, "Suggestions for reducing the prevalence of summer diarrheas in infants," *JAMA, 40* (1903), 1644; Charles Alfred Dukes, "Home modification of cow's milk," *Pac. Med. J., 48* (1905), 394–398; Charles Harrington, "The sanitary importance of clean milk," *Boston Med. & Surg. J., 154* (1906), 121–124; George W. Goler, "Municipal regulation of the milk supply," *JAMA, 49* (1907), 1077–1079; William Krauss commenting at the Tri-State Medical Association of Mississippi, Arkansas, and Tennessee, *JAMA, 55* (1910), 2091.

20 Thomas E. Cone, Jr., *History of American pediatrics* (Boston: Little, Brown, 1979), pp. 144–145; Alice Wood, "The history of artificial feeding of infants," *J. Am. Dietet. Assoc., 31* (1955), 479–480; Judith Walzer Leavitt, *The healthiest city: Milwaukee and the politics of health reform* (Princeton: Princeton University Press, 1982), pp. 152–189; "Public health: Milk for the poor," *JAMA, 23* (1894), 127; "Public health: To reduce infant mortality," *JAMA, 25* (1895), 38; "Medical notes: The distribution of sterilized milk," *Boston Med. & Surg. J., 135* (1896), 249; S. E. Getty, "Pasteurized milk: As dispensed in Yonkers and a study of the effect on infant mortality," *N. Y. Med. J., 66* (1897), 484–489, 508–510; "Public health: Death rates in Brooklyn reduced by the use of pasteurized milk," *JAMA, 29* (1897), 815; "Society proceedings: Medical Society of the State of New Jersey," *JAMA, 31* (1898), 240–241; "Editorial: The Straus Milk Depots in New York," *Boston Med. & Surg. J., 147* (1902), 362; "Medical news," *JAMA, 41* (1903), 42, 1213; Abt, *Baby doctor* (n. 5), pp. 130–133; George W. Goler, " 'But a thousand a year': The cost and the results in Rochester of feeding clean milk as food for the hand-fed baby," *Charities, 14* (1905), 966–973; "The Boston Milk Fund," *Boston Med. & Surg. J., 156* (1907), 859–860; S. E. Getty, "Infant mortality in the summer months: Methods adopted in Yonkers for its reduction and the results," *JAMA, 50* (1908), 1008–1011; Wilbur C. Phillips, "Infants' milk depots and infant mortality," *Am. Assoc. Study & Prev. Inf. Mort., 1* (1910), 77–88.

21 E. F. Brush, "Cow's milk for infant food," *JAMA, 13* (1889), 732–738; Fischer, *Infant-feeding* (n. 7), pp. 131–132. A representative sample of advertisements for Brush's milk may be found in various issues of *Babyhood* from 1894 to 1902.

22 Henry L. Coit, "A plan to procure cow's milk designed for clinical purposes," quoted in Robert H. Bremner, ed., *Children and youth in America: A documentary history,* vol. 2 (Cambridge: Harvard University Press, 1971), p. 868. Much of the information in the following two paragraphs has been drawn from Manfred J. Wasserman's thorough study, "Henry L. Coit and the certified milk movement in

the development of modern pediatrics," *Bull. Hist. Med., 46* (1972), 359–390. See also Leavitt, *The healthiest city* (n. 20); "Medical progress: Certified milk," *Babyhood, 12*, no. 137 (1896), xviii–xix; Richard Cole Newton, "The initial contamination of milk," *JAMA, 43* (1904), 1387–1391; C. W. M. Brown, "Certified milk in small cities," *JAMA, 48* (1907), 587–588; "Correspondence: Certified milk," *Boston Med. & Surg. J., 158* (1908), 467; Wilbur C. Phillips, "A plan for reducing infant mortality in New York City," *Med. Rec., 73* (1908), 890–894.

23 S. B. Sherry [*sic*], "A good infant food," *Am. J. Obst. & Dis. Women & Children, 16* (1883), 332; George B. Fowler, "A method of artificial infant feeding," *Med. Rec., 38* (1890), 42–43. See also Selden B. Sperry, "The best substitute for mother's milk," *JAMA, 7* (1886), 486–487; H. M. McClanahan commenting at AMA meeting, *JAMA, 31* (1898), 1105; George A. B. Hays, "Substitute for the mother's milk during infancy," *New Orleans Med. & Surg. J.,* n.s. *5* (1877–1878), 872–875; Bogardus, "Infant feeding" (n. 13); J. F. Gould, "Infant diet," *Arch. Ped., 1* (1884), 136–138; Binnie, "A plea for the artificial feeding" (n. 13): Curvier R. Marshall, "A practitioner's experience in infant-feeding," *N. Y. Med. J., 52* (1890), 237–238; Phelps, "Feeding the young" (n. 8).

24 Bogardus, "Infant feeding" (n. 13).

25 McClanahan commenting at AMA meeting (n. 23).

26 See, for example, Davis, "Hints" (n. 8); John M. Keating, "Clinical lectures: Infant feeding," *Arch. Ped., 1* (1884), 89–91.

27 Sherry, "A good infant food" (n. 23); Sperry, "The best substitute" (n. 23).

28 Gould, "Infant diet" (n. 23).

29 Binnie, "A plea for the artificial feeding" (n. 13).

30 Warner, "The sterilization of milk" (n. 5); Edmonds, *A treatise* (n. 7), p. 17; Marshall, "A practitioner's experience" (n. 23); W. S. Christopher, "Infant feeding," *JAMA, 18* (1892), 641–646; William Dickey, "Infant feeding," *Columbus Med. J., 15* (1895), 196–197.

31 Henry Dwight Chapin, "The question of gruels in the feeding of infants," *Med. Rec., 56* (1899), 181–183; Chapin, "The place of cereal in infant feeding," *Med. Rec., 60* (1901), 4–7; J. Frank Kahler, "Infant feeding and foods," *Med. Rec., 53* (1898), 335–336; "Medical Society of the State of New York, Jan. 1901," *Boston Med. & Surg. J., 144* (1901), 166; Gibbs, "Some observations" (n. 11); John D. Nourse, "Jacobi's food," *Clinic* (Cincinnati), *5* (1873), 287; Fowler, "A method of artificial infant feeding" (n. 23); Boggess at Falls City Medical Society (n. 12).

32 Chapin, *Theory and practice* (n. 14), p. 3; L. T. Royster commenting on Roger Dennett, "The teaching of infant feeding: Past and present," *Arch. Ped., 48* (1931), 236; August Caillé at the 1908 meeting of the American Pediatric Society, quoted in Harold Kniest Faber and Rustin McIntosh, *History of the American Pediatric Society, 1887–1965* (New York: McGraw-Hill, 1966), p. 75; Roland Freeman com-

menting on L. Emmett Holt, "A ready method of calculating milk formulas of various percentages and the caloric value of the same," *Tr. Am. Ped. Soc., 23* (1911), 282; Eugene A. Darling, "The use of whole milk and fat diminished milk in infant feeding," *Boston Med. & Surg. J., 165* (1911), 747.

33 Jason B. Bullitt commenting at the Falls City Medical Society, *Ped., 8* (1899), 169–170; John Howland, "Proprietary and predigested foods from the standpoint of the pediatrist," *JAMA, 54* (1910), 196–198; H. Lowenburg, "Why percentage feeding fails: A plea for its more frequent adoption by the general practitioner," *JAMA, 48* (1907), 588–590; Charles W. Townsend, "Remarks on infant feeding, with special reference to the home modification of milk," *Boston Med. & Surg. J., 140* (1899), 275–276; A. S. Everett, "The artificial feeding of infants," *Am. Med. Quart., 1* (1899), i–iii; Wells, "Some personal experiences" (n. 12); Dukes, "Home modification" (n. 19); Boorse, "Substitute feeding" (n. 5); Holliday, "Bottle-fed babies " (n. 3); Hugh N. Leavell, "Infant feeding," *Ped., 8* (1899), 161–170; Noer, "Substitute infant feeding" (n. 5).

34 See, for example, Townsend, "Remarks on infant feeding" (n. 33), p. 276.

35 Thompson S. Westcott, "The scientific modification of milk," *Internat. Clinics, 3* (1900), 235–237, 280–298.

36 L. Emmett Holt, *Diseases of infancy and childhood* (New York: D. Appleton, 1902), pp. 148–149; Holt, "A new method of calculating milk percentages," *Am. J. Obst. & Dis. Women & Children, 64* (1911), 555–558; Henry Dwight Chapin, "Infant feeding," *Am. J. Obst. & Dis. Women & Children, 43* (1901), 598, 603. See also Edward Hamilton, "Percentage modification of cow's milk for infant-feeding," *Am. J. Obst. & Dis. Women & Children, 44* (1901), 489–491; Chapin, *Theory and practice* (n. 14), pp. 213–216; Charles W. Townsend, "Cream for the home modification of milk," *Boston Med. & Surg. J., 148* (1903), 414–416. These analyses also ignored the problem of adulterated milk. Dairy farmers and dealers often diluted milk to increase its volume and added molasses, chalk, or plaster of Paris to improve its color. Physicians, especially in urban areas, were most aware of the sale of impure milk, and many were in the forefront of the fight for milk-control legislation. For more on this point, see Norman Shaftel, "A history of the purification of milk in New York; Or, 'How now, brown cow,'" *N. Y. St. J. Med.,58* (1958), 911–928; Leavitt, *The healthiest city* (n. 20), pp. 156–189; Thomas E. Cone, *Two hundred years of feeding infants in America* (Columbus, Ohio: Ross Laboratories, 1976), 30–31; Manfred J. Wasserman, "Henry L. Coit and the certified milk movement in the development of modern pediatrics," *Bull. Hist. Med., 46* (1972), 359–390; Harvey Levenstein, " 'Best for babies' or 'preventable infanticide'? The controversy over artificial infant feeding in America, 1880–1920," *J. Am. Hist., 70* (1983), 83–92.

37 For contemporary comments on these problems, see, for example, Charles

214

Gilmore Kerley, "Suggestions for infant feeding," *Med. Rec.,* 60 (1901), 328–329; David L. Edsall and Charles A. Fife, "Concerning the accuracy of percentage modification of milk for infants," *Tr. Am. Ped. Soc.,* 15 (1903), 58–75; G. E. Decker, "Artificial feeding of infants," *Ped.,15* (1903), 530–531; E. Kirkland Shelmerdine, "Ready methods of formulating modified milk mixtures," *N. Y. Med. J.,* 80 (1904), 587–590; G. W. Putnam, "Milk modification prescription blank," *JAMA, 49* (1907), 691; "Queries and minor notes: Establishment of proteids in milk," *JAMA, 51* (1908), 60.

38 A detailed description of the Walker-Gordon procedures may be found in Thomas Morgan Rotch, *Pediatrics: The hygienic and medical treatment of children* (Philadelphia: J. B. Lippincott, 1895), esp. pp. 245–263.

39 Taylor, "Recent improved methods" (n. 10), 603–606; L. Emmett Holt at the Cleveland Medical Society, Oct. 1900, *JAMA, 35* (1900), 1651–1652; Edwards A. Park and Howard H. Mason, "Luther Emmett Holt (1855-1924)," in Borden S. Veeder, ed., *Pediatric profiles* (St. Louis, Mo.: C. V. Mosby, 1957), pp. 39–40; Earle, "The sterilization of food" (n. 17), 474–475; William P. Northrup, "Modified milk; by prescription; milk laboratories, etc.," *Med. Rec., 44* (1893), 552–554; "Report of the 15 April 1896 meeting of Clinical Section of Suffolk District Medical Society," *Boston Med. & Surg. J.,* 135 (1896), 293–294; A. C. Cotton, "Has the milk laboratory come to stay?" *JAMA, 28* (1897), 1065–1067; Edwin E. Graham commenting at the Section on Diseases of Children at AMA, 1897, *JAMA, 29* (1897), 1020; William P. Northrup, "Exact infant feeding: Accidents and incidents," *Ped., 10* (1900), 106–107; Thomas Morgan Rotch, "The essential principles of infant feeding and the modern methods of applying them," *JAMA, 41* (1903), 416–421; idem, "Modern laboratory feeding and the wide range of resources which it provides," *Arch. Ped., 25* (1908), 641–654.

40 Dickey, "Infant feeding" (n. 30); J. A. Wessenger commenting on Anna Marion Cook and David Murray Cowie, "Rural city milk supplies; Their relation to infant feeding; Home modification versus laboratory feeding," *J. Michigan State Med. Soc., 5* (1906), 427; R. L. Duffus and L. E. Holt, Jr., *L. Emmett Holt: Pioneer of a children's century* (New York: D. Appleton-Century, 1940), pp. 168–169; Frank S. Churchill commenting on Alfred Hess, "Middle milk mixtures," *JAMA, 53* (1909), 524.

41 A. McAllister, "Whole milk versus laboratory milk," *JAMA, 47* (1906), 1087–1088; Louis Fischer, "Some practical points on infant feeding and infant feces," *JAMA, 29* (1897), 1200; Charles Townsend, "Infant feeding," *Am. J. Obst. & Dis. Women & Children, 39* (1899), 707; Louis Fischer, "Infant feeding," *Med. Rec., 58* (1900), 893–894; Louis Starr, "A clinical study of laboratory milk in substitute infant feeding," *Arch. Ped., 17* (1900), 1–7.

42 Chapin, *Theory and practice* (n. 14), pp. 244–245; J. P. Crozer Griffith, "Percent

age and laboratory feeding," *Phila. Med. J.*, 7 (1901), 526–530; Louis Fischer, "The management of infant feeding," *Ped.*, 2 (1896), 67–68.

43 Cook and Cowie, "Rural city milk supplies" (n. 40), 425.

44 A. H. Wentworth, "The importance of milk analysis in infant feeding," *Boston Med. & Surg. J.*, 146 (1902), 683–686; 147, 5–10. This work was summarized by the author in *Am. J. Obst. & Dis. Women & Children*, 46 (1902), 421–422.

45 Edwin Rosenthal, "Milk mixtures as food for infants," *JAMA*, 31 (1898), 1104.

46 A. H. Wentworth, "The importance of milk analysis in infant feeding," *Am. J. Obst.*, 46 (1902), 422; Oppenheim, *Care of the child* (n. 11), p. 81; Wells, "Some personal experiences" (n. 12), 1015.

47 C. E. Clark commenting on Henry A. Bunker, "The artificial feeding of infants," *Brooklyn Med. J.*, 10 (1896), 689; Leavell, "Infant feeding" (n. 33), 169–170; Jacobi, "Infant feeding—A review" (n. 17), 7–10; J. J. Thomas, "Laboratory feeding, with especial reference to the modified milk fund," *Cleveland Med. Gaz.*, 16 (1900–1901), 585–589; McAllister, "Whole milk versus laboratory milk" (n. 41).

48 Thomas Morgan Rotch, "An historical sketch of the development of percentage feeding," *N. Y. Med. J.*, 85 (1907), 535; Fischer, *Infant-feeding* (n. 7), p. 251. Rotch claimed in print that he never profited from the milk laboratories. Since I have been unable to locate Rotch's papers or records of the Walker-Gordon Company, I cannot prove or disprove the claim.

49 A few, however, remained active at least into the 1920s. Molly Ladd-Taylor, *Raising a baby the government way: Mothers' letters to the Children's Bureau, 1915–1932* (New Brunswick, N.J.: Rutgers University Press, 1986), p. 81–82.

50 L. W. Littig, "Modified milk: The principle not the rule," *Iowa Med. J.*, 12 (1906), 142–145; Noer, "Substitute infant feeding" (n. 5), 393–395; L. Emmett Holt, "Some phases of the feeding problem," *Tr. Am. Ped. Soc.*, 18 (1906), 23–25; Harold Kniest Faber and Rustin McIntosh, *History of the American Pediatric Society, 1887–1965* (New York: McGraw-Hill, 1966), pp. 69–70; "Society proceedings: Medical Society of the State of Pennsylvania, 1908," *JAMA* 51 (1908), 1630; J. Finley Bell commenting at the Association of American Teachers of the Diseases of Children, 1909, *JAMA*, 53 (1909), 587: Henry Dwight Chapin, "The relation between the science and art of infant feeding," *JAMA*, 53 (1909), 907–908; Daniel Rollins Brown, "The feeding of the infant in health," *Boston Med. & Surg. J.*, 160 (1909), 128–133; John Lovett Morse, "Some of the vagaries of the obstetrician from the standpoint of the pediatrician," *Boston Med. & Surg. J.*, 160 (1909), 93–96; George Reily Moffitt, "An accurate formula for use in the modification of cow's milk in the artificial feeding of infants," *JAMA*, 55 (1910), 1877–1879; H. Lowenburg, "Adaptability of scientific infant-feeding to general practice," *JAMA*, 55 (1910), 565–568.

51 Samuel A. Visanska, "Artificial feeding," *Ped.*, 13 (1902), 124–129.

216

52 Howland, "Proprietary and predigested foods" (n. 33); Fischer, *Infant-feeding* (n. 7), pp. 342–343; Lowenburg, "Why percentage feeding fails" (n. 33); Townsend, "Remarks on infant feeding" (n. 33); Everett, "The artificial feeding" (n. 33).

53 Examples of advertisements for infant foods may be found in the advertising sections of journals such as *JAMA, Boston Med. & Surg. J., Am. J. Obst. & Dis. Women & Children, Ped., and Pac. Med. J.* For companies' involvement in the AMA conventions, see the descriptions of exhibitors published in *JAMA* each year. The booklets, being somewhat ephemeral, are today often difficult to obtain. However, a scrapbook in box 3 of Horlick's Corporation Papers, 1873–1974, the State Historical Society of Wisconsin, Division of Archives and Manuscripts, Madison, Wisconsin, contains copies of many of the pamphlets this company sent to physicians. See also Rima D. Apple, " 'Advertised by our loving friends': The infant formula industry and the creation of new pharmaceutical markets, 1870–1910," *J. Hist. Med.,* 41 (1986), 3–23.

54 Charles Warrington Earle, "Infant feeding," *JAMA, 11* (1888), 152–153; Mellin's advertisement, *JAMA, 11* (1888), 14; Rosenthal, Milk-mixtures" (n. 45), 1105.

55 C. H. Routh, *Infant feeding and its influence on life; or the causes and prevention of infant mortality,* 3rd ed. (New York: William Wood, 1879), pp. 183–184; C. P. Putnam, "Nestlé's food for babies," *Boston Med. & Surg. J.,* 95 (1876), 551–552.

56 Haven, "A study of infant feeding" (n. 8), 545–546. For more on the use of condensed milk in infant feeding, see, for example, Hays, "Substitute for mother's milk" (n. 23); Edson, "Condensed milk" (n. 12); Charles Gilmore Kerley, "Condensed milk: Its use and limitations in infant feeding," *Med. News, 70* (1897), 736–738; Rima D. Apple, " 'How shall I feed my baby?' Infant feeding in the United States, 1870–1940," Ph.D. dissertation, University of Wisconsin–Madison, 1981, esp. pp. 160–162.

57 [Columbus G.] Slagle commenting at the 1898 AMA meeting, *JAMA, 31* (1898), 1105. Similar claims are found in Davis, "Hints" (n. 8), 183–184; "Report of Sub-Committee on Infant Feeding of the American Medical Association, May 1888," *JAMA, 11* (1888), 208; Edson, "Artificial feeding" (n. 5), 559; F. C. Morgan speaking at the Vermont State Medical Society, Oct. 1899, *JAMA, 33* (1899), 1225; Edmond Cantley, "Use and abuse of proprietary foods in infant feeding," *Am. J. Obst. & Dis. Women & Children,* 60 (1909), 360–361.

58 A. K. Bond, "Infant foods other than breast milk," *Maryland Med. J.,* 26 (1891–1892), 452; Ephraim Cutter, "Medical food ethics: Now and to come," *JAMA, 20* (1893), 239. See also A. E. Miller, "Hygienic management of children," *JAMA, 31* (1898), 1557.

59 S. W. Newmayer, "Erroneous ideas on infant mortality and methods of reducing it," *Am. Assoc. Study & Prev. Inf. Mort., 1* (1919), 228–234. See also C. F. Wahrer

commenting in *JAMA, 39* (1902), 253; Noer, "Substitute infant feeding" (n. 5), 384–393.

60 Cutter, "Medical food ethics" (n. 58), 239–240; Gibbs, "Some observations" (n. 11), 411; Gillham P. Robinson commenting at the Medical Association of Georgia, April 1899, *JAMA, 32* (1899), 996; George F. Still, "Use and abuse of condensed milk and patent foods in infant feeding," *Am. J. Obst. & Dis. Women & Children, 53* (1906), 140–141; H. Merriman Stelle, "Infant feeding with cow's milk," *Ped., 18* (1906), 626–628; Lowenburg, "Why percentage feeding fails" (n. 33), 890; Ira S. Wile, "Do medical schools adequately train students for the prevention of infant mortality?" *Am. Assoc. Study & Prev. Inf. Mort., 1* (1910), 218–223.

Chapter V. "Under the Supervision of the Physician"

1 William John Focke, interview, 17 October 1979. For a sample of writings that discuss the possible deficiencies of human milk and the necessity of supplements such as citrus juices and cod-liver oil, see Clifford G. Grulee, *Infant feeding,* 3rd ed. (Philadelphia: W. B. Saunders, 1917), p. 100; Charles F. Fisher, "The dangers of conservatism in infant feeding," *Arch. Ped., 41* (1924), 413–415; F. W. Schultz, "Infant feeding," *Journal-Lancet,* Minneapolis, *58* (1938), 486; W. A. McGee, "Suggestions for simplifying infant feeding," *Am. Med., 34* (1928), 867; C. Ulysses Moore, "Aids to adequate infant feeding," *Am. Med., 34* (1928), 853–854; C. Anderson Aldrich, "Science and art in child nutrition," *J. Ped., 1* (1932), 418; I. Newton Kugelmass, "Milk modification and infant constitution," *New Eng. J. Med., 215* (1936), 1285–1291.

2 J. I. Durand commenting on Harold K. Faber, "The food requirements of the new-born infant," *Med. Rec., 100* (1921), 36–37.

3 B. A. Melgaard, "Correspondence: Complementary feeding of new-born," *JAMA, 84* (1925), 1857–1858. For more on the advisability of bottle feeding newborns to avoid initial weight loss, see Edwin B. Cragin commenting at the New York Academy of Medicine, March 1916, *Med. Rec., 90* (1916), 351; Harold A. Backmann, "Observations on the effect of complemental feeding in new-born infants," *Am. J. Dis. Child., 26* (1923), 349–361; Charles K. Johnson, "Reduction of infant mortality," *New Eng. J. Med., 200* (1929), 1105–1106. See Chapter 7 for a discussion of supplementary bottles in hospitals.

4 A few examples include "Queries and minor notes," *JAMA, 86* (1926), 1091; Joseph Garland, "Maternal nursing," *Boston Med. & Surg. J., 194* (1926), 519; Richard M. Smith, "The important causes of infant mortality," *Child Health Bull., 5* (1929), 109; "Editorial: Breast-fed and bottle-fed babies," *JAMA, 96* (1931), 1231–1232; Paul L. Parrish, "A present-day conception of infant feeding," *Med. Times, 64*

218

(1936), 209; Richard S. Eustic, "Care of the new born," *New Eng. J. Med., 214* (1936), 681–683; Stuart Shelton Stevenson, "The adequacy of artificial feeding in infancy," *J. Ped., 31* (1947), esp. 628–629.

5 J. P. Sedgwick, "Establishment, maintenance, and reinstitution of breast feeding," *JAMA, 69* (1917), 417–418; idem, "Report of Breast Feeding Bureau at Minneapolis," *Tr. Am. Child. Hyg. Assoc.,* 1919, pp. 88–89; idem, "A preliminary report of the study of breast feeding in Minneapolis," *Tr. Am. Ped. Soc., 32* (1920), 279–291; J. P. Sedgwick and E. C. Fleischner, "Breast feeding in the reduction of infant mortality," *Am. J. Pub. Health, 11* (1921), 156; Mathilda Carson, "Breast feeding in private practice under ideal conditions," *Arch. Ped., 38* (1921), 568–571. Other examples include Thomas B. Cooley and Wyman Cole, "A study of breast feeding possibilities in a small industrial community," *Tr. Am. Ped. Soc., 33* (1921), 286–291; E. Blanche Sterling, "The milk feeding of children," *Pub. Health Reports, 44* (1929), 957–964; Samuel Stone and Harry Bakwin, "Psychologic aspects of pediatrics: Breast feeding," *J. Ped., 33* (1948), 660–667; "Round table discussion: Present day attitudes towards breast feeding," *Ped., 6* (1950), 656–659.

6 Karver L. Puestow, interview, 18 September 1980.

7 C. K. Johnson, "The management of breast feeding, with case reports," *Boston Med. & Surg. J., 173* (1915), 278–280; Garland, "Maternal nursing" (n. 4), 521; Frederick C. Irving, "The feeding of the newborn infant from the obstetrician's point of view," *Boston Med. & Surg. J., 194* (1926), 1167–1168; Julius H. Hess, "Mother's milk," *Hygeia, 1* (1923), 149–154; Joseph Garland, "Pediatrics in general practice," *Boston Med. & Surg. J., 195* (1926), 108–109; William Willis Anderson, "Infant feeding," *Arch. Ped., 50* (1933), 519; Joseph Brennemann, "Some neglected practical points in the technique of infant feeding," *Arch. Ped., 40* (1923), 359–366; Wilburt C. Davidson, *Pediatric notes,* 2nd ed. (Baltimore: n. p. [sold by the Student's Book Store], 1926), pp. 5–6; McGee, "Suggestions" (n. 1), 866; Aldrich, "Science and art" (n. 1), 418; "Society proceedings: Missouri State Medical Association, May 1930," *JAMA, 95* (1930), 151; Ruth Morris Bakwin and Harry Bakwin, "Psychologic care during infancy," *J. Ped., 12* (1938), 75–77; Lewis Webb Hill, *Practical infant feeding* (Philadelphia: W. B. Saunders, 1922), 109.

8 John Zahorsky commenting at the section on Diseases of Children of the American Medical Association, June 1912, *JAMA, 59* (1912), 1881. For similar comments describing the importance of bottle feeding in general medical practice, see George Dow Scott, "Science, wisdom and common sense in the artificial feeding of infants," *Am. Med., 24* (1918), 528–530; Lewis Webb Hill, "Some observations on the trend of modern pediatric teaching," *Boston Med. & Surg. J., 183* (1920), 477; Charles Anderson Aldrich, "The composition of private pediatric practice, including a method for keeping adequate clinical records," *Tr. Am. Ped. Soc., 45* (1933), 61–64; Channing Frothingham, "The trend of medicine in the twentieth century,"

New Eng. J. Med., 208 (1933), 1345; A. Hymanson, "A short review of the history of infant feeding," *Arch. Ped., 51* (1934), 9–10.

9 Sedgwick and Fleischner, "Breast feeding" (n. 5), 153. See also Harry Lowenburg, "Etiology of artificial feeding: A plea for the study of breast-milk problems," *JAMA, 61* (1913), 2124–2130; H. L. K. Shaw commenting on Sedgwick, "Report of Breast Feeding Bureau" (n. 5), 1–2; McClanahan commenting on Sedgwick, "A preliminary report" (n. 5), 289–290; Joseph Garland and Mabel B. Rich, "Duration of breast feeding: A comparative study," *New Eng. J. Med., 203* (1930), 1279, 1282; G. W. Haigh, "The problem of cracked nipples," *New Eng. J. Med., 213* (1935), 1153.

10 Moore, "Aids" (n. 1), 854.

11 For a few examples, see W. H. Crawford, "Infant feeding and summer," *Arch. Ped., 50* (1933), 642; Stafford McLean, "The feeding of normal infants," *Med. Rec., 98* (1920), 765–767; John Lovett Morse and Fritz B. Talbot, *Diseases of nutrition and infant feeding,* 2nd ed. (New York: Macmillan, 1920), p. 101; Davidson, *Pediatric notes* (n. 7), 5–12; A. H. Parmelee and W. C. C. Cole, "Round table discussion on the new born period, including asphyxia," *J. Ped., 17* (1940), 820–821.

12 S. Josephine Baker, *Fighting for life* (New York: Macmillan, 1939), pp. 128–129; idem, *Child hygiene* (New York: Harper & Brothers, 1925), p. 221.

13 Herman Schwarz, "Simple milk dilution feeding," *Am. Assoc. Study & Prev. Inf. Mort., 4* (1913), 86–87. See also Roger Dennett, "Simplified infant feeding," *Am. J. Obst. & Dis. Women & Children, 64* (1911), 694; Harry Rulison, "Some observations on infant feeding," *Arch. Ped., 30* (1913), 762.

14 Raymond Philip Schowalter, interview, 23 September 1980; Fritz B. Talbot, "Thomas Morgan Rotch (1849–1914)," in Borden S. Veeder, ed., *Pediatric profiles* (St. Louis: C. V. Mosby, 1957), p. 30; Dennett, "Simplified infant feeding" (n. 13), 694–698; Grulee, *Infant feeding* (n. 1), pp. 138–145, 157–164; Julius H. Hess, *Principles and practice of infant feeding,* 3rd ed. (Philadelphia: F. A. Davis, 1922), p. 119; Review of Hess's *Principles and practice, Boston Med. & Surg. J., 188* (1923), 402; James Burnet, "Infant feeding: Facts and fallacies," *Arch. Ped., 40* (1923), 127; "Editorial: Simplified infant feeding," *New Eng. J. Med., 208* (1933), 1061.

15 Schowalter, interview (n. 14); Julius H. Hess, "Infant feeding: Its present status," *J. Indiana St. Med. Assoc., 20* (1927), 419–422; H. Kent Tenney, Jr., interview, 24 September 1979; William F. Donlin, interview, 13 December 1979; Samuel X. Radbill, personal correspondence, dated 31 May 1979; Carl C. Fischer, "The artificial feeding of the healthy normal infant," *Hahneman. Month., 69* (1934), 533–534; medical notebook entitled "Few selected notes from Dr. C. H. Dunn's lectures at Boston, July, 1912," in box 4 of Henry Kleinpell Papers, the State Historical Society of Wisconsin, Division of Archives and Manuscripts, Madison, Wisconsin; J. E.

220

Baron to Kleinpell, dated 20 October 1939, in box 2, folder "Medical papers, 1938–1940," in Kleinpell papers; H. R. Litchfield, "Evaporated milk in infant feeding," *Arch. Ped.*, *61* (1944), 617–625; Harold Jacobziner, "A simple method for calculating formulae in infant feeding," *Arch. Ped.*, *64* (1947), 539–543.

16 William L. Waskow, interview, 16 September 1980.

17 N. Thomas Saxl, *Pediatric dietetics* (Philadelphia: Lea & Febiger, 1937), pp. 95–96, 118–123. See also Garland, "Pediatrics in general practice" (n. 7), 109; Franklin Gengenbach, "Infant feeding suggestions for the general practitioner," *Colorado Med.*, *27* (1930), 382–387; Eustic, "Care of the new born" (n. 4), 683; Kugelmass, "Milk modification" (n. 1), 1291; Arthur H. London, Jr., "The composition of an average pediatric practice," *J. Ped.*, *10* (1937), 762–771; C. A. Stewart, "The feeding of the child," *Journal-Lancet*, Minneapolis, *58* (1938), 239–244.

18 Mothers' perceptions from interviews at the Colonial Club, Sun Prairie, Wisconsin, 8 October 1969. For doctors' statements, see, for example, F. P. Gengenbach, "Recent interpretations of feeding disturbances in infants," *Ped.*, *25* (1913), 298–303; Schultz, "Infant feeding" (n. 1), 488–489; Stevenson, "Adequacy of artificial feeding" (n. 4), 616–630.

19 Tenney, interview (n. 15). Information for this paragraph came from my interview with Tenney and from his book, *Let's talk about your baby* (Madison: Kilgore Printing Co., 1934), a chatty presentation of infant-care advice that he wrote for his patients.

20 For Mead Johnson's appearances at the AMA meetings, see the list of exhibitors printed in *JAMA* each year. Advertisements for Dextri-Maltose appeared in almost every issue of *JAMA, Boston Med. & Surg. J.,* and other major medical journals, as well as smaller journals, in the first half of the twentieth century. Examples of the booklets and infant-feeding aids that the company sent to physicians and a copy of the sales training manual may be found in Mead Johnson & Company, Business Records, 1895–1971, Indiana State University-Evansville, Special Collections, Evansville, Indiana (hereafter referred to as MJC).

21 L. S. Johnson, "Your company—Past, present and future," typescript, undated, in folder "History-Documents," box 2C of MJC. A copy of the film is also in the MJC.

22 Mead Johnson advertisement, *JAMA*, *95* (1930), 22.

23 For S.M.A.'s appearances at the AMA meetings, see the list of exhibitors printed in *JAMA* each year. Advertisements for S.M.A. appeared consistently in most major general pediatric journals of the period. For a sample of advertisements directed to nonmedical readers, see various issues of *Hygeia*. Examples of literature sent to physicians and instructions to sales representatives on how to approach physicians may be found in "Master File, Research and Development," Mason Laboratories, Wyeth Laboratories, Inc., Mason, Ingham County, Michi-

gan. I wish to thank R. C. Stribley, Nutritional Director, Wyeth Laboratories, for sending me samples of this literature.

24 For Mellin's appearances at the AMA meetings, see the list of exhibitors printed in *JAMA* each year. Advertisements for Mellin's appeared in almost every issue of *JAMA, Boston Med. & Surg. J.*, and other major journals, as well as smaller journals such as *Hosp. Soc. Serv.*, in the period.

25 For Horlick's appearances at the AMA meetings, see the list of exhibitors printed each year in *JAMA*. Advertisements for Horlick's Malted Milk and Horlick's Milk Modifier appeared in many issues of *JAMA, Boston Med. & Surg. J.*, and other medical journals of the period. Examples of booklets, formula pads, and other aids sent to physicians are located in the Horlick's Corporation papers, 1873–1974, the State Historical Society of Wisconsin, Division of Archives and Manuscripts, Madison, Wisconsin (hereafter referred to as HCP). The company informed physicians of its policy of not supplying directions with packages of its Milk Modifier in a letter, undated, in box 3, Scrapbook, in HCP.

For Nestlé's appearances at the AMA meetings, see the list of exhibitors printed in *JAMA* each year. Advertisements for Nestlé's Milk Food and Lactogen may be found in most issues of medical journals from the period.

26 For appearances at the AMA meetings, see the list of exhibitors printed in *JAMA* each year. Advertisements for evaporated milks, both by brand name and by the Evaporated Milk Association, later the Irradiated Evaporated Milk Institute, may be found in most issues of medical journals of the period. For examples of booklets, see Carnation Company, *Infant feeding simplified with irradiated Carnation milk, unsweetened, evaporated* (Milwaukee: Carnation Co., 1943); Irradiated Evaporated Milk Institute, *Infant feeding with irradiated evaporated milk: A statement for physicians* (Chicago: EMI, 1935).

27 Martin L. Bell, *A portrait of progress: A business history of Pet Milk Company from 1885 to 1960* (St. Louis, Mo.: Pet Milk Company, 1962), pp. 102–104.

28 Mark S. Rueben, "Observations on milk station infants," *Arch. Ped., 31* (1914), 176–196. See also Joseph S. Wall, "The status of the child in obstetric practice," *JAMA, 66* (1916), 255–259; "Current medical literature: Abstract of A. A. Walker, 'Common sense and infant feeding,'" *JAMA, 88* (1927), 518.

29 H. M. McClanahan, "Supplemental breast-feeding in infants," *JAMA, 59* (1912), 1877–1878; Thomas A. Foster, "Patent foods in infant feeding," *J. Maine Med. Assoc., 11* (1920), 14; J. T. Marshall, "The growing prevalence in the rural districts of artificial feeding of infants," *Kentucky Med. J., 25* (1927), 369–371; John Lovett Morse, "Progress in pediatrics," *New Eng. J. Med., 206* (1932), 685.

30 See, for example, Grulee, *Infant feeding* (n. 1), p. 146; Williams McKim Marriott, *Infant nutrition: A text-book of infant feeding for students and practitioners of medicine* (St. Louis, Mo. C. V. Mosby, 1930), pp. 155–163.

31 L. Emmett Holt and Henry L. K. Shaw, *Save the babies,* Committee on Public Health Education among Women, Pamphlet no. 7 (Chicago: AMA Council on Health and Public Instruction, 1914), p. [10]; Foster, "Patent foods" (n. 29), 15–18; Richard M. Smith, "Acute gastrointestinal disease in infants," *New Eng. J. Med., 215* (1936), 701–702.

32 Crawford, "Infant feeding" (n. 11), 644–645; Samuel Friedman, "Infant feeding— The proprietary milk preparations," *Arch. Ped., 50* (1933), 261–271.

33 Tenney, interview (n. 15); Focke, interview (n. 1). See also David Forsyth, "The evolution of infant feeding," *Am. J. Obst. & Dis. Women & Children, 64* (1911), 393–395; Rulison, "Some observations" (n. 13), 767–768; "Queries and minor notes: S.M.A. and cow's milk," *JAMA, 91* (1928), 418; "Queries and minor notes: Rickets developing in child on S.M.A.," *JAMA, 94* (1930), 1939; J. B. Rogers commenting on Isador J. Raphael, "Practical points in infant feeding," *J. Indiana St. Med. Assoc., 24* (1931), 261. For more of the relationship between physicians and sales representatives, see John Pekkanen, *The American connection: Profiteering and politicking in the "ethical" drug industry* (Chicago: Follett, 1973), esp. pp. 64–75.

34 Roger H. Dennett, *The healthy baby: The care and feeding of infants in sickness and in health* (New York: Macmillan, 1912), p. xiii.

35 "Editorial: The present-day position of the 'milkstation,'" *Arch. Ped., 29* (1912), 721–723.

36 Michael M. Davis, "Relations of prenatal and postnatal work," *Boston Med. & Surg. J., 177* (1917), 294–297; Gustave Lippmann, "What the pediatrician can do to reduce the mortality in the first month of life," *Am. Assoc. Study & Prev. Inf. Mort., 8* (1917), 20–21; Isaac W. Brewer, "The next step in the campaign for infant welfare: The education of women of the nation for motherhood," *Boston Med. & Surg. J., 182* (1920), 276–277; Frederic H. Bartlett, *Infants and children: Their feeding and growth* (New York: Farrar & Rinehart, 1932), pp. 226–227; Henry F. Helmholz, "Presidential address," *J. Ped., 15* (1939), 745–746; Herman N. Bundesen, *Our babies: Their feeding, care, and training* ([Chicago]; n.p., 1939), p. 3. This rationale was not unique to the United States. On Britain, see Ann Oakley, *The captured womb: A history of the medical care of pregnant women* (New York: Basil Blackwell, 1984), esp. pp. 34–45.

37 Amos U. Christie commenting at "Roundtable discussion of nursing care in the new born infant," *Arch. Ped., 13* (1938), 440.

38 Charles Herman, "Premiums for nursing mothers and milk depots for infants," *Arch. Ped., 28* (1911), 518–522; S. Josephine Baker, "The infants' milk stations: Their relations to the pediatric clinics and to the private physician," *Arch. Ped., 31* (1914), 165–170; "Personals: The milkman of Milwaukee," *Survey, 26* (1911), 171–172.

39 Dennett, *The healthy baby* (n. 34), pp. vii–viii; Roger H. Dennett, *Simplified*

infant feeding (Philadelphia, J. B. Lippincott, 1915), 31–32; J. P. Crozer Griffith, "Demonstration and discussion of some methods of infant feeding and of food preparation," *Atlantic Med. J.*, 30 (1926–1927), 703–706.

40 Frank Howard Richardson, *Simplifying motherhood: Being a handbook on the care of the baby during the first year* (New York: G. P. Putnam's Sons, 1925), p. 9; Henry F. Helmholz, "The relation of heat to the morbidity and mortality of infants from gastro-intestinal diseases," *JAMA*, 63 (1914), 1373; Henry I. Bowditch, "Parental responsibility," *Boston Med. & Surg. J.*, *183* (1920), 518.

41 J. P. Crozer Griffith, *The care of the baby: A manual for mothers and nurses containing practical directions for the management of infancy and childhood in health and disease*, 6th ed. (Philadelphia: W. B. Saunders, 1915), pp. 146–147.

42. L. T. Royster, "The prevention of infant mortality from an educational point of view," *Am. J. Obst. & Dis. Women & Children*, 61 (1910), 581–585; Thomas B. Cooley, "Relation of the infant welfare movement to pediatrics," *JAMA*, 59 (1912), 2217–2221.

43 Henry E. Stafford, "The changing pediatric practice," *J. Ped.*, 8 (1936), 376.

44 Joseph Brennemann, "Vis medicatrix naturae in pediatrics," *Am. J. Dis. Child.*, 40 (1930), 5–6.

45 Isaac A. Abt, *Baby doctor* (New York: Whittlesey House, McGraw-Hill, 1944), pp. 290–291, 294; James M. Moser, "Details in infant feeding," *Arch. Ped.*, 39 (1922), 442–448; Jesse Robert Gerstley, *Clinical lectures on infant feeding* (Philadelphia: W. B. Saunders, 1917), p. 264.

46 Nancy Pottisham Weiss, "Mother, the invention of necessity: Dr. Benjamin Spock's *Baby and child care*," *Am. Quart.*, 29 (1977), 520, 529–530; Dorothy E. Bradbury, *Five decades of action for children: A history of the Children's Bureau*, U. S. Department of Health, Education and Welfare, Children's Bureau Publication no. 358 (Washington, D.C.: HEW, 1962), pp. 8–9; *The story of Infant Care* (Washington, D.C.: HEW, Children's Bureau, 1965), 5–22, which reprints the letters from the Advisory Medical Committee and West; "Report of the committee to cooperate with the Federal Children's Bureau," *Tr. Am. Ped. Soc.*, 27 (1915), 358; "Minutes of the American Pediatric Society," *Tr. Am. Ped. Soc.*, 26 (1914), 5; "Minutes of the American Pediatric Society: Executive session," *Tr. Am. Ped. Soc.*, 31 (1919), 5–6; "Editorial: Infant care," *Hygeia*, 8 (1930), 158; Molly Ladd-Taylor, *Raising a baby the government way: Mothers' letters to the Children's Bureau, 1915–1932* (New Brunswick, N.J.: Rutgers University Press, 1986).

47 Ralph R. Scobey, "The importance of infant feeding to the general practitioner," *Arch. Ped.*, 50 (1933), 111. See also Arthur H. Parmelee commenting at "Roundtable discussion on attitudes of and toward children," *J. Ped.*, 5 (1934), 133; "Queries and minor notes: Eagle Brand," *JAMA*, 87 (1926), 265; Norman M. MacNeill, "Can we retrieve breast-feeding?" *Pennsylvania Med. J.*, 51 (1947), 139.

48 "Section on Diseases of Children," *JAMA*, 65 (1915), 127–128; "Minutes of Section

224

on Diseases of Children," *JAMA, 82* (1924), 2042; 84 (1925), 1836; "Minutes of House of Delegates," *JAMA, 84* (1925), 1743; "Report of Section on Diseases of Children presented to House of Delegates," *JAMA, 84* (1925), 1744. The information in the following paragraphs has been drawn from "To investigate the general question of the advertising of proprietary foods in medical journals," *Tr. Sec. Dis. Child., AMA,* 1925, pp. 172–195. Dr. James Harvey Young has pointed out the important distinction between the "respectable wing" and the "quackish wing" of the infant-food industry. Most physicians, however, made little of this distinction until the twentieth century, when they differentiated between "ethical" and "non-ethical" products. For the development of the idea of "ethical" products, see James Whorton, " 'Thialion!!!': Anatomy of a pseudo-ethical proprietary," *Pharmacy in History, 23,* no. 3 (1981), 114–125.

49 "Committee on foods," *JAMA, 93* (1929), 1144, 1147–1148; Otis Pease, *The responsibilities of American advertising: Private control and public influence, 1920–1940* (New Haven: Yale University Press, 1958), pp. 93–95; James Harvey Young, *The toadstool millionaires: A social history of patent medicines in America before federal regulation* (Princeton: Princeton University Press, 1961), p. 224; J. R. Wilson, "Council on Foods and Nutrition," in Morris Fishbein, ed., *A history of the American Medical Association, 1847–1947* (Philadelphia: W. B. Saunders, 1947), pp. 936–939.

50 "Committee on Foods," *JAMA, 94* (1930), 485; 95 (1930), 595; 94 (1930), 1145.

51 Julius H. Hess commenting on Roger H. Dennett, "The teaching of infant feeding: Past and present," *Arch. Ped., 48* (1931), 232–233.

52 "Proceedings of the meeting: Executive session," *Tr. Am. Ped. Soc., 44* (1932), 10; "Committee on Foods: General committee decisions: Feeding formulas for infants in lay advertising," *JAMA, 99* (1932), 391. It would be interesting to analyze the deliberations that preceded this announcement; however, the AMA has closed these files to researchers.

53 "Committee on Foods: Mellin's Food," *JAMA, 99* (1932), 2266; "Commercial exhibits at 152nd Massachusetts Medical Society Meeting: Mellin's Food," *New Eng. J. Med., 208* (1933), 1082.

54 "The Massachusetts Medical Society commercial exhibits," *New Eng. J. Med., 218* (1938), 940–941; Williams McKim Marriott and P. C. Jeans, *Infant nutrition: A textbook of infant feeding for students and practitioners of medicine,* 3rd ed. (St. Louis: C. V. Mosby, 1941), pp. 216, 218–219.

55 "Committee on Foods: Acceptance withdrawn: Horlick's Malted Milk," *JAMA, 100* (1933), 1175.

56 Frank E. Hartman, typescript history of Horlick's, 1946, in the HCP.

57 Numerous Mead Johnson advertisements, such as the ones in *JAMA, 95* (1930), 22, and *J. Ped., 3* (1933), 26. See also Rima D. Apple, " 'To be used only under the

direction of a physician': Commercial infant feeding and medical practice, 1870–1940," *Bull. Hist. Med., 54* (1980), 402–417.

Chapter VI. "The Noblest Profession"

1 Child-care educators formed the largest class of scientific motherhood proponents, but other supporters included feminists like Charlotte Perkins Gilman and concerned mothers convinced of the value of science in the healthful rearing of children. Some advocates were medically trained persons interested in child care. In a few instances, promoters founded organizations such as the Home Economics Association to disseminate the ideology. Though home economists and other advocates rarely used the term "scientific motherhood" (they sometimes wrote of "trained motherhood"), their work clearly reflected the tenets of the ideology. At this time there is no comprehensive history of the development of scientific motherhood, though some scholars have discussed its significance in women's lives. See, for example, Kathleen Jones, "Sentiment and science: The late nineteenth-century pediatrician as mother's advisor," *J. Soc. Hist., 17* (1983), 79–96; Andrea Meditch, "In the nation's interest: Childcare prescriptions, 1890–1930," Ph.D. dissertation, University of Texas at Austin, 1981. For the parallel development of domestic science, the application of science to cooking, see Laura Shapiro, *Perfection salad: Women and cooking at the turn of the century* (New York: Farrar, Straus and Giroux, 1986).

2 Lucy White Palmer, "The coming guest," *Babyhood, 2* (1886), 313.

3 Mary R. Melendy, *Perfect womanhood for maidens-wives-mothers* ([Chicago?]: K. T. Boland, 1901) p. 7.

4 Charlotte Perkins Gilman, *Women and economics: The economic factor between men and women as a factor in social evolution* (1898; reprint ed., New York: Harper Torchbooks, 1966), pp. 178, 193–197; Lois W. Banner, *Women in modern America: A brief history* (New York: Harcourt Brace Jovanovich, 1974), p. 119.

5 The impact of these changes on women's lives has been explored in Ruth Schwartz Cowan, *More work for mother: The ironies of household technology from the open hearth to the microwave* (New York: Basic Books, 1983); Sheila M. Rothman, *Woman's proper place: A history of changing ideals and practices, 1870 to the present* (New York: Basic Books, 1978), esp. pp. 17–18, 21, 177–178, 209–218; Norton Juster, *So sweet to labor: Rural women in America, 1865–1895* (New York: Viking Press, 1979), esp. pp. 4–5; Adele Simmons, "Education and ideology in nineteenth-century America: The response of educational institutions to the changing role of women," in Berenice Carroll, ed., *Liberating women's history: Theoretical and critical essays* (Urbana: University of Illinois Press, 1976), pp.

226

115–126; Susan Strasser, *Never done: A history of American housework* (New York: Pantheon, 1982).

6 Ellen Battelle Dietrick, "A scientifically trained baby," *New Eng. Kitchen Mag. [Home Sci],* 2 (1895), 179–180.

7 Bettina Berch, "Scientific management in the home: The empress's new clothes," *J. Am. Culture, 3* (1980), 440–445. See also Shapiro, *Perfection salad* (n. 1); Barbara Ehrenreich and Deirdre English, *For her own good: One hundred fifty years of the experts' advice to women* (New York: Anchor, 1979), passim; Kathryn Kish Sklar, *Catharine Beecher: A study in American domesticity* (New York: W. W. Norton, 1973), 151–167; Barbara J. Harris, *Beyond her sphere: Women and the professions in American history* (Westport, Conn.: Greenwood Press, 1978), esp. pp. 32–72; Louise Michele Newman, *Men's ideas/women's realities: Popular Science, 1870–1915* (New York: Pergamon Press, 1985), xxiv–xxvi, 156–191.

8 Helen Watterson Moody, "The true meaning of motherhood," *Ladies' Home J., 16* (6) (1899), 12; Jane Stewart, "Is the mother ready for the baby? Training versus 'instinct' and 'experience,'" *Ladies' Home J., 30* (2) (1913), 76.

9 Gilman, *Women and economics* (n. 4), pp. 178, 193–197 (quotations from p. 196); "A trained mother," "Maternal instinct run riot," *Good Housekeeping, 52* (1911), 245–247

10 Anna Steese Richardson, *Making motherhood easy* (Philadelphia: Smith, Kline & French, 1915). Other examples include John Brisben Walker, "Motherhood as a profession," *Cosmopolitan, 25* (1898), 89–93; Anna Virginia Miller, "Food for children," *Am. Kitchen, 11* (1899), 42–46; Emma E. Walker, "Pitfalls of babyhood," *Good Housekeeping, 49* (1909), 435–437; Louise E. Hogan, *How to feed children: A manual for mothers, nurses and physicians,* 8th ed. (Philadelphia: J. B. Lippincott, 1906), pp. 9–10; Sarah Comstock, "Mothercraft: A new profession for women," *Good Housekeeping, 59* (1914), 672–678.

11 S. Josephine Baker, *Fighting for life* (New York: Macmillan, 1939), pp. 126–132; "Editorial: Summer milk stations in New York," *Arch. Ped., 28* (1911), 561–562; "The Attic Angels Association, 1889–1949," State Historical Society of Wisconsin, the Division of Archives and Manuscripts, Madison, Wisc., pp. 28–33.

12 (New York: Macmillan, 1907).

13 Baker, *Fighting* (n. 11), pp. 132–137.

14 Baker commenting on Wilbur C. Phillips, "Infants' milk depots and infant mortality," *Am. Assoc. Study & Prev. Inf. Mort. 1* (1910), 86; [Charles Herrman], "Instructing mothers and older girls in the care of babies," *Arch. Ped., 25* (1908), 617–618.

15 Information about Milwaukee's classes comes from various issues of *Healthologist,* a popular health magazine produced by the Milwaukee Board of Health, and annual reports of the Commissioner of Health, issued during 1912 and 1913. I wish to thank Evelyn Fine for directing me to these sources and for

allowing me to read her unpublished paper, "Educating girls for intelligent motherhood: Little mothers' roles in reducing infant mortality," University of Wisconsin-Madison, 1983. For similar courses outside New York City and Milwaukee, see Sarah Comstock, "Mothercraft: Feeding the baby," *Good Housekeeping, 60* (1915), 237–243; Philip Van Ingen, "Progress in pediatrics: Recent progress in infant welfare work," *Am. J. Dis. Child., 10* (1915), 212–221.

16 Vassar Female College, *Prospectus 1865,* p. 17, cited in Rothman, *Woman's proper place* (n. 5), p. 28; "Mrs. Kate Hunibee's diary," *Hearth and Home, 3* (1871), 29–30. See also Simmons, "Education and ideology" (n. 5); Rothman, *Woman's proper place* (n. 5), pp. 27–29, 106–112; Barbara Miller Solomon, *In the company of educated women: A history of women and higher education in America* (New Haven: Yale University Press, 1985); Juster, *So sweet to labor* (n. 5), pp. 213–236.

17 "Los Angeles Session," *JAMA, 57* (1911), 65. See also "Reduction of infant mortality," *Boston Med. & Surg. J., 151* (1904), 254; *Baby's health, nation's wealth* (Helena: Montana State Board of Health, 1916), p. 5.

18 *Our baby book: Mother's complete guide for the care of infant and baby's record,* 2nd ed. (Milwaukee: Baby Book Publishing Company, 1913), pp. 23–24; R. L. Duffus and L. E. Holt, Jr., *L. Emmett Holt: Pioneer of a children's century* (New York: D. Appleton-Century, 1940), pp. 115–118; Edwards A. Park and Howard H. Mason, "Luther Emmett Holt (1855–1924)," in Borden S. Veeder, ed., *Pediatric profiles* (St. Louis, Mo.: C. V. Mosby, 1957), pp. 37–38.

19 On the growing number of women's magazines, see Esther F. Stineman, "What the ladies were reading: Popular women's magazines in America, 1875–1975," Master's thesis, Graduate Library School, University of Chicago, 1976; Helen Rosen Woodward, *The lady persuaders* (New York: Ivan Obolensky, 1960); Vernetta Trenbeth Bartle, "Women's publications in America: Their influence and history," Master's thesis, University of Wisconsin, 1925.

20 *Babyhood, 9* (103) (1893), xii.

21 Elizabeth Robinson Scovil, "Mother's corner: Feeding a delicate baby," *Ladies' Home J., 9* (5) (1892), 20; "Mother's corner," *Ladies' Home J., 9* (6) (1892), 20.

22 Emelyn Lincoln Coolidge, "The young mother's guide," *Ladies' Home J., 28* (1) (1911), 37; Coolidge, "The young mother's guide," *Ladies' Home J., 29* (1) (1912), 65; Salme Harju Steinberg, *Reformer in the marketplace: Edward W. Bok and the Ladies' Home Journal* (Baton Rouge: Louisiana State University Press, 1979), p. 36. Similar articles and correspondence columns appear in other journals, such as *Babyhood, Mother's Friend, Home Sci.,* and *Farmer's Wife.*

23 Steinberg, *Reformer in the marketplace* (n. 22), pp. 61–63; *Am. Motherhood, 25* (1) (1907), 47. See also Rima D. Apple, " 'Advertised by our loving friends': The infant formula industry and the creation of new pharmaceutical markets, 1870–1910," *J. Hist. Med., 41* (1986) 2–23.

24 Mrs. Julian Heath, "The housewife and the advertiser," *Housewives Mag., 6* (2)

228

(1915), 14–20; "What our advertising means to you," *Housewives Mag.*, 7 (2) (1916), 95; "The endorsement of products by the National Housewives League," *Housewives Mag.*, 9 (3) (1917), 24–25.

25 Otis Pease, *The responsibilities of American advertising: Private control and public influence, 1920–1940* (New Haven: Yale University Press, 1958), pp. 81–82; Oscar E. Anderson, Jr., *The health of a nation: Harvey W. Wiley and the fight for pure food* (Chicago: University of Chicago Press, 1958), esp. pp. 260–263.

26 Advertisements and offers for booklets appeared in most contemporary women's magazines. See, for example, *Babyhood, 1* (4) (1885), v; *Babyhood, 9* (103) (1893), xi; *Modern Priscilla, 13* (7) (1899), 3; *Modern Priscilla, 13* (9) (1899), 13.

27 Some examples of these may be found in issues of contemporary magazines; see, for instance, *Cosmopolitan, 1908–1909.*

28 Marion Harland, *Our baby's first and second years* (New York: Reed & Carnrick, [1887?]), esp. pp. 9–10; emphasis in original.

29 Harland, *Our baby's first and second years* (n. 28), pp. 5–6, 8, 47.

30 Miller, "Food for children" (n. 10), p. 41; Hogan, *How to feed children* (n. 10), pp. 9–10.

31 Harland, *Our baby's first and second years* (n. 28), p. 5. Other examples include J. B. Dunham, *The baby: How to keep it well* (Chicago: Gross & Delbridge, 1885), pp. 26–27; Mrs. Prudence S. Saur, *Maternity: A book for every wife and mother* (Chicago: L. P. Miller & Co., 1888), pp. 249, 293; *Baby's health, nation's wealth* (n. 17), p. 17; Richard Mason Smith, *The baby's first two years* (Boston: n.p., 1915), pp. 21–30; D. A. Gorton, "Our babies," *Household Mag.*, 13 (1873), 269; W. Thornton Parker, "Feeding by the nursing bottle," *Babyhood, 2* (1886), 346.

32 "The decline of suckling power among American women," *Babyhood, 19* (1902), 5–8; Anna E. Richardson, "Suggestions for infant feeding," *Bulletin of the University of Texas*, no. 373 (1914); Mary Wood-Allen, "Preventable diseases of childhood: No. 1," *New Crusade, 4* (1897), 203; Mary A. Duns, *Practical care and feeding of children*, 2nd ed. (Chicago: Chicago Medical Book Co., 1909), pp. 9–10; Smith, *The baby's first two years* (n. 31), pp. 25–27.

33 Some examples of this include A. Shank, "Cream for infants," *Babyhood, 2* (1886), 382–383; Agnes Spaulding, "Clean milk saves money and lives," *Good Housekeeping, 42* (6) (1906), 632–634; Helene M. Pope, "Laying the foundations: How to plan the meals for little citizens," *Housewives Mag.*, 8 (2) (1916), 24; Emma Anzell Drake, *Maternity without suffering* (Philadelphia: Vir, 1902) p. 126; Smith, *The baby's first two years* (n. 31), pp. 106–134.

34 Emelyn Lincoln Coolidge, "The young mother's guide: What young mothers ask me," *Ladies' Home J.*, 26 (4) (1908–1909), 53.

35 L. Emmett Holt, *The care and feeding of children: A catechism for the use of moth-*

ers and children's nurses (New York: D. Appleton, 1894). Other editions include: 4th ed., 1906; 10th ed., 1922; and 13th ed., 1927 (the last revised by his son, L. Emmett Holt, Jr.).

36 Mellin's Food Company, *Mellin's food for infants and invalids* (Boston: Doliber, Goodale & Company, 1891), pp. 1–3. See also the 1884 edition of *Mellin's food for infants and invalids;* and the company's *Advice to mothers on the care and feeding of infants,* first copyrighted in 1884, which went through numerous editions in the 1890s and early decades of this century. Both the Collection of Business Americana, the National Museum of History and Technology, Smithsonian Institution, Washington, D.C. (in box labeled "Foods–Health Foods," folder labeled "Baby-Infant/Invalid foods"), and the Bella C. Landauer Collection of Business and Advertising Art, New York Historical Society, New York City (in scrapbook 6F: Ki-Me) have examples of tradecards, postcards, and pamphlets produced by Mellin's. I wish to thank James Harvey Young for directing me to these collections.

37 Harland, *Our baby's first and second years* (n. 28), p. 10.

38 Smith, *The baby's first two years* (n. 31), pp. 40–41.

39 Coolidge, "The young mother's registry: Giving the baby the right start," *Ladies' Home J., 33* (10) (1916), 62.

Chapter VII. "The Doctor Should Decide"

1 Mrs. John S. Reilly, *Common sense for mothers* (New York: Funk & Wagnalls, 1935), p. 348. Reilly's sentiments were not unusual. See also Grace F. Ellis, *The origin of life: A girl's physiology* (Grand Rapids, Mich.: Central High School, 1916), pp. 33–34; George A. Dorsey, "What every mother should know—and why," *Cosmopolitan, 84* (1928), 163; Park Jerauld White, Jr., "Expert mothers—Greatest of career women," *Hygeia, 15* (1937), 404; Carolyn Conant VanBlarcom, *Getting ready to be a mother,* 4th ed., rev. Hazel Corbin (New York: Macmillan, 1940), pp. 148–149. Recent historical studies have documented this also. See, for example, Susan Ware, *Holding their own: American women in the 1930s* (Boston: Twayne, 1982) and Susan M. Hartmann, *The home front and beyond: American women in the 1940s* (Boston: Twayne, 1982).

2 Mary Jacobs, "A course in practical motherhood," *Hygeia, 12* (1937), 416–418.

3 Mary Faulker in the introduction to *Home economics education* (Baltimore: Department of Education, Division of Vocational Education, 1925; rev. ed., 1930).

4 C. A. Harper in the introduction to Gertrude S. Hasbrouck, *Handbook for teachers of infant hygiene classes* (Madison: Wisconsin State Board of Health, Bureau of Child Welfare, 1927), p. 8.

5 Helen C. Goodspeed and Emma Johnson, *Care and training of children* (Philadelphia: J. B. Lippincott, 1929), quotation on p. vi. See also Ralph E. Blount,

Health: Public and personal (Boston: Allyn and Bacon, 1922); *Home economics education* (Baltimore) (n. 3); L. Thomas Hopkins and Kate W. Kinyon, *Home economics* (Denver: Public Schools, 1925); Annie Robertson Dyer, *The placement of home economics content in junior and senior high schools* (New York: Teachers College, Columbia University, 1927); Gertrude S. Hasbrouck, *Manual of infant hygiene* (Madison: Wisconsin State Board of Health, Bureau of Child Welfare, 1927); Kate W. Kinyon and L. Thomas Hopkins, *Junior home problems* (Chicago: Benj. H. Sanborn, 1929); *Home economics: Course of study, junior and senior high schools* (Augusta: Maine State Department of Education, Division of Vocational Education, 1929); "Health and the school: Training for parenthood," *Hygeia*, 9 (1931), 473–474; Robert S. Lynd and Helen Merrell Lynd, *Middletown: A study in contemporary American culture* (New York: Harcourt, Brace, 1929), esp. p. 196.

6 Mary H. Mayer, "Extension courses in public schools for adult women in the care and feeding of children," *Am. Assoc. Study & Prev. Inf. Mort.*, 8 (1917), 171–174; Walter R. Ramsey, "Are your children healthy?" *Farmer's Wife*, 29 (1926), 540; "Giving babies their birthright," *Farmer's Wife*, 31 (1928), 10. See also Agnes K. Hanna, "Analyses of child-care teaching in mothers' classes and little mothers' classes," *Child Health Bull.*, 3 (1927), 102–103; Steven L. Schlossman, "Notes toward a history of parent education in America, 1897–1929," *Harvard Ed. Rev.*, 46 (1976), 454.

7 William H. Chafe, *The American woman: Her changing social, economic, and political roles, 1920–1970* (New York: Oxford University Press, 1972), pp. 104–107; "Cornell's college course in child training," *Child Health Bull.*, 1 (1925), 43. See also Sheila M. Rothman, *Woman's proper place: A history of changing ideals and practices, 1870 to the present* (New York: Basic Books, 1978), esp. pp. 27–29, 106–112; Barbar Ehrenreich and Deirdre English, "The manufacture of housework," *Soc. Rev.*, 5 (4) (1975), 8–9; William D. Jenkins, "Housewifery and motherhood: The question of role change in the Progressive Era," in Mary Kelley, ed., *Woman's being, woman's place: Female identity and vocation in American history* (Boston: G. K. Hall, 1979), pp. 142–153; Emma Seifrit Weigley, "It might have been euthenics: The Lake Placid Conference and the home economics movement," *Am. Quart.*, 26 (1974), 79–96.

8 Information about the distribution of AMA booklets is found in the minutes of the House of Delegates Meeting, published each year in *JAMA;* Lillian R. Smith, "Prenatal work in Michigan," *Child Health Bull.*, 4 (1928), 93–96. Information about the booklets of other states may be found in Walter R. Ramsey, "Are your children healthy?" *Farmer's Wife,* various issues between 1924 and 1926.

9 Nancy Pottisham Weiss, "Save the children: A history of the Children's Bureau, 1903–1918," Ph.D. dissertation, University of California–Los Angeles, 1974; quotation from p. 209; *The story of Infant Care* (Washington, D.C.: HEW, Chil-

dren's Bureau, 1965), esp. pp. 30–34; James A. Toby, *The Children's Bureau: Its history, activities and organization,* Institute for Government Research, Service Monographs of the United States Government, no. 21 (Baltimore: Johns Hopkins Press, 1925); Lucille C. Birnbaum, "Behaviorism in the 1920s," *Am. Quart., 7* (1955), 15–30.

10 Anne Pierce, "What to feed the baby and why," *Parents' Mag., 3* (5) (1928), 16–17, 60, 61; Alma H. Jones, "New facts for old notions in child rearing," *Farmer's Wife, 32* (2) (1929), 41; *Modern Priscilla's* offers to send various Children's Bureau publications were appended to its regular monthly column "Our babies," written by Elizabeth MacDonald; in addition to the Health and Happiness Club, *Good Housekeeping* also conducted a correspondence column entitled "Dr. Wiley's question box," which answered queries from concerned mothers.

11 Charles S. Mohler, "Among *Hygeia* advertisers," *Hygeia, 6* (1928) 2; "Among Hygeia advertisers," *Hygeia, 12* (1934), 1058. See also the same column in *11* (1933), 1058. The AMA also used *Hygeia* to promote the importance of its Seal of Acceptance. See, for example, Doris W. McCray, "A housewife looks at the Committee on Foods," *Hygeia, 11* (1933), 881–884; *12* (1934), 319–321; and *13* (1935), 446–460, 477.

12 Bruce W. Brown, *Images of family life in magazine advertising: 1920–1970* (New York: Praeger, 1981); A. Michael McMahon, "An American courtship: Psychologists and advertising theory in the Progressive era," *Am. Studies, 13* (2) (1972), 5–18; Stuart Ewen, *Captains of consciousness: Advertising and the social roots of the consumer culture* (New York: McGraw-Hill, 1976).

13 The publishing history of Bundesen's manual is found in Herman N. Bundesen, *Our babies: Their feeding, care, and training* ([Chicago?]: n.p., [1939]); Lynn Z. Bloom, *Doctor Spock: Biography of a conservative radical* (Indianapolis: Bobbs-Merrill, 1972). Information about Baron Brothers is printed in a copy of Bundesen, *Our babies,* in my possession. Other physician-authored child-care manuals include Frank Howard Richardson, *Simplifying motherhood: Being a handbook on the care of the baby during the first year* (New York: G. P. Putnam's Sons, 1925); William M. Hanrahan, *General instructions to prospective mothers* (Chicago: Stewart Printing Co., 1927); H. Kent Tenney, *Let's talk about your baby* (Madison, Wisc.: Kilgore Printing Co., 1934); Frank Howard Richardson, *Feeding our children* (New York: Thomas Y. Crowell, 1937); W. Eugene Keiter, *Our new baby* (Kingston, N.C.: n.p., 1939); Louis W. Sauer, *From infancy through childhood* (New York: Harper & Bros., 1942); Herman N. Bundesen, *The baby manual* (New York: Simon and Schuster, 1944). On the growth in the number of child-care manuals published, see Joan Bel Geddes, *Small world: A history of baby-care from the Stone Age to the Spock Age* (New York: Macmillan, 1964), p. 10.

14 Bloom, *Doctor Spock* (n. 13), esp. pp. 101–124; Glenn Collins, "Heir apparent to

232

Dr. Spock," *New York Times*, 1 March 1985; Nancy Pottisham Weiss, "Mother, the invention of necessity: Dr. Benjamin Spock's *Baby and child care,"Am. Quart.*, 29 (1977), 519–546.

15 Benjamin Spock, *The common sense book of baby and child care* (New York: Duell, Sloan and Pearce, 1945, 1946). This sentence has been repeated in each subsequent edition of the book.

16 Alfred S. Traisman and Louis J. Halpern, "A modern nursery," *Arch. Ped.*, 57 (1940), 672–677. For more on the increase in hospitalized childbirth, see "Editorial: Hospital care for mothers," *JAMA, 124* (1944), 1258; Richard W. Wertz and Dorothy C. Wertz, *Lying-in: A history of childbirth in America* (New York: Free Press, 1977); Judith Walzer Leavitt, " 'Science' enters the birthing room: Obstetrics in America since the eighteenth century," *J. Am. Hist.*, 70 (1983), 281–304.

17 Joseph T. Smith, "Infections in the nursery," *Mod. Hosp.*, 50 (2) (1938), 53. For some statistics on diarrheal epidemics in hospital nurseries, see A. Daniel Rubinstein and George E. Foley, "Epidemic diarrhea of the newborn in Massachusetts," *New Eng. J. Med.*, 236 (1947), 87–94; Harry Bakwin, "Pseudodoxia Pediatrica," *New Eng. J. Med.*, 232 (1945), 694.

18 Smith, "Infections in the nursery" (n. 17). See also "Letters to the editor," *JAMA, 116* (1941), 550; Charles A. Weymuller et al., "Measures for the protection of newborn infants, I: Description of measures instituted in May 1937 at Long Island College Hospital," *JAMA, 133* (1947), 78–84.

19 Martin L. Bell, *A portrait of progress: A business history of Pet Milk Company from 1885–1960* (St. Louis, Mo.: Pet Milk Company, 1962), pp. 103–104.

20 John Zahorsky, "Some problems in the nursery of the newborn," *Arch. Ped.*, 54 (1937), 617–624; Clayton Ingwell, M.D., Deerfield, Wisconsin, interview, 14 October 1980; "The birth of a baby: Modern obstetric care as practiced in the Chicago Lying-In Hospital," *Hygeia, 16* (1938), 417–425; Irma and Gladys Fuehr, "Hospital baby," *Hygeia, 17* (1939), 189–190.

21 Joseph H. Marcus, "Nourishing the new-born," *Hygeia, 10* (1932), 140–143; C. Anderson Aldrich and Mary M. Aldrich, *Feeding our old fashioned children: A background for modern medicine* (New York: Macmillan, 1942), p. 78; Arnold Gesell and Frances L. Ilg, *Infant and child in the culture of today* (New York: Harper, 1943), pp. 86–87.

22 Edith Buxbaun, *Your child makes sense: A guidebook for parents* (New York: International Universities Press, 1949), p. 19.

23 See, for example, John Lovett Morse et al., *The infant and young child: Its care and feeding from birth until school age—A manual for mothers*, 2nd ed. (Philadelphia: W. B. Saunders, 1929), p. 72; "Science and health: Infant mortality controlled by sanitary progress," *Good Health*, 65 (12) (1930), 44; Frank Howard Richardson,

"You can nurse your baby," *Parents' Mag.*, *7* (12) (1932), 22, 44; "What is new in infant feeding," *New Eng. J. Med.*, *208* (1933), 273–274; Keiter, *Our new baby* (n. 13), pp. 20–24.

24 (Mrs.) E. E. Kellogg, "Diet for a nursing mother," *Good Health, 53* (1919), 730; Milton J. Senn and Phyllis Krafft Newill, *All about feeding children* (Garden City, N.Y.: Doubleday, Doran, 1944), pp. 10–12. Other examples include Lucy D. Cordiner, "Food for mother and child," *Farmer's Wife, 25* (1922), 14; Mary E. Bayley, "Maternal nursing," *Modern Priscilla, 40* (2) (1926), 44; Keiter, *Our new baby* (n. 13), pp. 17–18; *Kansas Mother's Manual*, 5th ed. (Topeka: Kansas State Board of Health, Division of Maternal and Child Health, 1939), pp. 36–37; Louise Zabriskie, *Mother and baby care in pictures* (Philadelphia: J. B. Lippincott, 1941), p. 132.

25 Sauer, *From infancy through childhood* (n. 13), p. 18.

26 Josephine Hemenway Kenyon, "Health and happiness club: The breast-fed baby," *Good Housekeeping, 86* (4) (1928), 106, 216; Frederic H. Bartlett, *Infants and children: Their feeding and growth (for mothers)* (New York: Farrar & Rinehart, 1932), p. 20; Frank Howard Richardson, "Complementary feeding," *Hygeia, 20* (1942), 70–72.

27 Morse et al., *The infant and young child* (n. 23) pp. 45–47; Bartlett, *Infants and children* (n. 26), p. 16; C. A. Aldrich, "Cultivating good appetites in babies," *Parents' Mag., 5* (6) (1931), 34, 76–77; Joseph H. Marcus, "From breast to bottle: An article on weaning the baby," *Hygeia, 10* (1932), 401–404. Various editions of *Infant Care* and other governmental pamphlets and child-care manuals offered the same advice.

28 Emelyn Lincoln Coolidge, "Must babies have colic?" *Parents' Mag., 11* (12) (1936), 25, 74, 76; Eleanor Gale Coles Carroll, "Home from the hospital," *Parents' Mag., 13* (1938), 22–23, 52–53; Abraham Tow, "The rationale of breast feeding: A modern concept," *Hygeia, 12* (1934), 406–408; Mary Grosvenor Ellsworth, "Babies must eat," *Parents' Mag., 11* (12) (1936), 19, 88–89.

29 Spock, *The common sense book* (n. 15), p. 34.

30 Hasbrouck, *Handbook for teachers* (n. 4), p. 10; Emeline S. Whitcomb, *Typical child care and parenthood education in home economics department* (Washington, D.C.: U.S. Bureau of Education, 1927), pp. 8–9. For other courses, see citations in n. 5.

31 Olive B. Cordua, "Human milk for human babies: A preliminary report on 250 infants, with commentary," *Arch. Ped, 52* (1935), 845–848; Edwin A. Riesenfield and H. L. Lichtenberg, "A comparative study of complementary feedings in 1,182 newborn infants," *Arch. Ped., 55* (1938), 553–559. See also Einar Robert Daniels, "Hospital standards for the care of obstetrical patients in general hospitals," M.D. thesis, University of Wisconsin, 1934.

234

32 Niles Rumley Newton and Michael Newton, "Relationship of ability to breast feed and maternal attitudes toward breast feeding," *Ped., 5* (1950), 870. For other examples, see "Letters to the editor," *JAMA, 120* (1942), 1147; "Medical news," *JAMA, 120* (1942), 1147; C. Anderson Aldrich, "The care of the full term infant," *Ped., 2* (1948), esp. pp. 108–109.

33 Colonial Club, interview, 8 October 1979.

34 *Good Housekeeping, 75* (11) (1922), 74, and *75* (12) (1922), 80. For KLIM advertisement, see *Good Housekeeping, 80* (12) (1925), 234, and other women's magazines of the period.

35 Hanrahan, *General instructions* (n. 13), pp. 1, 15.

36 Reilly, *Common sense* (n. 1), pp. 54–58, 15, 1–3.

37 Information for this paragraph has been drawn from Bundesen, *Our babies* (n. 13), pp. 5–35.

38 L. Emmett Holt, Jr., *The Good Housekeeping book of baby and child care* (New York: Popular Library, 1957), pp. 64–65.

Chapter VIII. "A Word of Comfort"

1 "Prairie croquet," in *To all inquiring friends: Letters, diaries, and essays in North Dakota, 1880–1910,* compiled by Elizabeth Hampsten (Grand Forks: Department of English, University of North Dakota, 1980), esp. pp. 244–245.2 See also Elizabeth Hampsten, *Read this only to yourself: The private writings of midwestern women, 1880–1910* (Bloomington: Indiana University Press, 1982), pp. 187–208. (For more on Ridge's Food, see Chapter 1, n. 21.).

2 For a sample of letters sent to women's magazines, see, for example, various issues of *Babyhood, Am. Motherhood, Farmer's Wife, Good Housekeeping, Ladies' Home J., Hygeia,* and *Modern Priscilla.* For the Children's Bureau, see U.S. Department of Labor, Children's Bureau, *The Children's Bureau: What it is, what it has done, and what it is doing for the children of the United States* (Washington, D.C.: Government Printing Office, 1928), pp. 4–5; Molly Ladd-Taylor, *Raising a baby the government way: Mothers' letters to the Children's Bureau, 1915–1932* (New Brunswick, N.J.: Rutgers University Press, 1986); Nancy Pottisham Weiss, "Save the children: A history of the Children's Bureau, 1903–1918," Ph.D. dissertation, University of California, Los Angeles, 1974, pp. 194–196; idem, "Mother, the invention of necessity: Dr. Benjamin Spock's *Baby and child care,*" *Am. Quart.,* 29 (1977), 522–527; quotation on p. 524.

3 Viola I. Paradise, *Maternity care and the welfare of young children in a homesteading county in Montana,* Children's Bureau Publication no. 34 (Washington, D.C.: Government Printing Office, 1919); reprinted in *Child care in rural America* (New York: Arno Press and the New York Times, 1972), p. 73.

4 For some cautions about using prescriptive literature as descriptions of actual

practice, see Michael Zuckerman, "Dr. Spock: The confidence man," in Charles E. Rosenberg, ed., *The family in history* (Philadelphia: University of Pennsylvania Press, 1975), p. 179; Jay Mechling, "Advice to historians on advice to mothers," *J. Soc. Hist., 9* (1975), 44–63; Carl N. Degler, "What ought to be and what was: Women's sexuality in the nineteenth century," *Am. Hist. Rev., 79* (1974), 1467–1490.

5 Cited in Weiss, "Mother, the invention of necessity" (n. 2), p. 527. See also Ladd-Taylor, *Raising a baby* (n. 2).

6 Urie Bronfenbrenner, "Socialization and social class through time and space," in Eleanor Maccoby, et al., eds., *Readings in social psychology,* 3rd ed. (New York: Holt, Rinehart and Winston, 1958), pp. 409–412, 424; idem, "The changing American child," in *Reference papers on children and youth, prepared for the 1960 White House Conference on Children and Youth* (n.p.: Golden Anniversary White House Conference on Children and Youth, Inc., 1960), pp. 1–8; Daniel R. Miller and Guy E. Swanson, *The changing American parent: A study in the Detroit area* (New York: John Wiley, 1958), pp. 5–23; Weiss, "Mother, the invention of necessity" (n. 2).

7 Daniel T. Nelson, "Some of the causes of the diseases of women," *JAMA, 7* (1886), 591; M. T. Runnels, "The physical degeneracy of American women," *Med. Era, 3* (1886), 301–302; "Infant foods," Am. Analyst, 5 (1889), 541; William J. Maybury, "The infant's food," *J. Med. & Sci.,* Portland, 4 (1897–1898), 219; Marks S. Rueben, "Observations on milk station infants," *Arch. Ped., 31* (1914), 176–196.

8 Salme Harju Steinberg, *Reformer in the marketplace: Edward W. Bok and the Ladies' Home Journal* (Baton Rouge: Louisiana State University Press, 1979), pp. 5–54. See also Esther F. Stineman, "What the ladies were reading: Popular women's magazines in America, 1875–1975," Master's thesis, Graduate Library School, University of Chicago, 1976, pp. 3–4, 18–19; Helen Rosen Woodward, *The lady persuaders* (New York: Ivan Obolensky, 1960), p. 5.

9 Annette Hills, "The baby and the bottle," *The Home-Maker, 2* (1889), 507–508; "A mother," "Mother and child: Proper feeding of infants," *Modern Priscilla, 23* (8) (1909), 44, 57. For a few specific examples of articles that assumed women were bottle feeding, see Harriet Lusk Childs, "Travelling with a baby," *Home Sci., 19* (1903), 169–170; Clare Brooks, "Baby talk: Concerning milk, whooping cough and other matters," *Good Housekeeping, 49* (1909), 75–76.

10 Elizabeth Robinson Scovil, "Suggestions for mothers," *Ladies' Home J., 16* (7) (1899), 41; "Discoveries," *Good Housekeeping, 53* (1911), 581–582.

11 Recent research has attempted to analyze the influence of advertising on modes of infant feeding. See Ted Greiner and Michael C. Latham, "The influence of infant food advertising on infant feeding practices in St. Vincent," *Internat. J. Health Services, 12* (1982), 53–75.

12 David L. Cohen, *The good old days: A history of American morals and manners as*

seen through the Sears, Roebuck catalogs, 1905 to the present (New York: Simon and Schuster, 1940), p. xxix; Daniel J. Boorstin, *The Americans: The democratic experience* (New York: Random House, 1973), pp. 127–128. Typical advertisements for infant foods and infant-feeding equipment may be found in various issues of the Sears, Roebuck catalogue from 1902 on.

13 "Nursery problems," *Babyhood, 14* (1898), 222; "Parents' problems," *Am. Motherhood, 24* (1907), 129; Mrs. L.O.B., "Talks with the doctor," *Am. Motherhood, 24* (1907), 265. For other examples, see E.W.W., "Nursery problems," *Babyhood, 9* (1892), 17–18; W.P., "Nursery problems," Babyhood, *9* (1893), 63–64; M.A., "Nursery problems," *Babyhood, 14* (1898), 143–144; "Talks with the doctor," *Am. Motherhood, 25* (1907), 55–56.

14 Mrs. J. F. Duggar, "The care of rubber nipples," *Babyhood, 10* (1894), 331–332; "Dr. Wiley's question box," *Good Housekeeping, 68* (2) (1919), 72.

15 "Nursery problems," *Babyhood, 4* (1887–1888), 30; F.W.P., "Nursery problems," *Babyhood, 2* (1886), 324–325; "A new reader," "Nursery problems," *Babyhood, 12* (1896), 126–127; and H.C., "Nursery problems," *Babyhood, 11* (1895), 180–181. See also M.R.S., "Mother's parliament," *Babyhood, 10* (1894), 244–245; "Nursery problems," *Babyhood, 1* (1895), 222; A.B. O'P., "Nursery problems," *Babyhood, 12* (1896), 211.

16 Emelyn Lincoln Coolidge, "The baby from birth to three," *Ladies' Home J., 19* (3) (1901–1902), 38; *19* (4) (1901–1902), 37; and *19* (6) (1901–1902), 36. See also "Mother's council," *Ladies' Home J., 8* (5) (1891), 17; ibid., 8 (9) (1891), 16; Elizabeth Robinson Scovil, "Suggestions for mothers," *Ladies' Home J., 11* (9) (1891), 27; ibid., *11* (11) (1891), 31; Coolidge, "The young mother's guide," *Ladies' Home J., 28* (9) (1911), 45.

17 E.V.D., "Pasteurization," *Babyhood, 9* (1893), 222–223; P.H.C., "Nursery problems," *Babyhood, 9* (1893), 348; F.B.S., "Various points of diet," *Babyhood, 10* (1894), 56–57.

18 H.E.H., "Successful use of artificial food," *Babyhood, 1* (1885), 246; Rosamond E., "Preparing and keeping baby's food," *Ladies' Home J., 9* (29) (1892), 18; "Mothers and the nursery," *Herald of Health, 41* (1891), 47–48; Mrs. J.J., "The care and feeding of children," *Am. Motherhood, 38* (1) (1914), 37. For numerous other examples, see various issues of *Babyhood, Home Sci., Am. Motherhood,* and *Ladies' Home J.*

19 F.F.S., "Mothers' council," *Ladies' Home J., 9* (1) (1891), 19.

20 See, for example, M.A., "Nursery problems," *Babyhood, 14* (1898), 143–144; W.P., "Nursery problems," *Babyhood, 9* (1893), 63–64; "The doctor's talks with mothers," *Home Sci., 19* (1903), 50–51; A.W., "Parents' problems," *Am. Motherhood, 24* (2) (1907), 129; "Parents' problems," *Am. Motherhood, 38* (6) (1914), 423–424.

21 E.B.W., "The doctor's talks with mothers," *Home Sci., 19* (1903), 49-50; Mrs. P.J.L., "The young mother and her child: Questions and answers about bottle fed babies," *Ladies' Home J., 22* (7) (1904-1905), 36. See also "Carnation milk," *Good Housekeeping, 57* (1913), 700.

22 S.M.L., "The blessed bottle," *Babyhood, 2* (1886), 175-176.

23 Ada E. Hazell, "Timely hints about baby," *Ladies' Home J., 5* (4) (1888), 5.

24 Lucy White Palmer, "In defense of the bottle-fed baby and his mother," *Babyhood, 5* (1889), 218-219.

25 "Hints for feeding a baby," *Ladies' Home J., 8* (2) (1891), 17. See also Helen Maxwell, "Baby's early days," *Ladies' Home J., 5* (7) (1888), 7; "A Baltimore mother," "Mother's council," *Ladies' Home J., 8* (8) (1891), 26.

26 Lola D. Wagner, "Personal experiences of mothers: How I raised my first baby," *Ladies' Home J., 29* (6) (1912), 36.

Chapter IX. "Count on Bottles"

1 Robert S. Lynd and Helen Merrell Lynd, *Middletown: A study in contemporary American culture* (New York: Harcourt, Brace, 1929), pp. 149-152; quotation on p. 151.

2 John E. Anderson, *The young child in the home: A survey of three thousand American families,* White House Conference on Child Health and Protection, section 3: Education and Training, Committee on the Infant and Preschool Child (New York: D. Appleton-Century, 1936), pp. 73-80.

3 Mrs. R.E.D., "Letters worth reading," *Farmer's Wife, 28* (1925), 355.

4 Mrs. P.O., Iowa, 23 July 1928 quoted in Molly Ladd-Taylor, *Raising a baby the government way: Mothers' letters to the Children's Bureau, 1915-1932* (New Brunswick, N.J.: Rutgers University Press, 1986), pp. 209-210.

5 J.B., "My $100 baby," *Cosmopolitan, 108* (6) (1940), 54.

6 Alice Dillon, "Escalator service," typescript, in box 2, file labeled "W.E.R.A. Child Health Nursing Project: Newspaper & Journal Publicity," Bessie Mae Beach, Summary report of 30 July 1937, county demonstration at De Forest, box 4, file labeled "Dane County (Center Narratives)," both in Program and Demonstration Materials, Wisconsin Department of Health and Social Services, Maternal and Child Health Bureau, Archives Division, State Historical Society of Wisconsin, Madison, Wisconsin.

7 For print media evidence, see, for example, Isadore Luce Smith, "We modern parents," *Atlantic Monthly, 152* (1933), 95; M. Beatrice Blakenship, "The enduring miracle," *Atlantic Monthly, 152* (1933), 412-413; Josephine Hemenway Kenyon, "Dressing and bathing babies," *Good Housekeeping, 96* (1933), 96; Marjorie F. Murray and Ruth I. Lyman, "A study of infant care in a rural community," *N. Y.*

238

St. J. Med., 35 (1936), 165–172; Ruth W. Washburn and Marian C. Putnam, "A study of child care in the first two years of life," *J. Ped., 2* (1933), 536. I conducted over fifty interviews between October 1979 and December 1981. Though the women interviewed do not represent a scientific sample, they do encompass a broad spectrum of experiences. Some had given birth in the late 1910s, but most had their children in the 1920s, 1930s, and 1940s. Though many of the women resided in or near Madison, Wisconsin, at the time of the interview, they had raised their children in diverse locales, ranging from urban environments, such as New York City, Chicago, Milwaukee, and Minneapolis, to farms and rural towns in the Midwest. Their educational backgrounds were similarly varied: almost all had at least graduated from high school; a few had attended college; one was a nurse. Some of the data cited were gathered in group interviews; references to this material specify the group name and date. Other information comes from individual conversations; this is cited by name of interviewee and date.

8 Ellen Plaenert, interview, 10 March 1980.

9 Westside Coalition, interview, 29 February 1980.

10 Interviews: Wanda Hila, 22 February 1980; Westside Coalition, 29 February 1980; Westside Coalition, 12 March 1980; 60 + Club, 10 April 1980.

11 Rural Kansas, Johnstown, Pa., Manchester, N.H., and Akron, Ohio, from Elizabeth Moore, *Maternity and infant care in a rural county of Kansas,* Children's Bureau Publication no. 2 (Washington, D.C.: Government Printing Office, 1917), reprinted in *Childcare in rural America* (New York: Arno Press and the New York Times, 1972), p. 42. Wisconsin, Saginaw, Mich., and New Bedford, Mass., from Florence Brown Sherbon and Elizabeth Moore, *Maternity and infant care in two rural counties in Wisconsin,* Children's Bureau Publication no. 46 (Washington, D.C.: Government Printing Office, 1919), reprinted in *Childcare in rural America,* p. 92. Boston, Mass., from Joseph Garland and Mabel B. Rich, "Duration of breast feeding: A comparative study," *New Eng. J. Med., 203* (1930), 1279–1282. Rural New York State from Rachael Sanders Bizal, "Our babies: What they are fed," *Med. Woman's J., 41* (1934), 158–162. Hospital births from Katherine Bain, "Incidence of breast feedings in hospitals in the United States," *Ped., 2* (1948), 313–320.

12 Frank Howard Richardson, "Feeding the baby in wartime," *Hygeia, 23* (1945), 220, 222.

13 Herman F. Meyer, "Breast feeding in the United States: Extent and possible trend," *Ped., 22* (1958), 116–121.

14 Eleanor Gale Coles Carroll, "Home from the hospital," *Parents' Mag., 13* (1938), 22–23, 52–53. For other articles that assumed mothers were bottle feeding, see Walter H. Eddy, "Milk plus: That is what you get when you buy milk with vitamin D added to it," *Good Housekeeping, 98* (1934), 136; Regina J. Woody, "Feeding the new baby," *Parents' Mag., 9* (9) (1934), 20, 63–65; Billee Wyer, "A schedule for the

new mother," *Parents' Mag.*, *12* (2) (1937), 22, 62–64; Doris Atkinson Karchevski, "Bottle for a baby," *Parents' Mag.*, *13* (1938), 29, 79; C. Anderson Aldrich and Mary M. Aldrich, "The baby learns to eat," *Parents' Mag.*, *14* (1939), 21, 44.

15 Paul T. Cherington, *The consumer looks at advertising* (New York: Harper & Brothers, 1928), pp. xiii, 177–189. See also Otis Pease, *The responsibilities of American advertising: Private control and public influence, 1920–1940* (New Haven: Yale University Press, 1958), pp. 20–25, 33–35, 169–173; Lois W. Banner, *Women in modern America: A brief history* (New York: Harcourt Brace Jovanovich, 1974), p. 143.

16 Claude Hopkins, *Scientific advertising* (with *My life in advertising*) (1923; reprint ed., Chicago: Advertising Publications, 1966), p. 282.

17 60 + Club, interview, 10 April 1980.

18 Anderson, *The young child* (n. 2), pp. 88–90.

19 "Questions & answers," *Hygeia*, *4* (1926), 422. See also "Infant feeding," *Hygeia*, *4* (1926), 486.

20 Janes Gilberth Heppes, "Easy does it with a baby," *Parents' Mag.*, *23* (11) (1948), 26, 168–169. For other examples, see Nathelie F. Gross, "Who's afraid of a baby?" *Parents' Mag.*, *21* (2) (1946), 24, 93–94; Lois Huntington, "Schedule for a new baby's mother," *Parents' Mag.*, *17* (9) (1942), 24–25, 61.

21 Doris Jackson, interview, 20 October 1981. See also Chapter 7.

22 Lenore Pelham Friedrich, "I had a baby," *Atlantic Monthly*, *163* (1939), 461–465; Thomas Sugrue, "To my unborn son," *American Magazine*, *125* (1938), 34–35, 137–140; Sarah M. Privette, letter published in *Atlantic Monthly*, *163* (1939), 769–771. See also Irma and Gladys Fuehr, "Hospital baby," *Hygeia*, *17* (1939), 189–190.

23 Mrs. Clayton Ingwell, interview, 14 October 1980.

24 J. C. Spence, "Modern decline of breast feeding," *Brit. Med. J.*, *2* (1938), 730–733. See also William Palmer Lucas, *Children's diseases for nurses* (New York: Macmillan, 1923), pp. 66, 108; Walter Lester Carr and Bret Ratner, "The results of follow-up work with infants in a maternity hospital," *Tr. Am. Ped. Soc.*, *35* (1923), 302–311.

25 Niles Rumely Newton and Michael Newton, "Relationship of ability to breast feed and maternal attitudes toward breast feeding," *Ped.*, *5* (1950), 869–875.

26 Clifford Sweet, "Essential points in the dietetic management of infants," *Arch. Ped.*, *45* (1928), 740–743; Rupert Rogers, "How to nurse your baby," *Parents' Mag.*, *15* (3) (1940), 25, 65–67.

27 Mary McCarthy, *The group* (New York: Harcourt, Brace & World, 1963), pp. 224–247.

28 Interviews: 60 + Club, 10 April 1980; Segoe Terrace group, 17 March 1980; Amy Wills, 10 April 1980.

29 Interviews: Westside Coalition, 12 March 1980; Dr. William F. Donlin, 13

240

December 1979; Dr. H. Kent Tenney, 24 September 1979; Dr. and Mrs. Clayton Ingwell, 14 October 1980.

30 Worth Tuttle, "A feminist marries," *Atlantic Monthly, 153* (1934), 74–75. See also Carr and Ratner, "The results of follow-up work" (n. 24).

31 Carroll, "Home from the hospital" (n. 14).

32 Katherine Burns, "The two weeks after the first ten days," *American Home, 24* (1940), 38, 54.

33 "Educated mothers, by one of them," *Commonweal, 23* (1936), 682–684.

34 Anne Swann, interview, 24 December 1981.

35 Betty Schwartz, interview, 15 December 1980.

36 Maybelle Hinton Osborne, "Eleven tips from a mother of three," *Better Homes & Gardens, 27* (3) (1948), 88.

37 J.B., "My $100 baby" (n. 5).

38 Ladd-Taylor, *Raising a baby* (n. 4), pp. 85–86.

39 Westside Coalition, interview, 29 February 1980; Ruth Normandy, "You can nurse your baby," *Parents' Mag., 10* (3) (1935), 23, 74; Charles F. Rennick, "Infant feeding in the first trimester," *Southwestern Med., 20* (1936), 96–98; Fuehr and Fuehr, "Hospital baby" (n. 22); J.B., "My $100 baby" (n. 5); Tenney interview (n. 29); Dr. William John Focke, interview, 17 October 1979; Donlin interview (n. 20); Dr. Karver L. Puestow, interview, 18 September 1980; 60 + Club, interview, 17 April 1980.

40 "They wanted to nurse their babies," *Parents' Mag., 25* (10) (1950), 36, 90–94.

41 Norma Starkweather, interview, 29 February 1980.

42 Interviews: Westside Coalition, 12 March 1980, 29 February 1980.

43 Garland and Rich, "Duration of breast feeding" (n. 11).

44 Interviews: 60 + Club, 17 April 1980; Ann Strain, 16 April 1980; Quaker Housing Group, 25 February 1980.

45 60 + Club, interviews, 10 April 1980.

46 60 + Club, interviews, 17 April 1980.

47 Interviews: Ellen Plaenert, 10 March 1980; Segoe Terrace Group, 17 March 1980; 60 + Club, 10 April 1980; Della Lewis, 14 March 1980; Colonial Club, 8 October 1979; 60 + Club, 17 April 1980; Quaker Housing Group, 25 February 1980; Edith Vandenburgh, 26 February 1980; Ann Strain, 16 April 1980.

48 Interviews: Quaker Housing Group, 25 February 1980; Westside Coalition, 12 March 1980; Segoe Terrace Group, 17 March 1980; Mrs. Clayton Ingwell, 14 October 1980; 60 + Club, 10 April 1980.

49 Amy Wills, interview, 10 April 1980.

Chapter X. "According to Your Own Preferences"

1. L. Emmett Holt and John Howland, *The diseases of infancy and childhood,* 7th ed. (New York: Appleton, 1920), pp. 42–47; L. Emmett Holt et al., *Holt's diseases*

of infancy and childhood, 10th ed. (New York: Appleton, 1936), pp. 44–47; L. Emmett Holt, Jr., and Rustin McIntosh, *Pediatrics,* 12th ed. (New York: Appleton-Century-Crofts, 1953), pp. 60–62; Herman Frederic Meyer, *Essentials of infant feeding for physicians* (Springfield, Ill.: Charles C. Thomas, 1952), pp. 9–10.

2 Recently several researchers have attempted to analyze the factors, primarily the environmental factors, contributing to the high rates of infant mortality due to diarrhea and gastrointestinal diseases in the late nineteenth and early twentieth centuries. Ian Buchanan, "Infant feeding, sanitation and diarrhoea in colliery communities, 1880–1911," in Derek J. Oddy and Derek S. Miller, *Diet and health in modern Britain* (London: Croom Helm, 1985), pp. 148–177; Rose A. Cheney, "Seasonal aspects of infant and childhood mortality: Philadelphia, 1865–1920," *J. Interdisciplinary Hist.,* 14 (1984), 561–585. Some epidemiologists have hypothesized that a change in the virulence of the microorganism was responsible; this suggestion is in line with the generally accepted explanation for the decline in scarlet-fever mortality over the last century. Bryan Gandevia, *Tears often shed: Child health and welfare in Australia from 1788* (Rushcutters Bay, New South Wales: Pergamon Press, 1977), pp. 123–134; Douglas Gordon, *Health, sickness and society: Theoretical concepts in social and preventive medicine* (Brisbane: University of Queensland Press, 1976), pp. 190–207.

3 John R. Williams, "A study of Rochester's infant mortality," *The Common Good,* 5 (4) (1912), 14–22; Robert Morse Woodbury, *Infant mortality and its causes* (Baltimore: Williams & Wilkins, 1926), esp. pp. 79–97; L. Emmett Holt, "Infant mortality and its reduction, especially in New York City," *JAMA,* 59 (1910), 682–691; S. Josephine Baker, *Child hygiene* (New York: Harper & Brothers, 1925), pp. 191–196, 210–213: Robert Morse Woodbury, "Relation between breast and artificial feeding and infant mortality," *Am. J. Hygiene,* 2 (1922), 668–687; Thomas E. Cone, Jr., *History of American pediatrics* (Boston: Little, Brown, 1979), esp. pp. 106–107, 131, 152, 159–160; George T. Palmer, "Infant mortality in 1922," *Mother & Child,* 4 (1923), 357–360; Charles K. Johnson, "Reduction of infant mortality," *New Eng. J. Med.,* 200 (1929), 1105–1106; Richard Smith, "Acute gastrointestinal disease in infants," *New Eng. J. Med.,* 215 (1936), 701–704.

Similar calls appeared in other industrialized countries. See Carol Dyhouse, "Working-class mothers and infant mortality in England, 1895–1914," *J. Soc. Hist.,* 12 (1979), 248–267; Milton Lewis, "The problem of infant feeding: The Australian experience from the mid-nineteenth century to the 1920s," *J. Hist. Med.,* 35 (1980), 174–187; Kerreen M. Regier, "Women's labour redefined: Child-bearing and rearing advice in Australia, 1880–1930s," in Margaret Bevege et al.,

242

eds., *Worth her salt: Women at work in Australia* (Sydney: Hale & Iremonger, 1982), pp. 72–83.

Comparative studies are needed to delineate the common factors underlying the promotion of artificial infant feeding and the development of scientific motherhood in these and other cultures. For example, it would be useful to have a history and content analysis of the many editions of the pamphlet *Child care* (issued by the Department of Health, Maternal and Child Welfare Branch, in Victoria, Australia), which includes statements such as "Good mothercraft is the loving common sense care of the child in light of recent scientific knowledge" (p. 14).

4 "Report of the Task Force on the Assessment of the Scientific Evidence Relating to Infant-feeding Practices and Infant Health," *Ped.*, 74 (1984), "Executive summary," pp. 580–581; Mary Grace Kovar et al., "Review of the epidemiological evidence for an association between infant feeding and infant health," pp. 615–638; quotations on p. 580. See also Armond S. Goldman, "Immunologic aspects of human milk," in Lucy R. Waletzky, ed., *Symposium on human lactation*, Department of Health, Education and Welfare Publication no. (HSA) 79-5107 (Washington, D.C.: HEW, 1979), pp. 55–56; Jane Pitt, "Immunologic aspects of human milk," in Dana Raphael, ed., *Breastfeeding and food policy in a hungry world* (New York: Academic Press, 1979), pp. 229–232; "Advantages of breast feeding to mother, to baby, and to his future," in *Good mothering through breastfeeding the world over,* transcript of the third Biennial Convention, Denver, 17–19 July 1968 (Franklin Park, Ill.: La Leche League International, 1970), pp. 224–231; Robin Marantz Henig, "The case for mother's milk," *New York Times Magazine,* 8 July 1979, pp. 40–42, 57; Jane E. Brody, "Why is breastfeeding better? Science starts finding the answers," *Milwaukee Journal,* 27 January 1980, Gail Bronson, "Breastfeeding advocates increasingly question safety, nutritional value of infants' formulas," *Wall Street Journal,* 21 March 1980.

5 On the history of childbirth, see Judith Walzer Leavitt, *Brought to bed: Child bearing in America, 1750–1950* (New York: Oxford University Press, 1986); Nancy Schrom Dye, "Review essay: History of childbirth in America," *Signs,* 6 (1980), 97–108; Richard W. Wertz and Dorothy C. Wertz, *Lying-in: A history of childbirth in America* (New York: Free Press, 1977); Margarete Sandelowski, *Pain, pleasure, and American childbirth: From twilight sleep to the Read method, 1914–1960* (Westport, Conn.: Greenwood Press, 1984). On the decline of the midwife in this country, see Judy Barrett Litoff, *American midwives, 1860 to the present* (Westport, Conn.: Greenwood Press, 1978). According to her study, by 1930 only 15 percent of all births were midwife-attended. My analysis in the following paragraphs owes much to the interpretations of Judith Walzer Leavitt, "Birthing and anesthesia: The debate over twilight sleep," *Signs,* 6 (1980),

147–164; idem, " 'Science' enters the birthing room: Obstetrics in America since the eighteenth century," *J. Am. Hist.*, 70 (1983), 281–304; Lawrence G. Miller, "Pain, parturition, and the profession: Twilight sleep in America," in Susan Reverby and David Rosner, eds., *Health care in America: Essays in social history* (Philadelphia: Temple University Press, 1979), pp. 19–44.

6 Ronald L. Numbers, ed., *The education of American physicians: Historical essays* (Berkeley: University of California Press, 1980); Rosemary Stevens, *American medicine and the public interest* (New Haven: Yale University Press, 1971), esp. pp. 34–55; Paul Starr, *The social transformation of American medicine* (New York: Basic Books, 1982).

7 Harold Kniest Faber and Rustin McIntosh, *History of the American Pediatric Society, 1887–1965* (New York: McGraw-Hill, 1966), pp. 19–20.

8 Kathryn M. Kram and George M. Owen, "Nutritional studies on United States preschool children: Dietary intakes and practices of food procurement, preparation and consumption," in Samuel J. Fomon and Thomas A. Anderson, eds., *Practices of low-income families in feeding infants and small children, with particular attention to cultural subgroups*, Proceedings of a National Workshop, Airlie Conference Center, Warrenton, Virginia, 17–19 March 1971 (Washington, D.C.: Department of Health, Education and Welfare, 1972), p. 13. See also Mary Ellen Wilcox, commenting on Jana W. Jones, "Child feeding in rural low-income families," ibid., pp. 46–47; Jones, "Child feeding," ibid., pp. 37–48; Norge W. Jerome, et al., "Infant and child feeding practices in an urban community in the north-central region," ibid., pp. 49–58.

9 For more on the mid-century explanations for the popularity of bottle feeding, see Derrick B. Jelliffe and E. F. Patrice Jelliffe, " 'Breast is best': Modern meanings," *New Eng. J. Med.*, 279 (1977): 912–915; Helen Starina, commenting on Jones, "Child feeding" (n. 8), p. 47; Lucy R. Waletzky, "Preface," *Symposium on human lactation* (n. 4), p. ii; Christine M. Olson and Donna L. Psiaki, "Imparting information on breast feeding to medical students," *J. Med. Ed.*, 53 (1978), 845–846; Niles Rumely Newton and Michael Newton, "Relationship of ability to breast feed and maternal attitudes toward breast feeding," *Ped.*, 5 (1950), 869–875; Benjamin Spock, *Baby and child care* (New York: Pocket Books, 1957), p. 81; *Feeding infants: A nutrition monograph for health professionals* (Madison: Wisconsin Department of Health and Social Services, Division of Health, 1979), p. 9; Herbert Ratner, "Foreword," *The womanly art of breastfeeding* (Franklin Park, Ill.: La Leche League International, 1963), pp. v–vii.

10 Marian Tompson, "The heart of the matter," *Good mothering* (n. 4), pp. 1–4.

11 Marian Tompson, quoted in Margot Edwards and Mary Waldorf, *Reclaiming birth: History and heroines of American childbirth reform* (Trumansburg, N.Y.: Crossing Press, 1984), p. 88.

12 Barbara Katz Rothman, *In labor: Women and power in the birthplace* (New York: W. W. Norton, 1982), pp. 204–205.

13 *Womanly art* (n. 9), esp. pp. 151–155. This need for a female network, the sense that new mothers need a support group of other mothers to "ease the transition into motherhood and decrease the isolation of new mothers," continues today. See, for example, Jill Muehrcke, "New mothers need to share experiences," *Sunshine/Madison Outlook,* 23 December 1981, p. 5.

14 Edith B. Jackson, "General reactions of mothers and nurses to rooming-in," *Am. J. Pub. Health, 38* (1948), 689–695.

15 American Academy of Pediatrics, Committee on Fetus and Newborn, *Standards and recommendations for hospital care of newborn infants* (Evanston, Ill.: American Academy of Pediatrics, 1949).

16 Dorothy Barclay, "Year's test of the 'rooming-in' plan," *New York Times Magazine,* 26 March 1950, p. 60. See also Rhoda Hanson, "You can nurse your baby," *Parents' Mag., 23* (5) (1948), 23, 136; "Babies welcome here," *Woman's Home Companion, 76* (1) (1949), 116–119; Marilyn Parks Davis, "The 'rooming-in' plan," *Hygeia, 26* (1948), 784–785, 827–828; Henry L. Barnett, "A note on experiences with a rooming-in arrangement for newborn infants in a small hospital," *J. Ped., 31* (1947), 49–53; Edith B. Jackson et al., "A hospital rooming-in unit for four newborn infants and their mothers," *Ped., 1* (1948), 28–43; Herbert Thoms et al., "The rooming-in plan for mothers and infants," *Am. J. Obst. & Gynec., 56* (1948), 707–711; Thaddeus L. Montgomery et al., "Observations on the rooming-in program of baby with mother in ward and private service," *Am. J. Obst. & Gynec., 57* (1949), 176–186; Myrtle Meyer Eldred, "Do you want to nurse your baby?" *Hygeia, 27* (1949), 392, 426–427.

17 Gilbert A. Martinez et al., "Milk feeding patterns in the United States during the first 12 months of life," *Ped., 68* (1981), 863–868; Gilbert A. Martinez and John P. Nalezienski, "1980 update: The recent trend in breast-feeding," *Ped., 67* (1981), 260–263; idem, "The recent trend in breast feeding," *Ped., 64* (1979), 686–692, and, in the American Academy of Pediatrics task force study, Gerry E. Hendershot, "Trends in breast-feeding" (n. 4), pp. 591–602. Though the percentage of breast-fed infants increased, Martinez and associates found that of the mothers who bottle fed, proportionately fewer used evaporated milk (EM) or whole milk (WCM) formulas and more used commercially prepared infant foods. For example, at age five to six months, the use of prepared formulas rose from 28 percent in 1971 to 60.8 percent in 1980; use of EM/WCM fell from 68.1 percent to 20.6 percent in the same time period.

18 Much of this information is summarized in the task force's study (n. 4); see esp. "Executive summary," pp. 579–583, and Artemis P. Simopoulos and Gilman D. Grave, "Factors associated with the choice and duration of infant-feeding prac-

tice," pp. 603–614. For interpretations published in the popular press, see Henig, "The case for mother's milk" (n. 4); Bronson, "Breastfeeding advocates" (n. 4); "Study on infant formula use," *New York Times*, 27 October 1981.

19 Mike Muller, *The baby killer* (London: War on Want, 1974); Barbara Garson, "The bottle baby scandal," *Mother Jones*, 2 (10) (1977), 32–34, 38–40, 60–62; Stephen Solomon, "The controversy over infant formula," *New York Times Magazine*, 6 December 1981, pp. 92, 94, 98–106. See also Ted Greiner, *The promotion of bottle feeding by multinational corporations: How advertising and the health professions have contributed*, Cornell International Nutritional Monograph Series, no. 2 (Ithaca, N.Y.: Cornell University, Division of Nutritional Sciences, 1975); idem, *Regulation and education: Strategies for solving the bottle feeding problem*, Cornell International Nutrition Monograph Series, no. 4 (Ithaca, N.Y.: Cornell University, Division of Nutritional Sciences, 1977); Barry M. Popkin et al., "Breast-feeding patterns in low-income countries," *Science*, *218* (1982), 1088–1093; Michael B. Bader, "Breast-feeding: The role of multinational corporations in Latin America," *Internat. J. Health Services*, 6 (1976), 609–626.

20 Task Force study, Janine M. Jason et al., "Mortality and infectious disease associated with infant-feeding practices in developing countries" (n. 4), 702–727; quotation on p. 717.

21 See in the Task Force's study Francis Notzon, "Trends in infant feeding in developing countries" (n. 4) 648–666; Michele R. Forman, "Review of research on the factors associated with choice and duration of infant-feeding in less developed countries" (n.4), 667–694, for summaries of this research. See also publications cited in n. 19.

22 Despite a proliferation of studies investigating contemporary infant-feeding practices in the Third World, their relation to infant mortality and morbidity, and the probable impact of infant-food advertising, few studies have examined the historical background. A notable exception is the work of Lenore Manderson, who shows that bottle feeding, particularly the use of manufactured foods, was practiced by certain groups of mothers as early as the late nineteenth century when products such as Nestlé's, Borden's, and Mellins' were imported into colonial Malaya. See Manderson, "Bottle feeding and ideology in colonial Malaya: The production of change," *Intern. J. Health Services*, *12* (1982), 597–616; idem., "Infant feeding practice, market expansion, and the patterning of choice, Southeast Asia 1880–1980," *New Doctor* (Journal of the Doctors' Reform Society) (Sydney), no. 26 (1982), 27–32.

23 Marie Pichel Warner, *A doctor discusses breast feeding* (Chicago: Budlong Press, 1970), pp. 1–6.

24 *Breast feeding your baby* (Columbus, Ohio: Ross Laboratories, 1977).

25 *Infant Care*, U.S. Department of Health, Education and Welfare Publication No.

246

(OHDS) 77-30015 (Washington, D.C.: Government Printing Office, 1972), pp. 2-3. This edition was still being distributed by the Government Printing Office in 1986. Even though congressional representatives send free copies of this pamphlet to constituents on request, *Infant Care* is also available from a trade publisher. See A. Frederick North, *Infant care* (New York: Arco Publishing, 1975).

Bibliographic Essay

Many aspects of American life, which changed dramatically between 1890 and 1950, affected the development, promotion and acceptability of bottle feeding. Changes in medical education and in medical practice, changes in the idealized image of motherhood and in women's experiences, changes in communications and transportation and in the commercial and industrial sectors of the United States: all contributed to shaping the various answers to the question "how shall I feed my baby?" The sources for investigating the social history of infant feeding are many and varied, but widely scattered and frequently difficult to locate. Though several secondary sources are particularly helpful in providing important background and contextual material, a more complete understanding of the shift from breast to bottle feeding emerges from study of a wide variety of sources. This essay focuses on some of the more significant published and unpublished sources used directly or indirectly in preparing this book. A fuller list of sources is found in the Notes section.

This monograph relies heavily on the words of those most directly involved in decisions about infant feeding, namely mothers and physicians. Data about them and their experiences are drawn from both the written record and interviews. I researched the runs of major medical journals and women's magazines such as *American Journal of Diseases of Children*, *American Journal of Obstetrics and Diseases of Women and Children*, *American Journal of Obstetrics and Gynecology*, *American Motherhood* (variously titled *Mother's Friend* and *New Crusade*), *Archives of Pediatrics*, *Babyhood*, *Boston Medical and Surgical Journal*, *Cosmopolitan*, *Good Health*, *Good Housekeeping*, *Hygeia*, *Journal of the American Medical Association*, *Journal of Pediatrics*, *Ladies' Home Journal*, *Modern Priscilla*, *Parents' Magazine* and *Pediatrics*. Close reading of the articles and of letters to the editor and other correspondence columns, as well as advertising matter, discloses both what was expected (prescriptions) and what mothers and physicians actually experienced (descriptions). Esther F. Stineman's "What the ladies were reading:

Popular women's magazines in America, 1875–1975" (unpublished master's thesis, Graduate Library School, University of Chicago, 1976) and indexes such as the *Index-catalogue of the Library of the Surgeon General,* ser. 1–4 (Washington, D.C.: Government Printing Office, 1880–1955) directed me to other pertinent periodical literature cited in the Notes section.

I conducted a series of interviews with physicians in practice before 1950 and with women who birthed in the same time period. The Wisconsin State Medical Society was able to give me the names of retired physicians. I approached several senior citizens' organizations and asked members to talk with me about their infant-care practices. Many women agreed to be interviewed. Some of these interviews were conducted at the organization's headquarters and in some instances volunteers convened a group of friends in their homes, thus enlarging the pool of interviewees. In other cases, the informant mailed me a description of her, or of her mother's, experiences or spoke with me informally about the topic. Though the interviews did not comprise a systematic and comprehensive survey, they did complement and give life to the data found in published sources.

In addition, a growing number of women's diaries and collections of women's letters are now being located and some have been published, making them available to a wider audience. Books such as Elizabeth Hampsten, *Read this only to yourself: The private writings of midwestern women, 1880–1910* (Bloomington: Indiana University Press, 1982) and Molly Ladd-Taylor, *Raising a baby the government way: Mothers' letters to the Children's Bureau, 1915–1932* (New Brunswick, N.J.: Rutgers University Press, 1986) are fascinating exemplars of this trend. Further documentation for the medicalization of infant feeding and the growing importance of bottle feeding was found in medical textbooks and medical advice manuals written by both physicians and laypersons, typically mothers, as well as in biographies and autobiographies of physicians. Many of these are cited in the Notes.

Within the period 1890 to 1950, the areas of medicine and mothering, in particular, were significantly transformed in this country; analyses of these transformations provide a backdrop against which one must interpret the move from breast feeding to medically supervised bottle feeding. Useful literature includes: on changes in medical practice, Judith Walzer Leavitt and Ronald L. Numbers, ed., *Sickness and health in America: Readings in the history of medicine and public health,* 2nd ed. (Madison: University of Wisconsin Press, 1985), Paul Starr, *The social transformation of American medicine* (New York: Basic Books, 1982), Susan Reverby and David Rosner, eds., *Health care in America: Essays in social history* (Philadelphia: Temple University Press, 1979), Morris J. Vogel and Charles E. Rosenberg, eds., *The therapeutic revolution: Essays in the social history of American medicine* (Philadelphia: University of Pennsylvania Press, 1979); on developments in medical education, Kenneth M. Ludmerer, *Learning to heal: The development of American medical education* (New York: Basic Books, 1985),

Ronald L. Numbers, ed., *The education of American physicians: Historical essays* (Berkeley: University of California Press, 1980); on professionalization, Rosemary Stevens, *American medicine and the public interest* (New Haven: Yale University Press, 1971), William G. Rothstein, *American physicians in the 19th century: From sects to science* (Baltimore: Johns Hopkins University Press, 1972), Harold Kniest Faber and Rustin McIntosh, *History of the American Pediatric Society, 1887–1965* (New York: McGraw-Hill, 1966); on the rise of hospitals, David Rosner, *A once charitable enterprise* (Cambridge: Cambridge University Press, 1982), Morris Vogel, *The invention of the modern hospital* (Chicago: University of Chicago Press, 1980), Dorothy Levenson, *Montefiore: The hospital as social instrument, 1884–1984* (New York: Farrar, Straus & Giroux, 1984).

What little secondary literature exists on the history of infant feeding is based almost exclusively on prescriptive and didactic medical literature and is useful primarily in identifying some of the early trends in the emerging profession of pediatrics around the turn of the century: most especially, Thomas E. Cone, Jr., *History of American pediatrics* (Boston: Little, Brown, 1979), Thomas E. Cone, Jr., *200 years of feeding infants in America* (Columbus, Ohio: Ross Laboratories, 1976).

In the last decade or so women's history has emerged as a fast growing and exciting field of research. Among the many works recently published, I found Laura Shapiro, *Perfection salad: Women and cooking at the turn of the century* (New York: Farrar, Straus and Giroux, 1986), Ruth Schwartz Cowan, *More work for mother: The ironies of household technology from the open hearth to the microwave* (New York: Basic Books, 1983), Susan Strasser, *Never done: A history of American housework* (New York: Pantheon Books, 1982), Shelia M. Rothman, *Woman's proper place: A history of changing ideals and practices, 1870 to the present* (New York: Basic Books, 1978) most useful. Within the general subject of women's history, the history of women and medicine has received a great deal of attention recently. My own work has been stimulated in particular by Judith Walzer Leavitt, *Brought to bed: Childbearing in America, 1750–1950* (New York: Oxford University Press, 1986), Regina Markell Morantz-Sanchez, *Sympathy and science: Women physicians in American medicine* (New York: Oxford University Press, 1985), Judith Walzer Leavitt, ed., *Women and health in America: Historical readings* (Madison: University of Wisconsin Press, 1984), Martha H. Verbrugge, "Women and medicine in nineteenth-century America," *Signs, 1* (1976), 957–972. Also of interest in analyzing the question of infant feeding are Ann Oakley, *Becoming a mother* (New York: Schocken Books, 1980), Margot Edwards & Mary Waldorf, *Reclaiming birth: History and heroines of American birth reform* (Trumansburg, N.Y.: The Crossing Press, 1984).

In the development of artificial infant feeding, the infant food industry was also party to the decision-making process. Data about the activities of many of these companies is not readily available. Company histories have been written for some firms, such as John

D. Weaver, *Carnation: The first 75 years, 1899–1974* (Los Angeles: Carnation Company, 1974), Martin L. Bell, *A portrait of progress: A business history of Pet Milk Company from 1885 to 1960* (St. Louis, Mo.: Pet Milk Company, 1952), Jean Heer, *World events, 1866–1966: The first hundred years of Nestlé,* A. Bradley et al., trans., (Lausanne, Switzerland: Nestlé, 1966), John Francis Marion, *The fine old house* (Philadelphia: Smith Kline Corporation, 1980), Typically, though these publications do not discuss the development of infant foods in any detail. The records of other companies have been preserved in archival collections open to the researcher, notably Mead Johnson & Company, Business records, 1895–1971 (at the Indiana State University–Evansville, Special Collection, Evansville, Indiana) and Horlick's Corporation papers, 1873–1974 (at the State Historical Society of Wisconsin, Division of Archives and Manuscripts, Madison, Wisconsin). While not establishing formal archival collections, several other manufacturers are supportive of historical investigations and will undertake some limited research for the historian. Still other companies claim to have no records at all.

Much information about the manufacture of infant foods must be gleaned from less direct sources. For instance, in endeavoring to attract the attention of mothers and physicians, especially in the early years, the companies advertised heavily and offered free child-care and infant-feeding booklets. An analysis of infant-food advertisements provides some gauge of the companies' activities and growth. Similarly, pamphlets prepared for mothers and physicians by the manufacturers tell much about the products and about the roles played by companies in the growing popularity of bottle feeding. Unfortunately, these sources can be extremely difficult to find. Most libraries do not bind medical journals with their advertising sections intact. Some institutions bind with no advertisements; others include the advertisements of one issue in each volume bound, thus making this aspect of research particularly frustrating. Fortunately for the historians, popular and women's magazines are more likely to integrate advertising matter and editorial matter throughout most of the journal. Consequently, bound volumes of these periodicals include most advertisements. Moreover, in the period under study home economics was a flourishing academic subject, particularly on the campuses of land-grant colleges. Therefore these institutions frequently continue to house complete runs of bound volumes of popular women's magazine such as *Good Housekeeping* and *Ladies' Home Journal.* Company-produced booklets are more difficult to find. Some are collected within company archives but the more likely, general sources are archival collections such as the Bella C. Landauer Collection of Business and Advertising Art (at the New York Historical Society, New York City) and the Collection of Business Americana (at the National Museum of American History, Smithsonian Institution, Washington, D.C.; especially "Folder: Baby-Infant/Invalid Foods" and "Box: Foods-Health Food (Medicinal), Infant (Baby) Food, Invalid (Ill) Food") and also the pamphlet files of medical and public libraries.

There are many similarities between the infant-food industry and that of patent medicines. Hence, any analysis of the history of bottle feeding has much to gain from work done in the history of patent medicines and quackery. Most useful for my work have been James Harvey Young, *The toadstool millionaires: A social history of patent medicines in America before federal regulation* (Princeton: Princeton University Press, 1961), James Harvey Young, *The medical messiahs: A social history of health quackery in twentieth-century America* (Princeton: Princeton University Press, 1967), Sarah Stage, *Female complaints: Lydia Pinkham and the business of women's medicine* (New York: W. W. Norton, 1979).

Finally, histories of advertising shine light on the advertising campaigns of some of the leading manufacturers of infant foods. Frank Presbrey, *The history and development of advertising* (Garden City, N.Y.: Doubleday, Doran, 1929) is still the first reference to check for nineteenth- and early twentieth-century advertising. Interesting, more recent analyses of advertising and its history include Michael Schudson, *Advertising, the uneasy persuasion: Its dubious impact on American society* (New York: Basic Books, 1984), Roland Marchard, *Advertising the American dream* (Berkeley: University of California Press, 1985), Stuart Ewen, *Captains of consciousness; Advertising and the social roots of the consumer culture* (New York: McGraw-Hill, 1976). Also helpful are Rima D. Apple, " 'Advertised by our loving friends': The infant formula industry and the creation of new pharmaceutical markets, 1870–1910," *Journal of the History of Medicine,* 41 (1986), 3–23; Samuel J. Thomas, "Nostrum advertising and the image of woman as invalid in late Victorian America," *Journal of American Culture,* 5 (1982), 104–112.

Index

COMPOSED BY CONNELL TYPESETTING COMPANY, KANSAS CITY, MISSOURI
MANUFACTURED BY EDWARDS BROTHERS, INC., ANN ARBOR, MICHIGAN
TEXT AND DISPLAY LINES ARE SET IN SABON

ⓊⓊ

Library of Congress Cataloging-in-Publication Data
Apple, Rima D. (Rima Dombrow), 1944–
Mothers and medicine.
(Wisconsin publication in the history of science
and medicine; no. 7)
Bibliography: pp. 247–251.
Includes index.
1. Infants—United States—Nutrition—History—19th
century. 2. Breast feeding—United States—History—
19th century. 3. Mothers—United States—History—
19th century. 4. Physicians—United States—History—
19th century. 5. Physician and patient—United States
—History—19th century. 6. Infants—United States—
Nutrition—History—20th century. 7. Breast feeding—
United States—History—20th century. 8. Mothers—
United States—History—20th century. 9. Physicians—
United States—History—20th century. 10. Physician
and patient—United States—History—20th century.
I. Title. II. Series. [DNLM: 1. Infant Care—
history—United States. 2. Infant Food—history—
United States. 3. Infant Nutrition. 4. Mothers.
5. Physician-Patient Relations.
WI WI805 no. 7 / WS 11 AAI A6m]
RJ216.A65   1987   362.1'9892   87-40137
ISBN 0-299-11480-5
ISBN 0-299-11484-8 (pbk.)